# Public Health Law and Ethics

California/Milbank Books on Health and the Public

# Public Health Law and Ethics

*A Reader*

Edited by Lawrence O. Gostin

UNIVERSITY OF CALIFORNIA PRESS
*Berkeley · Los Angeles · London*

THE MILBANK MEMORIAL FUND
*New York*

University of California Press
Berkeley and Los Angeles, California

University of California Press, Ltd.
London, England

Library of Congress Cataloging-in-Publication Data
    Public health law and ethics : a reader / edited by
    Lawrence O. Gostin.
    p. cm.—(California/Milbank books on health and
    the public)
    Includes bibliographical references and index.

    ISBN 978-0-520-23175-7

    1. Public health laws —United States. 2. Public
    health—Moral and ethical aspects. I.
    Gostin, Larry O. (Larry Ogalthorpe) II. Series.
    KF3775 .P83 2002
    344.73'04--dc21                    2001049172

09 08
10 9 8 7 6 5

# Contents

# List of Illustrations

PHOTOGRAPHS

FIGURES

# List of Tables

## A READER IN PUBLIC HEALTH LAW AND ETHICS: THE WEB SITE

To provide readers with the most comprehensive and timely information possible, I have launched a companion web site to complement this text. This site, which is integrated into the web site of the Center for Law and the Public's Health at Georgetown and Johns Hopkins Universities, is made possible with the generous support of the Milbank Memorial Fund. The *Reader* web site is designed to greatly enhance your reading experience and to provide an important resource for public health law students, scholars, and practitioners.

Throughout this book, readers are referred to materials posted on this site. The contents of the site are keyed to the chapters of the *Reader,* and include

- Full-text versions of selected court cases excerpted in the *Reader*
- Selected articles and reports discussed or cited in the *Reader*
- Recent public health law cases, statutes, regulations, and news updates
- Links to other sites of interest

Please visit the *Reader* web site at www.publichealthlaw.net/reader.

# Conventions Used
# in This Book

The excerpted materials in the *Reader* have been edited for clarity and reduced length. These edits have been made carefully so as not to compromise the meaning or substance of the readings. My intent is to communicate the substance of the case or article, in the words of the author(s), without interfering with its readability. The following editing and other conventions have been used consistently throughout the *Reader*.

The citation form for books and articles is taken from *The Chicago Manual of Style* (14th ed.). The citation form for judicial cases is taken from *The Bluebook: A Uniform System of Citation* (17th ed.). All original references or notes in the excerpts have been deleted, except where they support quotations. In these instances, the references have been added to the bibliography and indicated within the text of the reading. Headings and subheadings within articles or cases have been capitalized and italicized, respectively, regardless of how they appear in the original text. Brackets ([ ]) are used in the readings to introduce my own commentary or edits of the original excerpted material.

Omissions of text within articles and cases are indicated through the use of ellipses (. . .) in accordance with the following rules: three periods (. . .) indicate an omission within a sentence and four periods (. . . .) indicate an omission that includes a sentence break (and may consist of part of a paragraph or several paragraphs). Five asterisks within the text (* * * * *) indicate a break between the end of an article or case and my own written commentary, except where this break is clear (e.g., the excerpt is followed by a major subject header).

The term "companion text" refers to my public health law book, *Public Health Law: Power, Duty, Restraint* (New York: Milbank Memorial Fund and Berkeley: University of California Press, 2000). References to the "*Reader* web site" refer to the web site accessible at the following address: www.publichealthlaw.net/reader. This regularly updated web site offers supplemental information, cases, and updates to the *Reader* text.

Concerning abbreviations, the first time an abbreviation is mentioned in a chapter, I have included the full name or term to which the abbreviation pertains (e.g., Institute of Medicine [IOM]), unless the abbreviation is commonly known (e.g., AIDS). Each subsequent use of the name or term in the text or excerpt utilizes the abbreviation.

I welcome comments from readers about the comprehensiveness, readability, and clarity of the *Reader*. I would appreciate being informed if I have omitted major articles or cases important to public health law or ethics.

# Foreword

The Milbank Memorial Fund is an endowed national foundation that engages in nonpartisan analysis, study, research, and communication on significant issues in health care and public health. The fund makes available the results of its work in meetings with decision-makers, reports, articles, and books.

The purpose of the Fund's publishing partnership with the University of California Press is to encourage the synthesis and communication of findings from research and experience that could contribute to more effective health policy. The two volumes by Lawrence O. Gostin published by the Fund and the Press achieve this goal.

In 2000, the Fund and the Press published Gostin's *Public Health Law: Power, Duty, Restraint.* Reviewers of the manuscript of that book suggested we also publish a reader that could be used independently or as a companion to the first volume.

Gostin brings to both books vast experience as a lawyer and legal scholar on public health issues. For many years, in both the United Kingdom and the United States, Gostin has been a lawyer's lawyer as well as an adviser to policy makers on the most controversial issues in public health law. This combination of scholarship and experience leads Gostin to propose that public health law should be an instrument for developing as well as implementing public policy. In *Public Health Law* he offers a critical analysis and synthesis of law and science that promises to improve the effectiveness of public policy in enhancing the health of populations. The articles collected in this *Reader* and Gostin's commentary on them demonstrate the significance of law and the analysis of it for effective health policy.

*Daniel M. Fox*
*President*

*Samuel L. Milbank*
*Chairman*

# Preface

The field of public health is typically regarded as a positivistic pursuit and, undoubtedly, our understanding of the etiology and response to disease is heavily influenced by scientific inquiry. Public health policies, however, are shaped not only by science but also by ethical values, legal norms, and political oversight. *Public Health Law and Ethics: A Reader* offers a careful selection of government reports, scholarly articles, and court cases designed to illuminate the ethical, legal, and political issues in the theory and practice of public health.

Before examining law and ethics, it is helpful to explore the meaning of public health. The excerpts and commentaries in the *Reader* offer several alternative definitions of public health, but focus principally on the Institute of Medicine's (IOM) influential definition in *The Future of Public Health*: "Public health is what we, as a society, do collectively to assure the conditions for people to be healthy."

The IOM definition emphasizes the collective responsibility of organized society to promote the health of the population. Despite the richness of this definition, the IOM does not delineate the field's legitimate scope within a representational democracy. Should public health be confined to relatively discrete interventions to prevent immediate causes of injury and disease—for example, surveillance, health education, and infectious disease control? Alternatively, should public health be concerned with larger social and economic problems that play important, but not fully understood, roles in health and disease—such as livable cities, adequate housing, violence prevention, and reduction in socioeconomic disparities? The *Reader* does not resolve the tension between a narrow and a broad focus of public health, but it does frame the question and suggests potential benefits and disadvantages of each approach.

## THE PUBLIC HEALTH LAW INFRASTRUCTURE

The field of public health is grounded in law and cannot function effectively without a strong legal infrastructure. Law establishes the foundations for public health governance—for example, funding mechanisms, administrative structures, and workforce. Law empowers public health agencies to act, sets limits on those powers in order to protect individual rights, and requires health authorities to follow defined procedures. At the same time, law defines boundaries for acceptable behavior, both individual and organizational, and permits the deprivation of liberty, autonomy, privacy, and property to safeguard the public's health.

The IOM urged fundamental reform of state public health laws to achieve two objectives: (1) clearly delineate the basic authority and responsibility entrusted to public health agencies, and (2) support a set of modern disease control measures that address contemporary health problems. The U.S. Department of Health and Human Services report *Healthy People 2010* similarly recognized the importance of public health law: "The Nation's public health infrastructure would be strengthened if jurisdictions had a model law and could use it regularly for improvements."

The IOM and DHHS were concerned with a body of enabling laws and regulations that are highly antiquated; many state laws have not been significantly revised since the early twentieth century. As a result, these laws have failed to keep pace with the remarkable advances in public health sciences and constitutional doctrine. Indeed, most of these laws do not conform with modern thinking about the mission, core functions, and essential services of public health authorities.

The public health community is actively seeking to strengthen the public health law infrastructure. The IOM Board on Health Promotion and Disease Prevention established a study committee to provide a vision for public health in the twenty-first century, including law reform. Just as important, the Robert Wood Johnson and Kellogg foundations' *Turning Point* project launched a "Public Health Statute Modernization" initiative designed to write a comprehensive model state public health law. For a Model Emergency Health Powers Act written in response to the terrorist attacks on September 11, 2001, see www.publichealthlaw.net.

Public health laws not only provide the foundations for public health practice, but also provide a set of tools for public health authorities. There are at least five models for legal intervention designed to prevent injury and disease and promote the public's health. Although legal interventions can be effective, they often raise social, ethical, or constitutional concerns that warrant careful study.

*Model 1* is the power to tax and spend. This power, found in federal and state constitutions, provides government with an important regulatory technique. The power to spend enables government to set conditions for the receipt of public funds. For example, the federal government grants highway funds to states on condition that they set the drinking age at 21. The power to tax provides strong inducements to engage in beneficial behavior or refrain from risk behavior. For example, taxes on cigarettes significantly reduce smoking, particularly among young people. The spending and taxing power, however, can be seen as coercive and, in many cases, "sin" taxes are highly regressive.

*Model 2* is the power to alter the informational environment. Government can add its voice to the marketplace of ideas through health promotion activities such as health communication campaigns, provide relevant consumer information through labeling requirements, and limit harmful or misleading information through regulation of commercial advertising of unsafe products (e.g., cigarettes and alcoholic beverages). But even these interventions can be controversial. Not everyone believes that public funds should be expended, or the veneer of government legitimacy used, to prescribe particular social orthodoxies—unsafe sex, abortion, smoking, high-fat diet, or sedentary lifestyle, for example. Labeling requirements seem unobjectionable, but businesses strongly protest compelled disclosure of certain kinds of information. For example, should businesses be required to disclose that foods have been genetically modified (GM) or that dairy cows have received Bovine Growth Hormone (BGH)? GM foods and BGH have not been shown to be dangerous to humans, but the public demands a "right to know." Advertising regulations restrict commercial speech, thus implicating businesses' First Amendment rights. Should government be permitted to limit truthful information because it conveys adventuresome, healthful, or sexual images about harmful products?

*Model 3* is direct regulation of individuals (e.g., seatbelt and motorcycle helmet laws), professionals (e.g., licenses), or businesses (e.g., inspections and occupational safety standards). Public health authorities regulate pervasively to reduce risks to the population. Most people recognize the value of public health regulation, but coercive government action inevitably interferes with personal or economic liberty. Society faces a trade-off between the collective benefits of regulation and the diminution in individual interests in liberty, autonomy, privacy, free expression, and property.

*Model 4* is indirect regulation through the tort system. Tort litigation can provide strong incentives for businesses to engage in less risky activities. Litigation has been used as a tool of public health to influence manufacturers of automobiles, cigarettes, and firearms. Litigation has resulted in safer automobiles and in reduced advertising and promotion of cigarettes to young people. It has encouraged at least one manufacturer (Smith & Wesson) to develop safer firearms. At the same time, litigation may be antidemocratic and unfair. Critics claim that the policy-making branch of government, not the judiciary, should make judgments about unsafe products. They also point out that the financial benefits of litigation frequently go to a few plaintiffs and their attorneys rather than to the entire population that has been harmed.

The final model is deregulation. Sometimes laws are harmful to public health and stand as an obstacle to effective action. For example, criminal laws proscribe the possession and distribution of sterile syringes and needles. These laws, therefore, make it more difficult for public health authorities to engage in HIV prevention activities. Deregulation can also be controversial since it often involves a direct conflict with laws representing another set of values. For example, the criminal law represents society's disapproval of drug use and its intention to punish those who make it easier to inject unlawful drugs. Deregulation becomes a symbol of weakness in the fight against drugs that is often unpopular among the poor, minorities, and law enforcement.

The government, then, has many legal "levers" designed to prevent injury and disease and promote the public's health. Legal interventions can be highly effective and need to be part of the public health officer's arsenal. However, legal interventions can be controversial, raising important ethical, social, constitutional, and political issues. These conflicts are complex, important, and fascinating for students of public health law. The *Reader* systematically examines these kinds of legal interventions and the inevitable trade-offs between collective and individual interests.

## PUBLIC HEALTH ETHICS

The field of bioethics flourished during the late twentieth century. This was a time when scholars had great influence in shaping ideas about the salience of the individual in matters of health. Both ends of the political spectrum celebrated the values of freedom and choice—the political left emphasizing civil liberties and the political right emphasizing markets and free will. Personal interests in autonomy, self-determination, and privacy attained the status of "rights." Patients were transformed from passive recipients of medical treatment into rights holders. In this intellectual environment, the patient's view of his or her self-interests often prevailed over the interests of family or community.

Most observers recognize the importance of bioethics in improving the status and dignity of patients in the health care system. Personal interests and individual rights, however, are not always decisive factors in public health, and sometimes are harmful to critical thinking about healthy communities. The field of public health is concerned primarily with prevention rather than treatment, populations rather than individuals, and collective goods rather than personal rights or interests. Scholars in philosophy and ethics need to develop innovative ideas about the meaning and value of the common good. If individual self-interests—conceived as rights—are ever to give way to communal interests in healthy populations, it is important to understand the value of "the common" and "the good."

The field of public health would profit from a vibrant conception of "the common" that sees public interests as more than the aggregation of individual interests. A nonaggregative understanding of public goods recognizes that individuals exist within the context of culture, community, and society. There are interests that members of a society have in common, and seek to promote, even if they are not particularly self-interested. Individuals have a stake in healthy and secure communities where they can live in peace and well-being.

Suppose a person has sufficient wealth and status to secure adequate medical care, housing, and food. This person may still have an interest in ensuring that others in the community have access to these, and other, necessities of life. If one's neighbors feel sick, hungry, or vulnerable, it affects everyone. An unhealthy or insecure community may produce harms such as increased crime and violence, impaired social relationships, and a less productive workforce. Consequently, every person has a reason to support minimum levels of health and to reduce the sharp disparities in morbidity and mortality in the population.

There are important benefits, moreover, that even wealthy people cannot attain on their own and that require collective action. Without organized societal activities, people cannot assure many of the conditions for health such as clean air and water, safe roads and products, sanitation, and the control of infectious disease. Many of life's benefits, therefore, can be understood only as collective goods. In other words, individuals have a stake in living in a society that regulates risks that all share. People may have to forgo a little bit of self-interest in exchange for the protection and satisfaction gained from a healthier and safer community.

In the late twentieth century, bioethicists posed the question, What desires and needs do you have as an autonomous, rights-bearing individual? Now it is important to ask another kind of question: What kind of a community do you want and deserve to live in, and what personal interests are you willing to forgo to achieve a good society?

We also need to better understand the concept of "the good" or, more particularly, who decides which of these goods are preferable in any given case. In medicine, the meaning of "the good" is defined purely in terms of the individual's wants and needs. It is the patient, not the physician or family, who decides the appropriate course of action. For example, patients could decline medical treatment (e.g., an amputation or chemotherapy) even though it would improve their health and extend their lives.

In public health, the meaning of "the good" is far less clear. Who gets to decide in a given case which value is more important—freedom or health? One strategy for public health decision making would be to allow each person to decide, but this would thwart many public health initiatives. For example, if individuals could decide whether to acquiesce to a vaccination or permit reporting of personal information to the health department, it would result in a "tragedy of the commons." If enough people refused to participate in the public health program, the population would suffer. In the case of vaccination, herd immunity would break down, resulting in increased risks of infectious disease within the population; in the case of reporting, the surveillance system would not accurately track the incidence and prevalence of injury and disease. Consequently, collective interests may have to override individual interests if necessary to protect the population's health.

Another strategy for public health decision making is to allow the community to decide the merits of public health interventions. The problem, of course, is that the community is a complex abstraction, often without clearly identified leaders who can speak on its behalf. In a representative democracy, the government makes decisions on behalf of the population. Ideally, the government would set public health policy by reference to scientific or objective knowledge, maximizing the value of health and well-being within the population.

Many forward thinkers urge greater community involvement in public health decision making so that policy formation becomes a genuinely civic endeavor. Under this view, citizens would strive to safeguard their communities by civic participation, open fora, and capacity building to solve local problems. Public involvement should result in stronger support for health policies and encourage citizens to take a more active role in protecting themselves and the health of their neighbors. Public health authorities, for example, might practice more deliberative forms of democracy, involving closer consultation with consumers and the voluntary organizations that represent them (e.g., town meetings and consumer membership on government advisory committees). This kind of deliberative democracy in public health is increasingly evident in government-community partnerships at the federal, state, and local levels (e.g., AIDS action and breast cancer awareness). In summary, collective "goods" can be determined by public health authorities, using the best available scientific evidence of population health, and with active community participation.

## AN ANTHOLOGY AND INTERNET RESOURCES

*Public Health Law and Ethics: A Reader* provides a discussion and analysis of critical problems at the interface of law, ethics, and public health. It is intended as a stand-alone text for scholars, students, practitioners, and the informed public. The *Reader* offers a detailed commentary that defines a public health problem in each chapter, frames the relevant questions, and introduces the selected readings. The commentary also provides additional resources for readers interested in further pursuing the subject matter in the chapter.

The *Reader* can also be used as a companion to the book *Public Health Law: Power, Duty, Restraint* (University of California Press and Milbank Memorial Fund, 2000). The book offers a theory and definition of public health law, an explanation of its principal analytical methodologies, and an analysis of the major conflicts in public health theory and practice. The books are designed to be used together: *Public Health Law: Power, Duty, Restraint* provides a careful description and analysis of public health law, while the *Reader* offers cases and materials that provoke debate and informed discussion. The two books (used separately or as companions) provide resources for research, teaching academic courses and seminars, professional practice, and thinking about fascinating problems in public health theory and daily practice.

The books are supported by a wealth of resources available on the Internet: www.publichealthlaw.net/reader. The *Reader* web site contains the most recent court cases, articles, and reports providing insights on the theory and practice of public health law and ethics. The web site is updated on a regular basis to provide readers with modern developments in the field, such as new Supreme Court cases. The *Reader* web site is linked to other important web resources such as the Public Health Law Program at the CDC and the Center for Law and the Public's Health at Georgetown and Johns Hopkins universities.

## BUILDING A SYLLABUS
## FOR COURSES AND SEMINARS

Faculty in schools of law, public health, medicine, nursing, and public administration have adopted *Public Health Law: Power, Duty, Restraint* for courses and seminars on public health law and/or ethics. Some professors will prefer to use the *Reader* alone in their classes. Still others will use both books, as I do at Georgetown University.

If faculty members choose both books, the main text offers an accessible description and analysis of the field, while the *Reader* provides supplemental cases and articles. The accompanying table provides a basis for building a syllabus. One column contains the chapter headings for *Public Health Law: Power, Duty, Restraint*, and the other column contains the corresponding chapters in the *Reader*

## BUILDING A SYLLABUS

| Public Health Law: Power, Duty, Restraint | Public Health Law and Ethics: A Reader |
|---|---|
| Chapter 1. A Theory and Definition of Public Health Law | Chapters 1–4 |
| Chapter 2. Public Health in the Constitutional Design | Chapter 6 |
| Chapter 3. Constitutional Limits on the Exercise of Public Health Powers | Chapter 7 |
| Chapter 4. Public Health Regulation: A Systematic Evaluation | Chapter 5 |
| Chapter 5. Public Health Information: Personal Privacy | Chapter 10 |
| Chapter 6. Health, Communication, and Behavior: Freedom of Expression | Chapter 11 |
| Chapter 7. Immunization, Testing, and Screening: Bodily Integrity | Chapter 12 |
| Chapter 8. Restrictions of the Person: Autonomy, Liberty, and Bodily Integrity | Chapter 13 (see also chapter 12) |
| Chapter 9. Economic Behavior and the Public's Health: Direct Regulation | Chapter 8 |
| Chapter 10. Tort Law and the Public's Health: Indirect Regulation | Chapter 9 |
| Chapter 11. Public Health Law Reform | Chapter 14 |

that provide supplemental cases and articles. Model syllabi are posted on the *Reader* web site.

## ORGANIZATION OF THE *READER*

Chapter 1 of the *Reader* offers a discussion of the related fields of public health, law, ethics, and human rights. This chapter "maps" the relevant issues in these fields and describes the similarities and differences in goals, methods, and terminology.

The *Reader* is divided into four parts. Part One, "Foundations in Public Health Law and Ethics," takes a careful look at three ways of thinking about population health: the population perspective, the communitarian tradition of public health ethics, and the role of human rights in matters of health. Chapter 2 provides many of the classic analytical studies in public health, together with modern controversies about the field's appropriate role and scope. Chapter 3 examines the emerging field of public health ethics, explaining the differences between traditional bioethics and the values inherent in more communal ways of thinking about health. Chapter 4 discusses the synergies and conflicts between human rights and public health. This chapter features the pioneering work of the late Jonathan Mann and seeks to explore the meaning and functions of human rights in public health. Chapter 5 discusses the principal methods of reasoning in public health: philosophy, risk, and cost-effectiveness.

Part Two, "Law and the Public's Health," examines important doctrines and controversies in public health law. Chapter 6 discusses the powers and duties of public health authorities under the Constitution. Chapter 7 discusses the limitation of public health powers under the Constitution. Chapter 8 discusses the regulation of property and the professions (e.g., the law of nuisance, inspections, and regulatory "takings"). Chapter 9 discusses tort litigation for the public's health, including cigarette and firearm litigation.

Part Three, "Tensions and Recurring Themes," focuses on some of the major controversies and trade-offs involved in public health theory and practice. Chapter 10 discusses surveillance and the right to privacy. Chapter 11 discusses health promotion and commercial speech regulation, explaining the conflicts with freedom of expression. Chapter 12 discusses infectious disease powers such as immunization, screening, and treatment. Chapter 13 discusses restrictions of the person such as civil confinement and criminal punishment.

Part Four, "The Future of Public Health," focuses on a vision for public health in a new century. Chapter 14 offers case studies on three of the most important modern problems in public health: emerging infections, bioterrorism, and public health genetics.

A RENAISSANCE FOR PUBLIC HEALTH?
ACKNOWLEDGING LEADERS

Historians may look at the onset of the twenty-first century as a period of renaissance for public health law and ethics. The field of public health is reemerging from the shadows of high-technology medicine by expressing its own identity and importance.

Government and the private sector are engaged in a broad set of initiatives to reinvigorate the field. The following list describes many of the important projects together with the principal people leading the effort. I want to demonstrate the resurgence of interest in public health law and ethics and acknowledge the role of these public health leaders. I have the privilege of being personally involved in each of these projects and boards, so I have directly benefited from their activities. I am most grateful to the following people, who have shaped my thinking in the field of public health law and ethics.

*Milbank Memorial Fund* (www.milbankmemorialfund.org). The Milbank Memorial Fund, led by Daniel M. Fox, is an endowed national foundation that engages in nonpartisan analysis, study, research, and communication on significant issues in health policy. I appreciate the support of Kathleen S. Andersen, Gail Cambridge, Paul D. Cleary, John M. Colmers, and Jeffrey Edelstein.

*Turning Point Program* (www.turningpointprogram.org). The Turning Point Program, sponsored by the Robert Wood Johnson and Kellogg foundations, seeks to transform the public health system to make it more effective, community based, and collaborative. Notably, the Turning Point Program supports the Public Health Statute Modernization National Collaborative, a consortium of states and national public health organizations (www.hss.state.ak.us/dph/aphip/collaborative.htm). The Collaborative, led by Deborah Erickson, is conducting a comprehensive analysis of the structure and appropriateness of state public health statutes and developing a model state public health law. There are so many dedicated members of the Collaborative that I do not have space to acknowledge the important contribution that each person has made. I want to particularly thank Bobbie Berkowitz, Kristine M. Gebbie, Bud Nicola, and Jack Thompson. The Turning Point Program also supports the Public Health Governance Workgroup, led by Roz Lasker, which seeks to encourage local participation in public health decision making.

*Centers for Disease Control and Prevention, Public Health Law Program (PHLP)* (www.phppo.cdc.gov/phlawnet). Jeffrey P. Koplan, director of CDC, has exercised leadership in raising awareness of the vital role law plays in public health. The PHLP coordinates CDC's efforts to improve scientific understanding of the interaction between law and public health and to strengthen the legal foundation for public health practice. The PHLP is guided by Edward Baker,

Kathy Cahill, Richard Goodman, Paul Halverson, Heather Horton, Martha Katz, Paula Kocher, Gene Matthews, Anthony Moulton, and Verla Neslund.

*Center for Law & the Public's Health (CLPH)* (CDC's Collaborating Center Promoting Public Health Through Law) (www.publichealthlaw.net). The CLPH, at Georgetown and Johns Hopkins universities, is a primary resource on public health law, ethics, and policy for public health practitioners, lawyers, and policy makers. My colleagues at the Center are nationally known scholars: Scott Burris, James G. Hodge, Jr., Stephen P. Teret, and Jon Vernick.

*Institute of Medicine* (www.iom.edu). The Board on Health Promotion and Disease Prevention (HPDP) is broadly concerned with promoting the health of the public (physical, mental, and social), particularly through population-based interventions. The chair of HPDP is Robert B. Wallace and the director is Rose Marie Martinez. The 1988 IOM report *The Future of Public Health* proclaimed public health to be in disarray and prompted national discussion about the status of public health and steps necessary to strengthen its role. Since then, much has changed in the practice of public health improvement, in those participating in the work of building healthier communities, and in concepts of research and action in public health. While the public health system may no longer be in disarray, it is struggling to survive in a rapidly changing milieu of demands, expectations, opportunities, and resources. In recognition of these new challenges, the IOM conducted a new DHHS interagency-sponsored study entitled "Assuring the Health of the Public in the 21st Century." The committee's overarching goal is to describe a new, more inclusive framework for assuring population-level health that can be effectively communicated to and acted upon by diverse communities. The committee chairs are Jo Ivey Boufford and Christine Cassel, and its study director is Monica S. Ruiz. The committee report is due around the time of publication of the Reader in 2002.

*Hastings Center Project on Public Health Ethics.* The project, led by Daniel Callahan and Bruce Jennings, seeks to advance scholarship and practice on ethics and public health. Members of the study group include Ronald Bayer, Allan Brandt, Jan Malcolm, Donald R. Mattison, Thomas L. Milne, Margaret Pappaioanau, Ann Robertson, Dixie E. Snyder, Bonnie Steinbock, and Douglas L. Weed.

*Association of Schools of Public Health Project on Public Health Ethics Curricula Development.* The project aims to help develop model curricula on public health ethics. The project is led by Jeffrey Kahn, Wendy Katz, Anna Mastroianni, and Lisa Parker.

*Georgetown, Johns Hopkins, and the University of Virginia Project on Public Health Ethics.* The project seeks to advance scholarship on ethics and public health. Members of the study group include James Childress, Ruth Faden, Ruth Gaare, Nancy Kass, Jonathan Moreno, and Phillip Nieburg.

*Public Health Leadership Society (PHLS).* The PHLS is engaged in an important project to develop a code of ethics for public health professionals. The project, led by Jack Dillenberg, Michael Sage, Liz Schwarte, and James Thomas, is using a broad consultative process to develop the code.

I am indebted to my colleague James G. Hodge, Jr., and the research team he directs comprising students from Georgetown University Law Center and the Johns Hopkins Bloomberg School of Public Health. In addition to supervising the research, Professor Hodge provided important intellectual support for the text and images in the *Reader.*

The research team for this book project comprised the following students: Stephen Albrecht, Michael Chitwood, Daniel Cooper, Lance Gable, Kevin Greaney, Megan Guenther, Laura Kidd, Yon Lupu, David Maria, Marguerite Middaugh, Monique Nolan, William Tarantino, and Allison Winnike. I want particularly to express my gratitude to Mira S. Burghardt, Gabriel Baron Eber, Julia M. Rothstein, and Ahren S. Tryon. These talented students had valuable roles in the book and web projects.

I want to express my appreciation to two distinguished scholars who reviewed the manuscript: Richard Bonnie (University of Virginia) and Peter Jacobson (University of Michigan).

I am most grateful to my publishers Daniel M. Fox (Milbank Memorial Fund) and Lynne Withey (University of California Press) for their remarkable support for these book projects. I also wish to thank the deans and faculty at my two academic institutions, notably Dean Judith Areen (Georgetown University Law Center) and Dean Alfred Sommer (Johns Hopkins Bloomberg School of Public Health).

Finally, and most important, I express my love and devotion to my family: Jean, Bryn, and Kieran.

*Lawrence O. Gostin*
*Professor of Law, Georgetown University*
*Professor of Public Health, the Johns Hopkins University*
*Director, Center for Law and the Public's Health*
*CDC Collaborating Center Promoting Health Through Law*

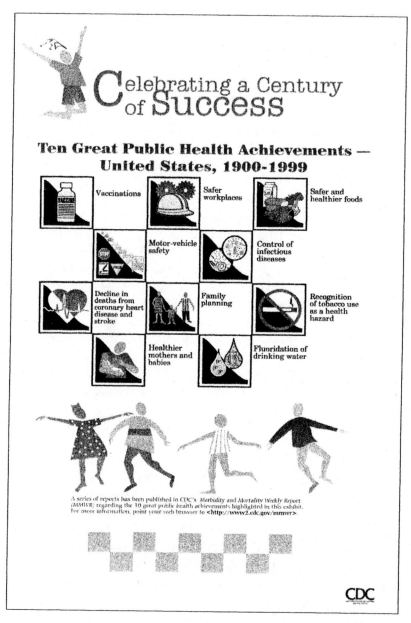

This illustration by the Centers for Disease Control and Prevention listing the ten great public health achievements of the twentieth century suggests a wide range of modern public health functions.

# ONE

# Public Health Law, Ethics, and Human Rights

*Mapping the Issues*

This *Reader* offers an organized selection of government reports, scholarly articles, and court cases on public health law, ethics, and human rights. The publication of a *Reader* on these subjects may suggest that a coherent, systematic understanding of the relationships between public health law, ethics, and human rights exists. Despite the deep traditions in these separate fields, they have rarely cross-fertilized. For the most part, each of these fields has adopted its own terminologies and forms of reasoning. To the extent that scholars in law, ethics, or human rights have engaged in sustained examinations of issues in health, they have written principally about medical care. This introductory chapter maps the important features of, and issues in, these respective fields as they pertain to the theory and practice of public health. Part One of the *Reader* explores public health, ethics, and human rights in more detail. Part Two examines major aspects of public health law, including constitutional, administrative, and tort law. Part Three focuses on some of the major controversies and trade-offs involved in public health theory and practice. And Part Four conceptualizes a vision for public health in a new century.

## I. PUBLIC HEALTH

In thinking about the application of ethics or human rights to problems in public health, it is important first to understand what we mean by public health. How is the field defined and what is its content—its mission, functions, and services? Who engages in the practice of public health—government, the private sector, charities, or community-based organizations? What are the principal methods or techniques of public health practitioners (Turnock 2001; Novick and Mays 2001)? In truth, finding answers to these fundamental questions is not easy because the field of public health is highly eclectic and conflicted (Beaglehole and Bonita 1997; Fielding 1999). For a summary of the definition, mission, functions, and jurisdiction of public health, see Table 1.

Definitions of public health vary widely, ranging from the World Health Organization's utopian conception of an ideal state of physical and mental health to a more concrete listing of public health practices. Charles-Edward A. Winslow (1920, 30), for example, defined public health as "the science and the art of preventing disease, prolonging life, and promoting physical health and efficiency through organized community efforts for the sanitation of the environment, the control of community infections, the education of the individual in principles of personal hygiene, [and] the organization of medical and nursing service for the early diagnosis and preventive treatment of disease." More recent definitions focus on "positive health," emphasizing a person's complete well-being (*Lancet* Editorial 1997, 229). Definitions of positive health include at least four constructs: a healthy body, high-quality personal relationships, a sense of purpose in life, and self-regard and resilience (Rowe and Kahn 1998).

The Institute of Medicine (IOM) (1988, 19), in its seminal report *The Future of Public Health,* proposed one of the most influential contemporary definitions: "Public health is what we, as a society, do collectively to assure the conditions for people to be healthy." The IOM's definition can be appreciated by examining its constituent parts. The emphasis on cooperative and mutually shared obligation ("we, as a society") reinforces that collective entities (e.g., governments and communities) take responsibility for healthy populations. Individuals can do a great deal to safeguard their health, particularly if they have the economic means to do so. They can purchase housing, clothing, food, and medical care (McKinlay and McKinlay 1977). Each person can also behave in ways that promote health and safety by eating healthy foods, exercising, using safety equipment (e.g., seatbelts, motorcycle helmets, or smoke detectors), and by refraining from smoking, using illicit drugs, or drinking alcoholic beverages excessively. Yet there is a great deal that individuals cannot do

TABLE I

PUBLIC HEALTH

| | |
|---|---|
| Definition | Society's obligation to assure the conditions for people's health |
| Mission | Promote physical and mental health; prevent disease, injury, and disability |
| Functions | *Assessment*—assemble and analyze community health needs<br>*Policy development*—informed through scientific knowledge<br>*Assurance*—services necessary for community health |
| Jurisdiction/Domain | *Narrow focus*—proximal risk factors (e.g., infectious disease control)<br>*Broad focus*—distal social structures (e.g., discrimination, homelessness, socioeconomic status) |
| Expertise/Skills | Epidemiology and biostatistics, education and communication, leadership and politics |

to secure their health, and therefore these individuals need to organize, build together, and share resources. Acting alone, people cannot achieve environmental protection, hygiene and sanitation, clean air and surface water, uncontaminated food and drinking water, safe roads and products, and control of infectious disease. Each of these collective goods, and many more, are achievable only through organized and sustained community activities (Gostin 2000a).

The IOM definition also makes clear that even the most organized and socially conscious society cannot guarantee complete physical and mental well-being. There will always be a certain amount of injury and disease in the population that is beyond the reach of individuals or government. The role of public health, therefore, is to "assure the *conditions* for people to be healthy." These conditions include a variety of educational, economic, social, and environmental factors that are necessary for good health.

Most definitions share the premise that the subject of public health is the health of populations—rather than the health of individuals—and that this goal is reached by a generally high level of health throughout society, rather than the best possible health for a few. The field of public health is concerned with health promotion and disease prevention throughout society. Consequently, public health is interested in devising broad strategies to prevent or ameliorate injury and disease.

Scholars and practitioners are conflicted about the "reach," or domain, of public health. Some prefer a narrow focus on the proximal risk factors for injury and disease. The role of public health agencies, according to this perspective, is to identify risks or harms and intervene to prevent or reduce them. This has been the traditional role of public health—exercising discrete powers such as surveillance (e.g., screening and reporting), injury prevention (e.g., safe consumer products), and infectious disease control (e.g., vaccination, partner notification, and quarantine).

Others prefer a broad focus on the socioeconomic foundations of health. Those favoring this position see public health as an all-embracing enterprise united by the common value of societal well-being. They claim that the jurisdiction of public health reaches "social ills rooted in distal social structures" (Meyer and Schwartz 2000, 1189). Ultimately, the field is interested in the equitable distribution of social and economic resources because social status, race, and wealth are important influences on the health of populations (Marmot and Wilkinson 1999; Syme 1998). Similarly, the field is interested in "social capital" because social networks of family and friends, as well as associations with religious and civic organizations, are important factors in public health (Cattell 2000).

This inclusive direction for public health is gaining popularity; many of the government's health objectives for 2010 seek reductions in health disparities and improved social cohesiveness. Figure 1 illustrates the determinants of health according to the Department of Health and Human Services (2000): physical environment, behavior and biology, and social environment. Using this vision, public health researchers and practitioners have ventured into areas of general social policy, ranging from city planning and safe housing (Hancock 2000; Maantay 2001) to violence, war, and discrimination (Breakey 1997).

The expansive view of public health may well be justified by the importance of culture, poverty, and powerlessness on the health of populations. Social epidemiologists have found an association between these factors and increased morbidity and mortality (Berkman and Kawachi 2000). Yet to many, this all-embracing notion is troublesome. First, there is the problem of excessive breadth. Almost everything human beings undertake impacts the population's health, but this does not justify an overly inclusive definition of public health. The field of public health appears less credible if it overreaches.

Second, there is the problem of expertise. Admittedly, the public health professions incorporate a wide variety of disciplines (e.g., occupational health, health education, epidemiology, and nursing) with different skills and functions (Gerzoff, Brown, and Baker 1999; Gebbie and Hwang 2000; HRSA 2000). But public health professionals do not possess all the skills necessary to intervene on behavioral, social, phys-

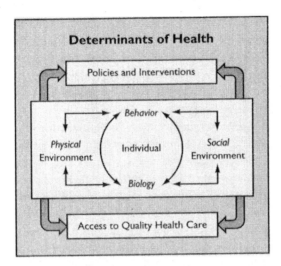

Figure 1. Determinants of health. (*Source:*
U.S. Department of Health and Human Services,
*Healthy People 2010.*)

ical, and environmental levels (e.g., competence in behavioral sciences, economics, and engineering).

Finally, there is the problem of political and public support. By espousing controversial issues of economic redistribution and social restructuring, the field risks losing its legitimacy. Public health gains credibility from its adherence to science, and if the field strays too far into political advocacy, it may lose the appearance of objectivity.

If public health has such a broad meaning, then who engages in the work of public health—government, the private sector, academia, charities, or community-based organizations? At the governmental level, public health has a significant jurisdictional problem. Even the most powerful public health agency cannot exercise direct authority over the full range of activities that affect health. Many of the determinants of health are normally the province of other agencies (e.g., agencies concerned with education, agriculture, transportation, housing, child welfare, and criminal justice). Furthermore, much of the behavior that public health authorities try to change (e.g., exercise and diet) is not subject to direct legal regulation at all. At the same time, many of the institutions that affect the public's health are outside government, such as managed care organizations, business and labor, community-based groups, and academic institutions (Keane, Marx, and Ricci 2001a,b; Béchamps, Bialek, and Caulk 1999;

Bowser and Gostin 1999). Thus, scholars need to consider the actors who carry out the work of public health. It matters a great deal in law and ethics to understand who is acting, with what authority, and with what resources. For example, society is prepared to allow government to wield powers to coerce (e.g., tax, inspect, license, and quarantine) that would be unacceptable in the private sector.

What are the principal methodologies of public health practitioners? Because of the field's broad sweep, the techniques of public health are highly diverse (Sommer and Akhter 2000). For example, public health practitioners monitor health status, which calls for skills in epidemiology and biostatistics; inform and educate the public, which calls for skills in education and communication; and create health policy and enforce laws, which calls for skills in leadership and politics. This description does not account for the many subjects in the field of public health requiring expertise in domains such as infectious diseases (e.g., virology and bacteriology), the environment (e.g., toxicology), and injuries (e.g., behavioral and social sciences). As the IOM (1988, 40) has observed, "Public health's subject matter . . . necessitate[s] the involvement of a broad spectrum of professional disciplines. In fact, . . . public health is a coalition of professions united by their shared mission."

As illustrated in Figure 2, the field of public health is caught in a dilemma. If it conceives itself too narrowly, then public health will be accused of lacking vision. It will fail to see the root causes of ill health and fail to utilize a broad range of social, economic, and behavioral tools necessary to achieve healthier populations (McGinnis and Foege 1993). At the same time, if it conceives itself too expansively, then public health will be accused of overreaching and invading a sphere reserved for politics, not science. It will lose the ability to explain its mission and functions in comprehensible terms and, consequently, to sell public health in the marketplace of politics and priorities (McGinnis 2001; Burris 1997b).

## II. PUBLIC HEALTH LAW

As we have just seen, the question "What is public health?" is much more difficult than it first appears. Despite the lack of conceptual clarity, it is important to study carefully the legal foundations of public health, its ethical dimensions, and its relationship to human rights.

The preservation of the public's health is among the most important goals of government. The enactment and enforcement of law, moreover, is

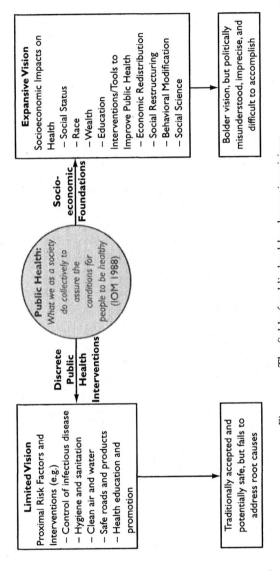

Figure 2. The field of public health: alternative visions.

a primary means by which government creates the conditions for people to lead healthier and safer lives. Law creates a mission for public health authorities, assigns their functions, and specifies the manner in which they may exercise their power (Gostin, Burris, and Lazzarini 1999). The law is a tool that is used to influence norms for healthy behavior, identify and respond to health threats, and set and enforce health and safety standards. The most important social debates about public health take place in legal fora—legislatures, courts, and administrative agencies—and in the law's language of rights, duties, and justice. It is no exaggeration to say that "the field of public health . . . could not long exist in the manner in which we know it today except for its sound legal basis" (Grad 1990, 4).

In *Public Health Law: Power, Duty, Restraint* (hereinafter the "companion text"), public health law is defined as "the study of the legal powers and duties of the state to assure the conditions for people to be healthy . . . and the limitations on the power of the state to constrain the autonomy, privacy, liberty, proprietary, or other legally protected interests of individuals for the protection or promotion of community health." Five characteristics help distinguish public health law from the vast literature on law and medicine (Figure 3): (1) the role of *government* in advancing the public's health, (2) the *population-based* perspective, (3) the *relationship* between the people and the state, (4) the *services* and scientific methodologies, and (5) the role of *coercion*.

Public health law scholars, therefore, are interested in government authority to prevent injury and disease and to promote the public's health, as well as in the constraints on state action to protect individual freedom (see chapters 6 and 7). Government has ample authority to act for the common good but must exercise that power within the constraints of the Constitution.

Law can be an effective tool to achieve the goal of improved health for the population. Law, regulation, and litigation, like other public health prevention strategies, intervene at a variety of levels, each designed to secure safer and healthier populations. First, government interventions are aimed at *individual* behavior through education (e.g., health communication campaigns), incentives (e.g., taxing and spending powers), and deterrence (e.g., civil and criminal penalties for risky behaviors). Second, the law regulates the *agents of behavior change* by requiring safer product design (e.g., safety standards and indirect regulation through the tort system). Finally, the law alters the informational (e.g., advertising restraints), physical (e.g., city planning and housing codes), and business (e.g., inspections and licenses) *environments*.

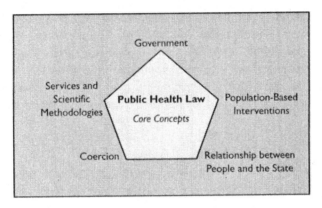

Figure 3.   Public health law: core concepts.

Government engages in the work of public health through three separate branches: legislative, executive, and judicial. The Constitution provides a system of checks and balances so that no single branch of government can act without some degree of oversight and control by another. Separation of powers is essential to public health, for each branch of government possesses a unique constitutional authority: (1) legislatures create health policy and allocate the resources necessary to effect it; (2) executive agencies implement health policy, promulgate health regulations, and enforce regulatory standards; and (3) courts interpret laws and resolve legal disputes. As a society, we forgo the possibility of bold public health governance by any single branch in exchange for constitutional checks and balances that prevent government from overreaching and ensure political accountability.

Public health law is concerned with the trade-offs entailed in the exercise of government power. Under what circumstances should government be permitted to act to achieve a public good when the consequence of that act is to invade a sphere of individual liberty? This is the kind of question that intrigues scholars interested in law and the public's health. Rather than using ethical discourse to resolve these conflicts, the law uses the language of duties, powers, and rights.

It is clear from the foregoing description that public health law is a vast field incorporating thinking from a variety of legal subspecialties—constitutional, civil, administrative, and tort law. The Constitution affords the federal government certain powers and limits the authority of all governments to protect a sphere of freedom. Civil and administrative law is concerned with the body of statutes and regulations that set health and safety standards, together with agency powers to interpret and enforce those standards. Tort law provides a method of indirect regulation through the courts. By levying damages for certain kinds of harm, tort law can provide powerful disincentives to risk behaviors (e.g., litigation against cigarette and firearm manufacturers). As the chapters in this *Reader* unfold, these legal dimensions are explored (see Part Two).

## III. PUBLIC HEALTH ETHICS

The field of bioethics has richly informed the practice of medicine and decisions about the allocation of health care resources. Bioethicists have not devoted the same sustained attention to problems in public health, but this is beginning to change with some interesting and important scholarship in public health ethics (Steinbock and Beauchamp 1999; Bradely and Burls 2000; Coughlin and Beauchamp 1996). A critical unanswered question is whether public health ethics have features distinguishing them from conventional bioethics. Are ethical principles, or the methods of ethical analysis, materially different when applied to populations than when applied to individual patients? In thinking about this question it will be helpful to consider public health ethics from at least two perspectives: the ethics *of* public health professionals (professional ethics) and ethics *in* public health theory and practice (applied ethics) (Callahan and Jennings 2002). See Table 2.

The ethics *of* public health are concerned with the ethical dimensions of professionalism and the moral trust that society bestows on public health professionals to act for the common welfare (Callahan 2000). This form of ethical discourse stresses the distinct history and traditions of the profession, seeking to create a culture of professionalism among public health students and practitioners. It instills in professionals a sense of public duty and trust (Weed and McKeown 1998). Professional ethics are role oriented, helping practitioners to act in virtuous ways as they undertake their functions.

Many professional groups, such as physicians and attorneys, hold themselves accountable through a set of ethical guidelines, but public health professionals have no code of ethics. Perhaps the explanation is that there is no single public health profession, but rather a variety of different disciplines. Indeed, some public health disciplines have their own ethical codes—for example, epidemiologists and public health educators (links to these codes of ethics are provided in the *Reader* web site: www.publichealthlaw.net).

TABLE 2
PUBLIC HEALTH ETHICS

| | |
|---|---|
| Ethics *of* Public Health (i.e., Professional Ethics) | Ethical dimensions of professionalism<br>Moral trust society bestows on professionals to act for the common good |
| Ethics *in* Public Health (i.e., Applied Ethics: Situation or Case Oriented) | Ethical dimensions of public health enterprise<br>Moral standing of population's health<br>Trade-offs between collective goods and individual interests<br>Social justice: equitable allocation of benefits and burdens |
| Advocacy Ethics (i.e., Goal-Oriented, Populist Ethic) | Overriding value of healthy communities<br>Serves interests of populations, particularly powerless and oppressed<br>Methods: pragmatic and political |

SOURCE:  Hastings Center Project on Ethics and Public Health.

A code of ethics, or at least a well-articulated values statement, could be helpful to the field. A code could give the profession a moral compass, providing concrete guidelines to help clarify distinctive ethical dilemmas. Public health professionals work in a field of considerable moral ambiguity where guidance could be instructive. A code could also give moral credibility to the field and a higher professional status. The Public Health Leadership Society has developed a code of ethics for the field. The code, based on a broad consultation process, is posted on the *Reader* web site.

A public health code of ethics would have to confront the salient issue of fiduciary responsibility. To whom do public health professionals owe a duty of loyalty, and how can these professionals know what actions are morally acceptable? Physicians, attorneys, and accountants have a fiduciary duty to their clients that informs their moral world. For example, client-centered professions usually adhere to the principle that the professional serves the client, advises the client fully and honestly, takes instructions from the client, and avoids acting against the client's best interests.

In the context of public health, the community might be regarded as the "client." The problem is that it is unclear what constitutes a "community"; the notion is often vague and fragmented. In any given situation, different groups may claim to represent community interests. If the community's wants and needs are not easily ascertained, should public health professionals make their own judgments about communal interests? Public health professionals may, at times, coerce some members of the community—not necessarily in the community's best interests, but in the interests of others. In thinking about public health's complex relationship to populations, is the concept of fiduciary duty helpful as an ethical value?

Do public health professionals have a duty to tell the full truth and, if so, under what standard should they be judged? Public health professionals may earnestly believe that their mission requires vigorous interventions to prevent risk behaviors (e.g., smoking) or encourage health-promoting behaviors (e.g., screening and treatment). To achieve these beneficent objectives, public health professionals may exaggerate the risks or benefits or make claims that are insufficiently grounded in science (Wikler and Beauchamp 1995). Suppose public health professionals know that the risk of sexual transmission of HIV in middle-class, low-prevalence areas is relatively low. Are they obliged to disclose this fact when advising men to wear condoms? How would an ethical code address the nuanced question of "truth telling" by public health professionals?

A second form of public health ethics might be called ethics *in* public health theory and practice. Ethics in public health are concerned not so much with the character of professionals as with the ethical dimensions of the public health enterprise itself. Here, scholars study the philosophical knowledge and analytic reasoning necessary for careful thinking and decision making in creating and implementing public health policy. This kind of "applied" ethics is situation or case oriented, seeking to understand morally appropriate decisions in concrete cases. Scholars can helpfully apply general ethical theory and detached analytical reasoning to the societal debates common in public health.

The application of general ethical principles to public health decisions can be difficult and complicated. Since the mission of public health is to achieve the greatest health benefits for the greatest number of people, it draws from the traditions of utilitarianism or consequentialism. The "public health model," argue Buchanan et al. (2000), uncritically assumes that the appropriate mode of evaluating options is some form of cost-benefit (or cost-effectiveness) calculation—the aggregation of goods and bads (benefits and costs) across individuals. Public health, according to this view, appears to permit, or even require, that the most fundamental interests of individuals be sacrificed in order to produce the best overall outcome.

This characterization misperceives, or at least oversimplifies, the public health approach. The field of public health certainly is interested in securing the greatest benefits for the most people. But public health does not simply aggregate benefits and burdens, choosing the policy that produces the most good and the least harm. Rather, the overwhelming majority of public health interventions are intended to benefit the whole population without knowingly harming individuals or groups. When public health authorities work in the areas of tobacco control, the environment, and occupational safety, for example, their belief is that everyone will benefit from smoking cessation, clean air, and safe workplaces. Certainly, public health focuses almost exclusively on one vision of the "common good" (health, not wealth or prosperity), but this is not the same thing as sacrificing fundamental interests to produce the best overall outcome.

The public health approach, of course, does follow a version of the harm principle. Thus, public health authorities regulate individuals or businesses that endanger the community. The objective is to prevent unreasonable risks that jeopardize the public's health and safety—for example, polluting a stream, practicing medicine without a license, or exposing others to an infectious disease. More controversially, public health authorities often recommend paternalistic interventions such as mandatory seat belt or motorcycle helmet laws. Public health authorities reason that the sacrifice asked of individuals is relatively minimal and the communal benefits are substantial. Few public health experts advocate denial of truly fundamental individual liberties in the name of paternalism. In the public health model, individual interests in autonomy, privacy, liberty, and property are taken seriously, but they do not invariably trump community health benefits.

The public health approach, therefore, differs from modern liberalism primarily in its preferences for balancing; public health favors community benefits, whereas liberalism favors liberty interests. Characterizing public health as a utilitarian sacrifice of fundamental personal interests is as unfair as characterizing liberalism as a sacrifice of vital communal interests. Both traditions would deny this kind of oversimplification.

Scholars in bioethics have demonstrated convincingly the power and importance of individual freedom. However, until recently they have given insufficient attention to the equally strong values of partnership, citizenship, and community (Beauchamp 1998). As members of a society in which we have a common bond, we also have an obligation to protect and defend the community against threats to health, safety, and security. Members of society owe a duty—one to another—to promote

the common good. A new public health ethic should advance the idea
that individuals benefit from being part of a well-regulated society that
reduces risks that all members share.

There remains much work to do in public health ethics. What is the
moral standing that should be attached to the collective good? Does the
health of a community have a moral standing that is independent of the
health of individuals within that population? Under what circumstances should individual interests yield to achieve an aggregate benefit
for the population?

At the same time, ethics in public health raise the important issue of
social justice. How can society equitably allocate benefits or services,
on the one hand, and burdens or costs, on the other (Powers and Faden
2000)? Does an otherwise effective policy become unfair if it disproportionately disadvantages a racial, ethnic, or religious group? For example, public health professionals often advocate primary enforcement
of seatbelt laws so that police can stop a driver simply for failure to
comply with the law. But what if primary seatbelt laws are enforced disproportionately against African Americans? Similarly, agencies advocate an increase in the cigarette tax, knowing that the tax is highly regressive. Is it fair to disproportionately burden the poor who use
tobacco products to achieve generally lower levels of smoking in the
population?

Public health professionals routinely face these and many other
kinds of dilemmas that could be informed by ethics scholarship. Think
about the dilemmas that occur in the everyday practice of public
health. When do educational messages cross the line to become persuasion or propaganda? When does surveillance or research unaccept-
ably interfere with privacy? Under what circumstances—consistent
with free expression—can agencies restrict commercial advertising? In
regulating professionals and businesses (e.g., through licenses, inspections, and nuisance abatements), how much deference should agencies
give to property interests?

In addition to "professional" and "applied" ethics, it is possible to
think of an "advocacy" ethic informed by the single overriding value of
a healthy community (Callahan and Jennings 2002). Under this rationale, public health authorities think they know what is ethically appropriate and their function is to advocate for that social goal. This pop-
ulist ethic serves the interests of populations, particularly the powerless
and oppressed, and its methods are principally pragmatic and political.
Public health professionals strive to convince the public and its repre-

sentative political bodies that healthy populations and reduced inequalities are the preferred social responses.

Public health ethics, therefore, can illuminate the field of public health in several ways. Ethics can offer guidance on (1) the meaning of public health professionalism and the ethical practice of the profession, (2) the moral weight and value of the community's health and well-being, (3) the recurring themes of the field and the dilemmas faced in everyday public health practice, and (4) the role of advocacy to achieve the goal of safer and healthier populations.

There needs to be a much more sustained, sophisticated discussion of ethics among students, practitioners, and scholars in public health (Callahan and Jennings 2002). For example, ethics instruction in schools of public health is scarce and targeted primarily to biomedical ethics (Coughlin and Katz 2000). Further, few public health employers in the public and private sectors offer continuing education that includes ethical issues. Government and academic institutions should consider the value of including ethics in accreditation of schools, credentialing of professionals, and the promotion of public health research.

## IV. HUMAN RIGHTS

The language of human rights is used in different, but overlapping, ways. Some use human rights to mean a set of entitlements under international law. Others use human rights to mean a set of ethical standards that stress the paramount importance of individuals. Still others use human rights language for its aspirational, or rhetorical, qualities (see Table 3). A scholar is bound to be concerned when the terminology of human rights is invoked without clarification of the sense in which it is intended (Marks 2001).

Legal scholars and practitioners use human rights to refer to a body of international law that originated in response to the egregious affronts to peace and human dignity committed during World War II. The main source of human rights law within the United Nations system is the international Bill of Human Rights, comprising the Universal Declaration of Human Rights (UDHR) and two international covenants on human rights. Human rights are also protected under regional systems, including those in the Americas, Europe, and Africa.

In its preamble, the United Nations Charter articulates the international community's determination "to reaffirm faith in fundamental human rights, [and] in the dignity and worth of the human person." The

TABLE 3
HUMAN RIGHTS

| | |
|---|---|
| International Law | International Bill of Human Rights: civil and political/economic, social, and cultural<br>Treaty obligations: text and precedent |
| Philosophical | Reasoning and argumentation<br>Import of individual interests |
| Aspirational/Rhetorical | Appeal to fundamental rights of people<br>Symbol commanding reverence and respect<br>Tool of advocacy |

Charter, as a binding treaty, pledges member states to promote universal respect for, and observance of, human rights and fundamental freedoms for all without distinction as to race, sex, language, or religion (arts. 55–56).

The UDHR, adopted in 1948, built upon the promise of the Charter by identifying specific rights and freedoms that deserve promotion and protection. The UDHR was the organized international community's first attempt to establish "a common standard of achievement for all peoples and all nations" to promote human rights (preamble). The UDHR has largely fulfilled the promise of its preamble, becoming the "common standard" for evaluating respect for human rights. Although it was not promulgated to legally bind member states, its key provisions have so often been applied and accepted that they are now widely considered to have attained the status of customary international law.

The adoption of the UDHR set the stage for a binding, treaty-based scheme to promote and protect human rights. The International Covenant on Civil and Political Rights (ICCPR) and the International Covenant on Economic, Social, and Cultural Rights (ICESCR) were adopted in 1966 and entered into force in 1976. The United States has ratified the ICCPR but not the ICESCR. The rights contained in the ICCPR are principally negative or defensive in character, affording individuals a sphere of protection from government restraint. These rights, which are to be respected without discrimination, include the following: the right to life, liberty, and security of person; the prohibition of slavery, torture, and cruel, inhuman, or degrading treatment; the right to an effective judicial remedy; the prohibition of arbitrary arrest, detention, and exile; freedom from arbitrary interference with privacy, family, or home; freedom of movement; freedom of conscience, religion, expression, and association; and the right to participate in government.

The UDHR characterizes economic, social, and cultural rights as "indispensable for [a person's] dignity and the development of his personality" (art. 22). The ICESCR forms the foundation for "positive rights," that is, those requiring affirmative duties of the state to provide services. Such positive rights include the right to social security, the right to education, the right to work, the right to receive equal pay for equal work and to remuneration ensuring "an existence worthy of human dignity," and the right to share in the cultural life of the community and "to share in scientific advancement and its benefits" (arts. 22–27). Article 12 of the ICESCR requires governments to recognize "the right of everyone to the highest attainable standard of physical and mental health." Article 25 of the UDHR also expressly recognizes a right to health: "Everyone has the right to a standard of living adequate for the health and well-being of himself and his family, including food, clothing, housing and medical care and necessary social services, and the right to security in the event of unemployment, sickness, disability, widowhood, old age or other lack of livelihood in circumstances beyond his control."

The two covenants diverge in their treatment of permissible derogations and limitations. The ICCPR recognizes that certain rights are so fundamental as to be absolute and proscribes any derogation of them. Nonderogable rights include the right to life (art. 6); freedom from torture and from cruel, inhuman, or degrading treatment or punishment (art. 7); freedom from slavery or servitude (art. 8); the right to recognition as a person before the law (art. 16); and freedom of thought, conscience, and religion (art. 18). The ICCPR states that other rights may be justifiably limited under certain conditions. Freedom of movement, for example, may be justifiably limited where restrictions are "provided for by law, are necessary to protect national security, public order, public health or morals or the rights and freedoms of others" (art. 12). The ICESCR, on the other hand, permits "such limitations as are determined by law only in so far as this may be compatible with the nature of these rights and solely for the purpose of promoting the general welfare in a democratic society" (art. 4).

Human rights law follows a set of internationally agreed rules specified in the text of treaties and other instruments, is informed by precedent, and is interpreted by tribunals and commissions. International human rights law seldom provides easy answers; rather, it struggles to define and enforce human rights in the context of the legitimate powers of governments and the needs of communities.

Ethicists use the language of human rights for related but different purposes. The fields of ethics and human rights share an abiding belief in the paramount importance of individual rights and interests, but beyond that their perspectives diverge. Whereas human rights scholars stress the importance of treaty obligations, ethicists seldom refer to international law doctrine. Whereas human rights scholars rely on text and precedent, ethicists employ philosophical reasoning and argumentation. When ethicists adopt the language of international human rights, there is bound to be a certain amount of confusion. For example, if ethicists claim that health care is a "human right," do they mean that a definable and enforceable right under international law exists, or simply that philosophical principles such as justice support this claim?

Finally, public health students, as well as the lay public, often use the language of human rights for its aspirational, or rhetorical, qualities. Major public health schools, such as the Johns Hopkins University and Harvard University, give their students a copy of the UDHR at commencement or offer special certificates in human rights. When "rights" language is invoked, it is intended to convey the fundamental importance of the claim. It expresses the idea that government should adhere to certain standards, or provide certain services, because it is right and just to do so. Human rights as a symbol commands reverence and respect. Used in this aspirational sense, human rights need not be supported by text, precedent, or reasoning; they are self-evident, and government's responsibility simply is to conform.

Human rights, then, have features in common with ethics, but they are different fields. Human rights, like ethics, are often concerned with individual rights and interests, and like advocacy ethics, human rights convey a sense of moral certainty. However, international human rights are also quite distinct from ethics. The field of human rights is based on a body of rules and precedents intended to express binding duties. It is complex and evolving, usually rejecting easy resolutions to the conflict between individual interests and collective goods.

The field of human rights has much work to do if it is to contribute usefully to health policy analysis. For example, human rights scholars and advocates have not clarified the meaning of the right to health (Gostin and Lazzarini 1997; Jamar 1994). The conceptualization of health as a human right, and not simply a moral claim, suggests that states possess binding obligations to respect, protect, and fulfill that entitlement (Leary 1994). Considerable disagreement, however, exists as to whether "health" is a meaningful, identifiable, operational, and enforceable right, or whether it is merely aspirational or rhetorical (Kinney 2001). A right to health that is too broadly defined lacks clear content and is less likely to have a meaningful effect. If health is, in WHO's words, truly "a state of complete physical, mental, and social well-being," then it can never be achieved. Even if this definition were construed as a reasonable, as opposed to an absolute, standard, it remains difficult to implement and is unlikely to be justiciable. Vast scholarship and litigation in international fora have been necessary to define and enforce civil and political rights. Social and economic rights, notably the right to health, deserve the same rigorous and sustained attention (Gostin 2000c). This is beginning to happen in international fora (Toebes 1999b). For example, the United Nations Committee on Economic, Social, and Cultural Rights offered detailed guidance on the meaning of the right to health (Gostin 2001), which is discussed further in chapter 4.

## THE *READER*'S OBJECTIVES

The *Reader* probes the interrelated fields of public health, law, ethics, and human rights. The goal is to raise the most important and enduring intellectual issues and practical problems. In so doing, it should provoke discussion and debate among students, scholars, and practitioners. More important, the *Reader* provides a framework for rigorous analysis of the philosophical, political, economic, and jurisprudential dimensions of government intervention to assure the health of the populace. Nothing is so important to the security and vibrancy of a nation as the well-being of its people.

# PART ONE

# Foundations of Public Health Law and Ethics

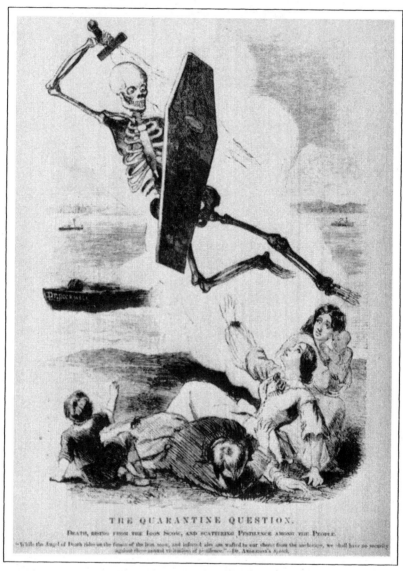

This drawing, which appeared in *Harper's Weekly* on October 2, 1858, portrays the threat from incoming vessels, demonstrating the role of quarantine in shielding populations from infectious disease.

# TWO

# Public Health

*The Population-Based Perspective*

The readings in this chapter examine the origins, theories, and practices of public health. The first section, "History," discusses the evolution of American traditions in public health. The reading by the famous Sanitary Commission of Massachusetts, authored by an early pioneer of public health, Lemuel Shattuck, highlights the importance of legal systems supporting disease prevention and health promotion, as well as the challenges and tensions within the field in the mid-nineteenth century. The reading by Elizabeth Fee, former Johns Hopkins professor and now at the National Library of Medicine, traces the history of American public health—the major epidemics, the social responses, and the important social movements.

The second section, "Mission and Functions," emphasizes the goals, services, and roles of public health. The Institute of Medicine's (IOM) influential 1988 report *The Future of Public Health* provided the foundations for modern public health programs. The IOM expressed concern about the lack of leadership and visibility in the field of public health. Scott Burris, a leading public health law scholar from Temple University, explains why the field of public health often does not receive the public and political support it deserves (see also McGinnis 2001).

The final section, "The Population Focus," discusses one of the most distinctive aspects of the field of public health relative to other health professions: the emphasis on the well-being of the population as opposed to clinical benefits for individuals. The primary objective of public health is to improve the community's overall health and wellness. These two readings advance this notion through distinct analytical frameworks. By reasoning "backward" from traditional medical causes of death, two well-known modern public health policy researchers, J. Michael McGinnis and William Foege, effectively show that social and behavioral factors contribute most to lost years of life. Through his discussion of the prevention paradox, the late British epidemiologist Geoffrey Rose analyzes how public health interventions often require significant commitment from the individual (such as improved diet and exercise) and offer the greatest benefit to the community, while often offering little concrete "return" to the individual. Rose's prevention paradox may help explain the difficulty of public health in selling behavior change in the marketplace of ideas.

## I. HISTORY

The industrial revolution of the nineteenth century created an expanding market for urban jobs. As a result, much of the American population, including large groups of newly arrived immigrants, migrated to the cities for work. Industrialization and urbanization, combined with a lack of planned growth, resulted in overcrowding, slum conditions, homelessness, squalor, and violence. Among the working community, there existed a growing realization that garbage, sewage, pollution, poorly stored food, and unclean drinking water had negative effects on the health of their children and families.

It was within this context that citizens began to think of the control of disease as being properly within the sphere of government control. Government's concern with the health of populations—in England and then in the United States—was often expressed through commissions created to study the problem. The most prominent American public health commission of the time, the Sanitary Commission of Massachusetts, commenced with a call for sanitary legislation (Shattuck 1850, 9–10):

> The condition of perfect public health requires such laws and regulations as will secure to man associated in society the same sanitary enjoyments that he would have as an isolated individual, and as will protect him from injury from any influences connected with his locality, his dwelling house, his occupation, or those of his associates or neighbors, or from any other social causes. It is under the control of public authority, and public administration;

and life and health may be saved or lost, as this authority is wisely or unwisely exercised.

The following reading from the Sanitary Commission report, written by Shattuck, expresses an early vision of the power and duty of government to assure the conditions for the health of the populace. Notice the Sanitary Commission's emphasis on statistical approaches to help measure and understand the sources of injury and disease (a precursor of modern biostatistics and epidemiology) as well as on the importance of disease prevention. The commission also recognized the inherent conflict between personal liberties and the common good, a conflict that remains at the heart of American public health law and ethics. The Shattuck report addresses two specific issues: state collection of information regarded as private and infringements on basic civil and economic liberties, such as restrictions on personal behavior and private property.

The reading following the Sanitary Commission report, by Fee, offers a broad historical account of public health in America from early to modern times. Fee's perspective emphasizes the connectedness of public health policy to major social, economic, scientific, and political conditions of the time. The readings by Shattuck and Fee introduce themes that will be discussed throughout the *Reader*. (For an illuminating account of the relationship between public health and medicine during the twentieth century, see Brandt and Gardner [2000].)

---

## Introduction and Private Rights and Liberties*
*Lemuel Shattuck*

We believe that the conditions of perfect health, either public or personal, are seldom or never attained, though attainable; that the average length of human life may be very much extended, and its physical power greatly augmented; that in every year, within this Commonwealth, thousands of lives are lost which might have been saved; that

---

*Reprinted from *Report of the Sanitary Commission of Massachusetts* (1850; reprint, Cambridge: Harvard University Press, 1948).

tens of thousands of cases of sickness occur, which might have been prevented; that a vast amount of unnecessarily impaired health, and physical debility exists among those not actually confined by sickness; that these preventable evils require an enormous expenditure and loss of money, and impose upon the people unnumbered and immeasurable calamities, pecuniary, social, physical, mental, and moral, which might be avoided; that means exist, within our reach, for their mitigation or removal, and that measures for prevention will affect infinitely more than remedies for the cure of disease.

But whom does this great matter of public health concern? By whom is this subject to be surveyed, analyzed, and practically applied? And who are to be benefitted by this application? Some will answer, the physician, certainly. True, but only in a degree; not mainly. It will assist him to learn the causes of disease; but it will be infinitely more valuable to the whole people, to teach them how to prevent disease, and to live without being sick. This is a blessing which cannot be measured by money value. The people are principally concerned, and on them must depend, in part, at least, the introduction and progress of sanitary measures. . . .

It may be said, "[Sanitary measures] will interfere with private matters. If a child is born, if a marriage takes place, or if a person dies, in my house, it is my own affair, what business is it to the public? If the person dies at one age or at another, if he dies of one disease or of another, contagious or not contagious, it's my business, not another's, these are private matters."

Men who object and reason in this manner have very inadequate conceptions of the obligations they owe to themselves or to others. No family, no person liveth to himself alone. Every person has a direct or indirect interest in every other person. We are social beings—bound together by indissoluble ties. Every birth, every marriage, and every death, which takes place, has an impact somewhere; it may not be upon you or me now; but it has upon some others, and may hereafter have upon us. In the revolutions of human life it is impossible to foretell which shall prosper, this or that, whether I shall be a pauper or have to contribute to support my neighbor. Or, whether I shall inherit his property or he inherit mine. . . .

It may be said, "This will interfere with private rights. If I own an estate, haven't I a right to do with it as I please? To build upon it any kind of house, or to occupy it in any way, without the public interference? Haven't I a right to create or continue a nuisance—to allow disease of any kind on my own premises, without accountability to others?"

Different men reason differently, in justification of themselves, on this matter. One man owns real estate in an unhealthy locality; and if its condition were known, it might affect its value. Another has a dwelling house unfit for the residence of human beings; and he will oppose any efforts to improve it because it will cost money, and he can have tenants in its present condition. Another does business in a place where, and at a time when, an epidemic prevails; and his occupation may tend to increase it; and, if these facts were known, it might affect his profits. These and similar reasons may lead different minds to oppose this measure. How extensively such opinions prevail we will not attempt to state. Some twelve years since one of this commission introduced into the city council of Boston, an order of inquiry relating to a certain locality supposed to be unhealthy; but it was strongly opposed, because, as was stated, it would impair the value of the real estate in the neighborhood! There may be individuals who place dollars and cents, even in small amounts, by the side of human health and human life, in their estimate of value, and strike a balance in favor of the former; but it is to be hoped that the number of such persons is not large.

---

### The Origins and Development of Public Health in the United States*
*Elizabeth Fee*

What is public health? . . . The broader one's definition of health, the grander the scope of public health—the public responsibility to create the conditions under which all members of the population can experience the maximum degree of good health, within the limits that may be imposed by economics, genetics, or the state of our knowledge. . . . Clearly, public health defined in this manner embraces virtually all aspects of social and economic policies from the tax code to environmental regulations and will include social welfare policies, the provision of health services,

---

*Reprinted from *Oxford Textbook of Public Health: Volume I: The Scope of Public Health,* edited by Roger Detels, Walter W. Holland, James McEwen and Gilbert Omenn (3rd edition, 1997), by permission of Oxford University Press. © Roger Detels, Walter W. Holland, James McEwen, and Gilbert S. Omenn 1997.

and the prevention of war. . . . As people working in public health are well aware, there is, in most times and places, a great disjunction between what the more visionary public health leaders believe could or should be done to promote the public health and their ability to realize these ideals in practice [taking into account political and economic realities].

## THE ORIGINS OF PUBLIC HEALTH IN THE NEW WORLD

The first colonists had found a healthy land of bracing air, clean water, and acres of fertile soil. Duffy (1990) recounted the enthusiastic reports of the first settlers and their subsequent struggles with hunger and malnutrition, as well as endemic and epidemic diseases. The new arrivals brought scurvy, smallpox, cholera, measles, diphtheria, typhoid fever, and influenza. The deadliest of the European imports was smallpox, a constant threat to the colonists, but a devastation to the Indian tribes with whom they came into contact. The colonists arrived with some immunity to diseases such as smallpox and measles but, in epidemiological terms, Native Americans were a virgin population; disease thus played an essential part in the European conquest. . . .

In the colonies, public health consisted of activities deemed necessary to protect the population from the spread of epidemic diseases, by the enactment of sanitary laws and regulations governing such matters as the construction of toilets, the disposal of wastes, and the disposition of dead animals. Public health was, in the main, an urban affair. Towns and cities appointed inspectors and levied fines against the sellers of putrid meat and property owners who refused or neglected to drain their swamps. Public health, when organized at all, was a strictly local matter.

By the eighteenth century, quarantine laws had been passed in all the major towns along the eastern seaboard—laws that admittedly tended to be enforced only during the immediate threat of epidemic diseases. Pesthouses were built for the immigrants arriving on infected ships and in Boston, Cotton Mather and Zabdiel Boylston introduced the practice of inoculation for smallpox. Smallpox inoculation, while controversial, was perhaps the most successful specific preventive against disease and, when Jenner's vaccine was later announced, it was almost immediately accepted. . . .

## THE CIVIL WAR

The Civil War enforced a national consciousness of epidemic disease: two-thirds of the 360,000 Union soldiers who died were killed by infectious diseases rather than by enemy fire. Joseph Jones, a surgeon in the medical department of the Confederate Army, estimated that three-quarters or 150,000 of the Confederate soldiers' deaths were due to disease; others believed he had underestimated these losses. In either case, contemporary accounts reported the main causes of death on both sides as "typhomalaria" (perhaps a combination of typhoid fever and malaria), camp diarrhoea, and "camp measles." Scurvy, acute respiratory diseases, venereal diseases, rheumatism, and epidemic jaundice were widespread and the ravages of dysentery, spread by inadequate or non-existent sanitary facilities in army encampments, were appalling. . . .

## INDUSTRIALIZATION AND THE DEVELOPMENT OF PUBLIC HEALTH

In the period after the Civil War, northern industrialists began to transform the country into a single national market. Agricultural and industrial mechanization irrevocably altered the traditional patterns of production and consumption and small companies were merged or collapsed into large corporations. Between 1860 and 1894, the value of manufactured goods multiplied by five. The United States was moving into first place as the most powerful industrial country in the world, bypassing England, Germany, and France. . . .

At this time, there were no formal requirements for public health positions, no established career structures, and no job security for health officials. Public health positions were usually part-time appointments at a nominal salary; those who devoted much effort to public health typically did so on a voluntary basis. Until the mid-nineteenth century, public health, like other governmental functions, was considered the responsibility of the social élite. . . . [L]ocal élites regarded public health with a certain complacency; they believed the American environment was much healthier than that of Europe—and the social order more egalitarian. Poverty and disease could largely be attributed to individual weakness, wickedness, or laziness. The belief that epidemic diseases posed only occasional threats to an otherwise healthy social order was, however, shaken by the economic transformation of the late nineteenth century. The burgeoning social problems of the industrial cities could not then be ignored: the overwhelming influx of immigrants crowded into narrow alleys and tenement housing, the terrifying death and disease rates of working class slums, the total inadequacy of water supplies and sewage systems for the rapidly growing population, the spread of endemic and epidemic diseases from the tenements to the homes of the wealthy, the escalating squalor and violence of the streets—all impressed members of the social élite that urban problems required concerted attention. Poverty and disease could no longer be treated simply as individual failings; they were becoming social and political problems of massive proportions.

As cities grew in size, as the flow of immigrants continued, and as public health problems became ever more obvious, city health departments mounted rearguard actions against the filth and congestion generated by anarchic urban development. . . . In the aftermath of the Civil War, most states created boards of health. . . .

## PUBLIC HEALTH AS SOCIAL REFORM

With the industrialization of America, the older concerns with quarantines and the threat of disease from without soon paled in comparison with the perceived threats from within. America no longer fitted its own self-image as a republic of independent farmers and craftsmen; like the European countries, it now displayed extremes of wealth and privilege, social misery, and deprivation. Labour agitation and political unrest forced awareness of social inequalities and widespread distress. . . .

An increasing number of reform groups devoted themselves to social issues and improvements of every variety. At the levels of both city and state, health reformers, physicians, and engineers urged sanitary improvements. Medical men were prominent in these reform organizations, but they were not alone. Rosenkrantz (1974, 57) contrasted public health in the late nineteenth century with the internecine battles within general medicine: "the field of public hygiene exemplified a happy marriage of engineers, physicians and public spirited citizens providing a model of complementary comportment under the banner of sanitary science." . . .

Middle- and upper-class women, seizing an opportunity to escape from the narrow bounds of domestic responsibilities, joined in campaigns for improved housing, the abolition of child labour, maternal and child health, and temperance. Active in the settlement house movement, trade union organizing, the suffrage movement, and municipal sanitary reform, they declared "municipal house-keeping" a natural extension of women's training and experience as "the housekeepers of the world" (Ryan 1975). Beginning by cleaning up their homes, neighbourhoods, and cities, reforming women announced themselves ready to take on the nation as a whole. Across the country, volunteers and public health nurses established infant feeding centres, well baby clinics, and school health services. Indeed, national voluntary health organizations—largely organized and staffed by women—supplied much of the impulse and energy behind public health.

Progressive groups in the public health movement advocated reform on political, economic, humanitarian, and scientific grounds. Although sharing the revolutionaries' perception of the plight of the poor and the injustices of the system, they usually counselled less radical solutions. Politically, public health reform seemed to offer a middle ground between the cutthroat principles of entrepreneurial capitalism and the revolutionary ideas of the socialists, anarchists, and Utopian visionaries. . . .

## THE PROFESSIONALIZATION OF PUBLIC HEALTH

These developments led to an increasing demand for people trained in public health to direct the new programmes being created at the local, state, and national levels. Those responsible for such activities became increasingly critical of the lack of properly trained personnel; part-time public health officers were simply not adequate to staff the ambitious new programmes being planned and implemented. Public health reformers agreed that full-time practitioners, specially trained for the job, were needed. . . .

Public health had been defined in terms of its aims and goal—to reduce disease and maintain the health of the population—rather than by any specific body of knowledge. Many different disciplines contributed to effective public health work: physicians diagnosed contagious diseases, sanitary engineers built water and sewage systems, epidemiologists traced the sources of disease outbreaks and their modes of transmission, vital statisticians provided quantitative measures of births and deaths, lawyers wrote sanitary codes and regulations, public health nurses provided care and advice to the sick in their homes, sanitary inspectors visited factories and markets to enforce compliance with public health ordinances, and administrators tried to organize everyone within the limits of health department budgets. Public health thus involved economics, sociology, psychology, politics, law, statistics, and engineering, as well as the biological and clinical sciences. However, in the period immediately following the brilliant experimental work of Louis Pasteur and Robert Koch, the bacteriological laboratory became the first and primary symbol of a new, scientific public health.

## BACTERIOLOGY AND THE NEW PUBLIC HEALTH

The clarity and simplicity of bacteriological methods and discoveries gave them tremendous cultural and ideological importance: the agents of particular diseases had been made visible under the microscope. The identification of specific bacteria seemed to have cut through the misty miasmas of disease to define the enemy in unmistakable terms as a series of microscopic foreign invaders. Bacteriology became an ideological marker, sharply differentiating the "old" public health, the province of untrained amateurs, from the "new" public health, which would belong to scientifically trained professionals. . . .

The public health laboratory demonstrated the scientific and diagnostic power of the new public health. The approach of locating, identifying, and isolating bacteria and their human hosts seemed to provide a more elegant, effective, and easier way of dealing with disease than environmental reform. The powerful new methods of identifying diseases through the microscope therefore tended to draw attention away from the larger and more diffuse problems of urban sanitation, street cleaning, housing reform, and the living conditions of the poor. . . .

## PUBLIC HEALTH ORGANIZATION AND PRACTICE

The practical importance of public health was well recognized by the early decades of the twentieth century. Mortality rates from tuberculosis, diphtheria, and other infectious diseases were falling, apparently in response to energetic public health campaigns. Public health nurses established school health clinics and promoted maternal and child health programmes. In many cities, health education efforts increased the visibility of public health departments. . . .

A major stimulus to the development of public health practice came in response to the Depression, with the New Deal legislation and in particular the Social Security Act of 1935. The Social Security Act expanded financing of the Public Health Service and provided federal grants to the states for public health initiatives. . . .

## PUBLIC HEALTH AND THE WAR

With the mobilization for war, public health was declared a national priority for the armed forces and the civilian population engaged in military production. . . . Major population shifts had occurred with the mobilization for war, the movement of troops, and the migration of workers to defence industry plants. Army training camps had often been placed in areas with warm climates, where the *Anopheles* mosquito bred in profusion and malaria was endemic. Responding to this threat, the Public Health Service established the Center for the Control of Malaria in War Areas. After the war, when substantial funds were made available for malaria eradication efforts, this organization was gradually transformed into the Centers for Disease Control and Prevention, which would come to play a major national role in the effort to control both infectious and non-infectious diseases. . . .

## THE DECLINE OF PUBLIC HEALTH IN THE POSTWAR ERA

There are many reasons why the United States moved towards ever more sophisticated biomedical research and high technology medicine in the postwar era. . . . In retrospect, it seems clear that public health failed to claim sufficient credit for controlling infectious diseases. The major scientific achievements of the war in relation to health—the discovery of penicillin and the use of DDT—were particularly relevant to public health. In popular perception, however, scientific medicine took credit for both the specific wartime discoveries and the longer history of combating epidemic disease: in public relations terms, medicine and biomedical research seized the public glory, the political interest, and the financial support given for further anticipated health improvements in the postwar world. . . .

## SOCIAL AGITATION AND CIVIL RIGHTS

Throughout the 1950s, the Civil Rights movement had been growing, igniting passions across the southern states and industrial cities across the land. . . . The renewed political mobilization of the country seemed to extend in all directions—to the women's movement and the gay and lesbian movement, Native American rebellions, environmentalists, hippies, and yippies, and new organizations of the elderly, prisoners, welfare mothers, and the mentally ill. The antipoverty effort of Great Society programmes, the Environmental Protection Agency, and the Occupational Health and Safety Act of 1970 were among the responses to these popular movements. The organization and financing of medical care again became a matter of political debate, culminating in Medicare and Medicaid legislation in 1965 to cover medical care costs for those on social security and for the poor. Medicare and Medicaid reflected the usual priorities of the medical care system in

favouring highly technical interventions and hospital care while failing adequately to provide for preventive services. . . .

## THE EXPANSION OF PUBLIC HEALTH EDUCATION

In the 1980s, the Reagan administration cut funding for public
health programmes clustered together in block grants. . . . By 1988,
almost three-quarters of all state and local health department expenditures went on personal health services. . . . [D]irect provision of
medical care absorbed the limited resources—in personnel, money,
energy, time, and attention—of public health departments, leading to
a slow starvation of public health and preventive activities. The
problem of care for the uninsured and the indigent loomed so large
that it eclipsed basic public health needs in the minds of many legislators and the general public.

The AIDS epidemic and the resurgence of tuberculosis added to the
burdens of state and city health departments and gave new visibility
and urgency to their efforts. . . . Public health officials, gay leaders, and
community advocates urged a major national effort in education and
prevention. However, most of the AIDS funding, when it did come,
went into research and medical care; education and prevention proved
too controversial to receive adequate political support.

## THE PRESENT AND FUTURE OF PUBLIC HEALTH

To public health professionals, it is obviously desirable to devote more
significant resources to disease prevention and health promotion.
Surely prevention is preferable to cure. As Waitzkin (1983) and others
have argued, we are spending "billions for band-aids." In the political
climate of 1995, however, when the health reform effort collapsed and
social programmes were under attack, establishing prevention as a priority was to prove difficult.

Political struggles and economic constraints are nothing new to public health. Public health professionals at the local, state, and national
levels and in schools of public health will have to make a more effective case for the importance of prevention. . . . In this climate of cost
containment, it may be argued that public health and preventive services will prove cost-effective by reducing the need for expensive cura-
tive and hospital care. . . .

One problem with cost-benefit analyses in relation to public
health is that those who pay the costs are not necessarily those who

most directly benefit. In addition to these types of economic calculations are the social benefits to be gained from happier and healthier lives. Political and ethical values are therefore intrinsic to the debate over prevention policies and the future of public health. The overarching challenge ahead is to create the conditions under which all people—irrespective of status, class, race/ethnicity, gender, cultural background, or sexual preference—can enjoy a state of "physical, mental, and social well-being."

## II. MISSION AND FUNCTIONS

As Fee and other historians explain, the field of public health became invigorated during the late nineteenth and early twentieth centuries. This was the time of the so-called Sanitarian movement, where community activists powerfully advocated the importance of hygiene, controls on industry, and social regulation (Duffy 1990). Somehow, America lost its commitment to public health in the latter part of the twentieth century. Part of the reason may have been the sheer success of public health. For example, in 1972 the surgeon general informed Congress that it was time to "close the book on infectious diseases" (Bloom and Murray 1992, 1055). The late twentieth century has also been a time of distrust of government and citizen antipathy toward excessive taxation and regulation.

In its foundational report *The Future of Public Health,* the IOM (1988, 19) concluded that "this nation has lost sight of its public health goals and has allowed the system of public health activities to fall into disarray." The IOM vigorously urged fundamental reform of the public health infrastructure, the training capacity, and the body of enabling laws and regulations. The mission and functions of public health have clearly changed from the Shattuck report in the mid-nineteenth century, to the IOM report in 1988, to the present day.

The Public Health Functions project (a coalition of national public health organizations), the Department of Health and Human Services (DHHS) report *Healthy People 2010,* and the Centers for Disease Control and Prevention report *Public Health's Infrastructure* (CDC 2000f) responded to the IOM's critique. These groups set about the task of reinvigorating the field of public health. Figure 4

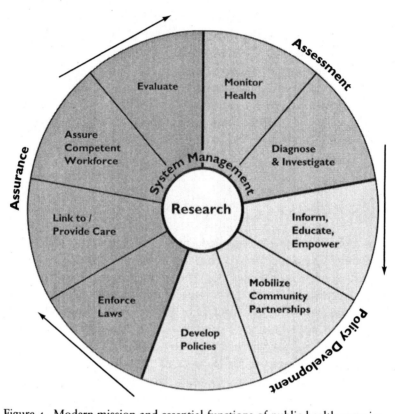

Figure 4. Modern mission and essential functions of public health agencies. (*Source:* Public Health Functions Steering Committee, July 1995.)

presents an illustration of the modern mission and functions of public health agencies.

Congress also responded to IOM's call for an improved public health infrastructure by enacting the Public Health Threats and Emergencies Act of 2000 (also known as the Frist-Kennedy Act) (42 U.S.C. § 247d to d-7). The law authorizes expenditures for updated public health capacity at the state level, together with specific programs to combat antimicrobial resistance and bioterrorism (see chapter 14). The Senate Appropriations Committee (1999, 244–45) expressed concern over "the disparities of quality and capabilities of the American public health infrastructure . . . and the insufficient capital funding of hospitals, laboratories, clinics, information networks, and other essential public health services." Table 4 describes the goals and recommendations of the CDC (2000f) for a strong public health infrastructure.

### TABLE 4
### GOALS AND RECOMMENDATIONS
### FOR PUBLIC HEALTH'S INFRASTRUCTURE

1. A Skilled Workforce
   *Goal:* Each community will be served by a fully trained, culturally competent public health team, representing the optimal mix of professional disciplines.

2. Robust Information and Data Systems
   *Goal:* Each health department will be able to electronically access and distribute up-to-date public health information and emergency health alerts, monitor the health of communities, and assist in the detection of emerging public health problems.

3. Effective Health Departments and Laboratories
   *Goal:* Each health department and laboratory will meet basic performance and accountability standards that recognize their population base, including census, geography, and risk factors, with specific needs identified through state public health improvement plans.

SOURCE: CDC (2000f): "Every Health Department Fully Prepared; Every Community Better Protected."

## The Functions of Public Health*
*Institute of Medicine*

A MISSION OF PUBLIC HEALTH

[P]ublic health is "public" because it involves "organized community effort." It is not simply the outcome of isolated individual efforts. Its mission is to ensure that organized approaches are mobilized when they are needed. For example, both smallpox vaccination of countless individuals and treatment of unvaccinated patients would not have rid us of smallpox without strategies aimed specifically at the communitywide (in this case, the worldwide) level, such as epidemiologic studies, consistent reporting of cases, and organized distribution of vaccine. In a similar way, neither treatment of lung disease nor exhorting individuals to avoid smoking could have achieved the reduction of smoking in public places made possible by organized community effort to adopt laws and regulations restricting smoking. Seat belt legislation is still another instance in which a communitywide approach has augmented individual effort.

*Reprinted from *The Future of Public Health* (Washington, D.C.: National Academy Press, 1988), 39–46.

Public health is also public in terms of its long-range goal, which is optimal health for the entire community. This goal encompasses both the sum of the health status of individual community members and communitywide benefits such as clean air and water. Our shared sense of what "complete well-being" might be, though none of us has ever experienced it, serves as a focus for commitment to extend community efforts beyond the narrow concerns of special interests and the boundaries of any one professional discipline. . . .

[For these reasons,] the committee defines the *mission* of public health as: the fulfillment of society's interest in assuring the conditions in which people can be healthy.

## THE SUBSTANCE OF PUBLIC HEALTH

Within this mission fall a number of characteristic themes, which over the course of a long historical tradition have coalesced around the goal of the people's health. . . . Over time, the substance of public health has expanded. . . . [A] commitment to multidimensional well-being implies the need to address factors that fall outside the normal understanding of "health," including decent housing, public education, adequate income, freedom from war, and so on. While encouraging a holistic approach, this tendency to widen the boundaries of public health has the effect of forcing practitioners to make difficult choices about where to focus their energies and raises the possibility that public health could be so broadly defined so as to lose distinctive meaning.

Even restricting public health's subject matter to disease prevention and control, health promotion, and environmental measures necessitates the involvement of a broad spectrum of professional disciplines. In fact, it is frequently pointed out that public health is a coalition of professions united by their shared mission; their focus on disease prevention and health promotion; their prospective approach in contrast to the reactive focus of therapeutic medicine; and their common science, epidemiology. . . .

Epidemiology is the "glue" that holds public health's many professions together. It is by means of the application of scientific and technical knowledge, above all else, that public health practitioners strive to improve the lot of humankind, to understand the causes of disease, to identify populations at risk, and to develop new approaches to prevention.

Thus, the committee defines the *substance* of public health as: organized community efforts aimed at the prevention of disease and promotion of health. It links many disciplines and rests upon the scientific core of epidemiology. . . .

## THE ROLE OF GOVERNMENT IN PUBLIC HEALTH

. . . In general, Americans are skeptical about the role of government. Concern for individual rights shapes the public philosophy and attitudes of policymakers and ordinary citizens alike. From this perspective, society is made up of individual persons with "inalienable rights." The purpose of government is to protect those rights and ensure the basic conditions necessary for their exercise—civil order, a free market, and equal individual opportunity. Government, in other words, ensures that the basic means to the good life are available, but it refrains from specifying what the content of that life should be or how individuals should behave, except to prevent them from infringing on the rights of others.

This mainstream perspective is tempered somewhat by another long-standing tradition in American political philosophy, rooted in concern for the community as a whole. This view emphasizes the social ties that bind people together, including the values they share. It sees government as a facilitator of the social bond and the policy process as a means of defining positive goals and taking concerted action. These two themes are reflected in the history of American governance. In general, the philosophy of limited government implied by a concern for individual rights has prevailed. But the theme of positive values and community effort has persisted, and deliberate government steps to combat acknowledged social ills have become increasingly acceptable to most Americans, remaining so even during the renewed stress on individualism in recent years. . . .

## THE FUNCTIONS OF GOVERNMENT IN PUBLIC HEALTH

The committee sees the government role in public health as made up of three functions: assessment, policy development, and assurance. These functions correspond to the major phases of public problem-solving: identification of problems, mobilization of necessary effort and resources, and assurance that vital conditions are in place and that crucial services are received.

### Assessment

Under this heading are all the activities involved in the concept of community diagnosis, such as surveillance, identifying needs, analyzing the causes of problems, collecting and interpreting data, case-finding, monitoring and forecasting trends, research, and evaluation of outcomes.

Assessment is inherently a public function because policy formulation, in order to be legitimate, is expected to take in all relevant available information and to be based on objective factors—to the extent possible. Private sector entities are expected to have self-interests.

Therefore the information they generate, while frequently quite useful to the policy process, is not judged by its fairness. In contrast, although public agencies in practice do not always weigh all sides of a question, in principle they are obligated to do so.

Moreover, public decisions take place in the context of limited resources. Society cannot do everything it would like to do or with the intensity it might prefer. Thus trade-offs among competing uses of resources are necessary. The wisdom, justice, and perceived legitimacy of public decisions are crucially affected by the quality of the information on which they are based. A function of government is to provide a central mechanism by means of which competing proposals can be assessed equitably.

In addition, the government has an important responsibility to develop a broader base of knowledge in order to ensure that policy is not driven by purely short-range issues constrained by current knowledge. Public sector assessment activities should include supporting and conducting research into fundamental determinants of health—behavioral, environmental, biological, and socioeconomic—as well as monitoring health status and trends. . . .

### Policy Development

Policy formulation takes place as the result of interactions among a wide range of public and private organizations and individuals. It is the process by which society makes decisions about problems, chooses goals and the proper means to reach them, handles conflicting views about what should be done, and allocates resources. Government provides overall guidance in this process. In contrast to private entities, it alone has the power to give binding answers. Therefore, although it joins with the private sector to arrive at decisions, government has a special obligation to ensure that the public interest is served by whatever measures are adopted. As with other governmental entities, the public health agency bears this responsibility. . . .

### Assurance

A core public sector function is to make sure that necessary services are provided to reach agreed upon goals, either by encouraging private sector action, by requiring it, or by providing services directly.

The assurance function in public health involves seeing to the implementation of legislative mandates as well as maintaining statutory responsibilities. It includes developing adequate responses to crises and supporting crucial services that have worked well for so long that they are now taken for granted. It includes regulation of services and products provided in both the private and public sectors, as well as maintaining accountability to the people by setting objectives and reporting on progress. Assurance implies the maintenance of a level of service needed to attain an intended impact or outcome that is achievable given the resources and techniques available.

Carrying out the assurance function requires the exercise of authority. This is not a responsibility that can be delegated to the private sector. Members of society expect government to make certain that they enjoy at least adequate safety and security. The public health agency must be able to exercise authority consistent with fulfilling citizens' expectations and must account to them for its actions with equal energy.

As a part of the assurance function, in the interest of justice public health agencies should guarantee certain health services. Such a guarantee expresses a measurable public commitment to each member of society. In operational terms, this implies guaranteeing both that the services are available (present somewhere in the community) and, in the case of services to individuals, that the costs will be borne by the government for those unable to afford them. When these services are not and cannot be present in the larger community, it is the public health agency's responsibility to provide them directly.

Such a guarantee reflects a community consensus that access to certain health services is necessary to maintain our notion of a decent society. A guarantee acts as a barrier to service cuts in hard times, which tend to fall on the most vulnerable. Such a step also serves as a stimulus to improvement, as has happened in the case of public education, where community efforts have moved from ensuring universal coverage to enriching the quality of the service.

---

## The Invisibility of Public Health: Population-Level Measures in a Politics of Market Individualism*
Scott Burris

Modern public health work is informed by a recognition of the important role of culture, particularly political culture, in defining the meaning of disease and setting limits on what government can do in the

---

*Reprinted from *American Journal of Public Health* 87 (October 1997): 1607–10.

name of promoting the public's health. The success of Surgeon General Thomas Parran's fight against venereal disease surely depended in substantial part on the ascendancy of New Deal Democrats. Surgeon General Joycelyn Elders, by contrast, was undone by her frank talk about sex, characterized in a conservative political climate as a government attack on family values. . . .

The tendency among public health advocates is to accommodate the prevailing mood. To win support for its programs, public health must, to some extent, frame its goals in language that will be broadly acceptable to politicians and their constituents. But I want to suggest . . . that there is a long-term danger in an excessive devotion to short-term pragmatism, which does little to change the habits of thought in politics and the larger culture that essentially exclude public health from serious consideration. A good example is the IOM's 1988 report on the future of public health. The book, often cited as the authoritative prescription for public health reform, spoke of the need to convince Americans of the value of public health work but itself offered a narrow, uninspiring account of the enterprise painted in the drab palette of the Reagan years: mistrust of government, preference for the market, and a focus on the individual. There was nowhere a recognition that both the health problems we face and the barriers to addressing them are tied to the very market individualism the report embraces.

Public health is, in its essence, the collective response to the health threats a society faces. While much of the most important public health work is done in the private sector and the work of the state must take a wide variety of forms beyond direct regulation, "public health" without the dynamic leadership of government in deploying the nation's wealth against the ills arising from individual choices in the market is a contradiction in terms. Yet it is precisely this collective stake and government role that prevailing political dogma obscures.

To show how this is so, I offer an analysis of the conservative platform, not as a detailed blueprint for actual changes in the workings of government but as a heuristic, a judgmental strategy for simplifying complex phenomena to allow easier intellectual and emotional digestion. . . . As a heuristic, market individualism offers three closely related concepts for analyzing the problems of governing: the supremacy of the free market as a regulatory device, a concomitant belief in individual freedom of choice and personal responsibility, and the elevation of individual satisfaction as the chief goal of society. I argue here that public health advocates must forcefully oppose the social vision expressed in this heuristic, if only for the reason that to accept the rhetorical structure of market individualism is to accept a political language that has no words for public health.

## THE MARKET AS THE SOLUTION, OR THE MARKET AS THE PROBLEM

Casting the market as a tool for solving health problems fools the user into assuming that the market is outside the process of disease creation, when, in fact, the way in which we produce and distribute wealth is crucial to the health of Americans.

For the market individualist, the market is virtually always the best protector of health. Communicable disease control is often used as the exception that proves the rule, the archetype of the common good for which the market makes no provision. A few other functions—such as water purification and sanitation—move on and off the list in keeping with the spirit of the age. More significant in recent times has been the debate over how to use government and the market to regulate the externalities of industrial production, such as pollution and occupational injury. This is a useful debate in terms of efficient regulation, but it does not go to the heart of the issue of the market as a solution to public health problems. The market does not simply produce health problems as an accidental by-product; illness is virtually a primary product of market activity. Many of the things the economy generates are in themselves dangerous to some degree: cigarettes, alcohol, cars, planes, Big Macs, Laz-E-Boy chairs. We do not, for the moment, live in a society in which most people die from communicable diseases. We live in a society in which people die from exposure to the fruits of affluence (fatty diets, excessive leisure, fast cars) or the bitter harvest of social stresses (drug use, violence). Beyond the instances in which specific products are linked to ill health is the large amount of data showing a correlation between socioeconomic status and health, between social harmony and health, and even between racism and health. Even the emergence of new infectious diseases is closely tied to economic activity.

The invisible hand conjures ill health along with wealth. The long-term and subtle health costs of production are easily externalized and tend to fall most heavily on those socially vulnerable people with the least market power. For rich and poor alike, the economy substantially determines the sort of health threats a society will face. Market

individualism affords a happy vision of a society getting richer but obscures the prospect of the ills even riches entail.

## INDIVIDUAL RESPONSIBILITY AND CHOICE

The heuristic of market individualism seems to fit snugly in the dominant explanation of health in this country in this century. According to
this view, "health" is a personal, medical matter, a state of freedom
from pathology achieved by an individual through the mediation of a
doctor. Improvements in health flow from the application of science to
specific ills of the body, and access to medical care is the chief determinant of health. Seen this way, one's health is one's own business and is
largely in one's own hands. Everything from starting smoking to using
a condom to wearing a motorcycle helmet is a personal choice, privileged with all of the liberal or libertarian appurtenances thereunto. Individual actors are rational (if not always very smart or well informed),
and their choices, freely made, are entitled to respect and should not be
lightly interfered with by government. Their bad choices are their responsibility.

Public health, by contrast, has tended to adopt an ecological
model under which health is understood as an attribute of communities in social and physical environments. Health takes its shape in
large numbers—in morbidity and mortality statistics—and, ideally,
includes not just a high level of well-being for some but its even distribution throughout a society. In this view, improvements in health
arise from healthful changes in the social and physical environment.

From this ecological point of view, individual "free" choice depends
on the social options available to the chooser and, more deeply, on the
way in which different options are socially constructed. The sense that
smoking is sexy, or a taste for beef rather than sushi, is a function of
cultural conditioning, not choice. Public health assumes that rational
choosers start with a heavily inscribed slate and tend to align their behaviors and values with peer groups whose attitudes they adopt and use
to measure their conduct.

This account provides the warrant for purposeful action to change
choices. And that means changing the background world. Whether
the behavior is smoking or unsafe sex or too sedentary a lifestyle, improving public health inevitably entails an attempt to influence the
social values and conditions that support dangerous choices by individuals. In the United States, this work is often done by private organizations such as the American Cancer Society, but government

has also traditionally played a role as both funder and speaker. Government, as the representative of our collective interests, arguably speaks with a special moral authority (although certainly not to everyone). Moreover, government's persuasive powers go beyond mere speech. Through taxation and other regulatory actions, government has unique powers to make unsafe activities more burdensome and less desirable. . . .

The individual choice heuristic powerfully impedes this public health work. It explains why the market is not a problem: the market is simply giving people what they want. And it provides a vocabulary to oppose government intervention to modulate choices: government manipulation of values and behaviors invades the private sphere and undermines freedom. The heuristic works to establish a rule that private actors motivated by profit can pervasively and expensively work to manipulate choices and mold society but the people, through their government, working in the name of health, cannot.

INDIVIDUAL SATISFACTION

If we are rational actors making free choices in a free market, it can be neither surprising nor inherently problematic that many of us make choices that others regard as bad or stupid. People find smoking to be a very satisfying activity, worth the risks, and there are many other activities—like riding cycles without helmets or watching TV instead of jogging—that are much less personally risky than smoking. As long as we are happy and prepared to accept the consequences of our own actions, what business is it of anybody else? So goes the heuristic of individual satisfaction.

The public health perspective is different. On one level, we are simply talking about a different measure: public health is concerned with the health of the population as a whole, as expressed in phenomena measurable on a large scale. But there is something even deeper going on. How we see determines what we see. The public's health, I suggest, is not simply the aggregation of individual satisfactions, it is a different way of experiencing and defining health: a relation between a population and its environment that does not express itself in individual cases in a meaningful way.

Individuals are naturally concerned with their own state of health. We want to feel well and to believe that our wellness will last. We want a measure of control over our health, which we may get by following prevailing prescriptions for a healthy lifestyle, avoiding certain arbitrarily selected threats, or going to the doctor. We tend to look for personalized information that seems to define our health: the leading example is the "risk factor," the genetic, physiologic, or behavioral marker that purports to measure our personal risk of various kinds of ill health against the population's average risk.

The premises of this individualized perspective on health are largely alien to public health. Relative risk alone, for example, is a poor predictor of the distribution of an illness in the population, because a high relative risk in a small population does not create as many cases as a low risk in a much larger one. From the population perspective, the best explanation—and by and large the only one needed—for why a particular person dies the way she or he does is chance. The biological, social, and environmental causes of cancer in the population are public health's concern. The particular cause of Joe's case of cancer is not. . . .

## CONCLUSION

I aim to get past the notion that market individualism is an immutable trait deep in the "American character" that must be accepted as "reality." The important question, I suggest, is not what people think now, but how they came to think it, and the answer is the same as for other attitudes and behaviors: they were taught. Individualism is not genetic. There is no market miasma emanating from the North American continent. Ideas like the ones that dominate American politics are inculcated consciously and unconsciously in school, work, family, and the social interaction of daily life. The purveyors of the political heuristic I have described in this paper have worked for long years to bring their ideas from the unthinkable to the statute books.

Seen in this way, the task for public health advocates is a familiar one: the slow, diffuse job of changing social attitudes, in this case by developing effective alternative ways of understanding the social and physical ecology. . . . In the political field, it entails showing at every opportunity how the market puts our health at risk, how individual choices are mediated by social and cultural conditions, and how the welfare of the community can diverge from the welfare of the individual. Even before the first step is taken, however, the project requires that public health advocates themselves recognize the way in which modes of thought, such as market individualism, have made public health unthinkable and how alternative ways of thinking are a necessary, if not sufficient, condition to revitalizing it.

---

## III. THE POPULATION FOCUS

Public health interventions are designed to prevent injury and disease among populations. This section offers two foundational articles explaining the population-based focus of the field of public health. The groundbreaking article by McGinnis and Foege introduces the different forms of thinking in medicine and public health. Medical explanations of death, often in the form of code numbers from the International Classification of Disease (ICD-10) on death certificates, point to discrete pathophysiological conditions, such as cancer, heart disease, cerebrovascular disease, and pulmonary disease.

The biomedical model of record keeping and the societal need to explain a cause of death with a discrete medical condition distract the public from real contributors to mortality. Public health explanations instead examine the root causes of disease. Seen in this way, the leading causes of death are environmental, social, and behavioral factors. Although the statistics cited by McGinnis and Foege are dated, they are not offered here for their currency. The numbers show the magnitude of the mortality associated with preventable causes of death and the potential implications of successful public health campaigns. For more recent data on the leading causes of death, see Table 5.

Like McGinnis and Foege, Rose offers a comparison of medicine and public health. In his authoritative article, Rose compares the scientific methods and objectives of medicine with those of public health. "Why did *this* patient get *this* disease at *this* time?" is a prevailing question in medicine, and it underscores a physician's central concern for sick individuals and an individual etiology. By contrast, those interested in public health seek knowledge about why ill health occurs in the population and how it can be prevented.

Under Rose's "prevention paradox," measures that have the greatest potential for improving public health (such as seatbelt use) offer little absolute benefit to any individual, whereas measures that heroically save individual lives (such as heart transplants) make no significant contribution to the population's health. This article introduces another unique aspect of public health and the population focus: the emphasis on the

TABLE 5
## TEN LEADING CAUSES OF DEATH BY AGE GROUP: 1997

| | | | Age Group | | |
|---|---|---|---|---|---|
| Rank | <1 | 1–4 | 5–9 | 10–14 | 15–24 |
| 1 | Congenital anomalies 6178 | Unintentional injuries 2005 | Unintentional injuries 1534 | Unintentional injuries 1837 | Unintentional injuries 13,367 |
| 2 | Short gestation 3925 | Congenital anomalies 589 | Malignant neoplasms 547 | Malignant neoplasms 483 | Homicide 6146 |
| 3 | SIDS 2991 | Malignant neoplasms 438 | Congenital anomalies 223 | Suicide 303 | Suicide 4186 |
| 4 | Respiratory distress syndrome 1301 | Homicide 375 | Homicide 174 | Homicide 283 | Malignant neoplasms 1645 |
| 5 | Maternal complications 1244 | Heart disease 212 | Heart disease 128 | Congenital anomalies 224 | Heart disease 1098 |
| 6 | Placenta cord membranes 960 | Pneumonia and influenza 180 | Pneumonia and influenza 76 | Heart disease 185 | Congenital anomalies 420 |
| 7 | Perinatal infections 777 | Perinatal period 75 | HIV 62 | Bronchitis emphysema asthma 79 | HIV 276 |
| 8 | Unintentional injuries 765 | Septicemia 73 | Bronchitis emphysema asthma 50 | Pneumonia and influenza 65 | Pneumonia and influenza 220 |
| 9 | Intrauterine hypoxia 452 | Benign neoplasms 65 | Anemias 38 | Cerebro-vascular 51 | Bronchitis emphysema asthma 201 |
| 10 | Pneumonia and influenza 421 | Cerebro-vascular 56 | Benign neoplasms 35 | Benign neoplasms 41 | Cerebro-vascular 188 |

SOURCE: Centers for Disease Control and Prevention, National Center for Injury Prevention and Control, National Center for Health Statistics.

| | | Age Group | | | |
|---|---|---|---|---|---|
| 25–34 | 35–44 | 45–54 | 55–64 | 65+ | Total |
| Unintentional injuries 12,598 | Malignant neoplasms 17,099 | Malignant neoplasms 45,429 | Malignant neoplasms 86,314 | Heart disease 606,913 | Heart disease 726,974 |
| Suicide 5672 | Unintentional injuries 14,531 | Heart disease 35,277 | Heart disease 65,958 | Malignant neoplasms 382,913 | Malignant neoplasms 539,577 |
| Homicide 5075 | Heart disease 13,227 | Unintentional injuries 10,416 | Bronchitis emphysema asthma 10,109 | Cerebro vascular 140,355 | Cerebro-vascular 159,791 |
| Malignant neoplasms 4607 | HIV 7073 | Cerebro-vascular 5695 | Cerebro-vascular 9676 | Bronchitis emphysema asthma 94,411 | Bronchitis emphysema asthma 109,029 |
| HIV 3993 | Suicide 6730 | Liver disease 5622 | Diabetes 8370 | Pneumonia and influenza 77,561 | Unintentional injuries 95,644 |
| Heart disease 3286 | Homicide 3677 | Suicide 4948 | Unintentional injuries 7105 | Diabetes 47,289 | Pneumonia and influenza 86,449 |
| Cerebro-vascular 678 | Liver disease 3508 | Diabetes 4335 | Liver disease 5253 | Unintentional injuries 31,386 | Diabetes 62,636 |
| Diabetes 620 | Cerebro-vascular 2787 | HIV 3513 | Pneumonia and influenza 3759 | Alzheimer's disease 22,154 | Suicide 30,535 |
| Pneumonia and influenza 534 | Diabetes 1858 | Bronchitis emphysema asthma 2838 | Suicide 2946 | Nephritis 21,787 | Nephritis 25,331 |
| Liver disease 516 | Pneumonia and influenza 1394 | Pneumonia and influenza 2233 | Septicemia 1852 | Septicemia 1852 | Liver disease 25,175 |

measurement of the health of populations as an indicator of success. The answer to the question "Did this person survive?" indicates success for the physician. For the public health professional the question is "How many person-years of life were saved?" Public health is in the position of controlling negative externalities and inducing behavior change in pursuit of improved mortality rates. Although Rose acknowledges that medical interventions appear more heroic and have a higher chance of patient compliance, he favors the broad and powerful impact of successful population-based campaigns. For further discussion of public health from the population perspective, see Green and Ottoson (1999).

---

## Actual Causes of Death in the United States*
*J. Michael McGinnis and William H. Foege*

In 1990, approximately 2,148,000 U.S. residents died. Certificates filed at the time of death indicate that their deaths were most commonly due to heart disease (720,000), cancer (505,000), cerebrovascular disease (144,000), accidents (92,000), chronic obstructive pulmonary disease (87,000), pneumonia and influenza (80,000), diabetes mellitus (48,000), suicide (31,000), chronic liver disease and cirrhosis (26,000), and HIV infection (25,000). Often referenced as the 10 leading causes of death in the U.S., they generally indicate the primary pathophysiological conditions identified at the time of death, as opposed to their root causes. These conditions actually result from a combination of inborn (largely genetic) and external factors.

Because most diseases or injuries are multifactorial in nature, a key challenge is sorting out the relative contributions of the various factors. For heart disease, well-established external risk factors include tobacco use, elevated serum cholesterol levels, hypertension, obesity, and decreased physical activity; for various cancers, such risk factors include tobacco use, dietary patterns, certain infectious agents, and environmental or occupational exposure to carcinogenic agents. Even motor vehicle injuries can be associated with multiple factors, including alcohol use, failure to use passenger protection systems, poor roadway de-

---

*Reprinted from *Journal of the American Medical Association* 270 (November 10, 1993): 2207–12.

ACTUAL CAUSES OF DEATH IN
THE UNITED STATES IN 1990

| | Deaths | |
| --- | --- | --- |
| Cause | Estimated No. | Percentage of Total Deaths |
| Tobacco | 400,000 | 19 |
| Diet/Activity patterns | 300,000 | 14 |
| Alcohol | 100,000 | 5 |
| Microbial agents | 90,000 | 4 |
| Toxic agents | 60,000 | 3 |
| Firearms | 35,000 | 2 |
| Sexual behavior | 30,000 | 1 |
| Motor vehicles | 25,000 | 1 |
| Illicit use of drugs | 20,000 | <1 |
| Total | 1,060,000 | 50 |

sign, and inadequate law enforcement. These factors may act independently of each other, the risks being additive according to the effect of each, or they may act synergistically; the interaction of factors presenting a greater total risk than the sum of their individual effects.

Available analyses of the roles of various external factors in these conditions suggest that the most prominent identifiable contributors to death among U.S. residents are tobacco, diet and activity patterns, alcohol, microbial agents, toxic agents, firearms, sexual behavior, motor vehicles, and illicit use of drugs. When these contribute to deaths, those deaths are by definition premature and are often preceded by impaired quality of life. Although mortality is but one measure of the health status of a nation, the public health burden imposed by these contributors offers both a mandate and guidance for shaping health policy priorities. . . .

RESULTS

*Tobacco*

Tobacco accounts for approximately 400,000 deaths each year among Americans. It contributes substantially to deaths from cancer (especially cancers of the lung, esophagus, oral cavity, pancreas, kidney, and bladder, and perhaps of other organs), cardiovascular disease (coronary artery disease, stroke, and high blood pressure), lung disease (chronic obstructive pulmonary disease and pneumonia), low birth weight and other problems of infancy, and burns. . . . Using a specially developed software package, the Centers for Disease Control and Prevention (CDC) estimated that 418,690 deaths were caused by tobacco in 1990, including approximately 30% of all cancer deaths and 21% of cardiovascular disease deaths. The CDC estimates have been widely accepted and provide the basis for the 400,000 figure included in the table.

### Diet and Activity Patterns

Dietary factors and activity patterns that are too sedentary are together accountable for at least 300,000 deaths each year. Dietary factors have been associated with cardiovascular diseases (coronary artery disease, stroke, and high blood pressure), cancers (colon, breast, and prostate), and diabetes mellitus. Physical inactivity has been associated with an increased risk of death for heart disease and colon cancer. The interdependence of dietary factors and activity patterns as risk factors for certain diseases is illustrated by the case of obesity, which is associated with increased risk for cardiovascular disease, certain cancers, and diabetes, and is clearly related to the balance between calories consumed and calories expended through metabolic and physical activity. Similarly, high blood pressure, a major risk for stroke, can be affected by dietary sodium, obesity, and sedentary lifestyle. . . . Half of all type II diabetes (non-insulin-dependent diabetes mellitus) is estimated to be preventable by obesity control. A 50% reduction in consumption of animal fats might result in a proportionate reduction in risk for colon cancer. . . . Because of the complexity of the issues and the difficulty of the analyses relating diet and activity patterns to disease outcomes, [a conservative estimate of 300,000 deaths is] presented in the table.

### Alcohol

Misuse of alcohol accounts for approximately 100,000 deaths each year, but the related health, social, and economic consequences of alcohol extend far beyond the mortality tables. An estimated 18 million U.S. residents suffer from alcohol dependence, and some 76 million are affected by alcohol abuse at some time. Estimates of alcohol's death toll range from 3% to 10% of deaths. . . . The CDC used clinical case studies and analytic epidemiologic studies to determine alcohol-attributable fractions of various diagnoses and concluded that a total of 105,095 deaths were caused by alcohol in 1987, including approximately 30,000 deaths from unintentional injuries, 19,600 from digestive diseases including liver cirrhosis, 17,700 from intentional injuries, and

16,000 from cancers. Because the CDC estimate is the one most often reported, it has been applied to 1990 death rates and serves as the basis for the 100,000 alcohol-related deaths included in the table.

### Microbial Agents

Infectious agents—apart from those counted elsewhere with causes of HIV infection or consequent to use of tobacco, alcohol, or drugs—currently account for approximately 90,000 deaths per year. Infections were once the leading killer in the U.S., and they are still a prominent threat, especially to persons with other health impairments. Infectious agents also exert great influence on society through an estimated 740 million nonfatal illnesses caused by symptomatic infections that occur annually among Americans. . . .

The major contributors to death from infectious agents are pneumococcal pneumonia, nosocomial infections (in both acute and chronic care facilities), legionellosis, *Staphylococcus aureus* infection, hepatitis, and group A streptococcal infections. . . . The 90,000 deaths included here for microbial agents represent the sum of 1990 deaths from key International Classification of Diseases codes 001 through 139 (infectious and parasitic diseases), 320 through 323 (meningitis and encephalitis), and 480 through 482 (pneumonia and influenza), and not including those from codes 042 through 044 (HIV infection), and those otherwise estimated to be attributable to tobacco use, alcohol use, sexual behavior, and illicit use of drugs.

### Toxic Agents

Estimates of the deaths attributable to toxic agents vary widely, and because measurement techniques and the recognition of health effects are still evolving, the number of 60,000 per year included in the table may be the most uncertain of the figures indicated for the various causes.

Toxic agents may pose a threat to human health as occupational hazards, environmental pollutants, contaminants of food and water supplies, and components of commercial products. They can contribute to conditions that are potentially lethal, including cancer and other diseases of the heart, lungs, liver, kidneys, bladder, and neurological system. Estimates of the total cancer deaths caused each year by synthetic chemicals in the environment or occupational settings range upward from about 30,000, including an estimated 9,000 from asbestos exposure. Occupational exposures alone have been estimated to cause 1% to 3% of all cardiovascular, chronic respiratory, renal, and neurological disease deaths, as well as all pneumoconioses. In addition, occupational exposures have been linked with about 4% to 10% of all cancer deaths, and pollutants with approximately another 2% of all cancer deaths. Although evidence is generally unavailable for the long-term effects of ambient pollutants on cardiovascular or pulmonary death rates, significant elevations of respirable pollutants such as particulates, sulfur dioxide, and carbon monoxide have been associated with transient increases in daily mortality rates of 4% to 16%.

Indoor air may present a greater burden of pollutants than outdoor air. Environmental tobacco smoke is an established carcinogen, and estimates of radon's contribution to lung cancer deaths range from about 7,000 deaths per year to nearly 24,000 deaths per year. In all, geophysical factors such as background ionizing radiation and ultraviolet light may be accountable for some 3% of cancer deaths. . . .

### Firearms

Firearms caused more than 36,000 deaths among Americans in 1990, including about 16,000 homicides, 19,000 suicides, and 1,400 unintentional deaths. The number of deaths caused by firearms is now higher than those caused by motor vehicle crashes in five states and the District of Columbia. Comparison data indicate that firearm-related homicide rates for young males in the U.S. are 12 to 273 times the rates in other industrialized nations, whereas non-firearm-related homicide rates are 1.4 to 9.2 times greater than those elsewhere. For example, in 1986 there were 1,043 firearm-related homicides among U.S. males aged 15 to 19 years, compared with 6 such deaths in Canada and 2 in Japan. Firearm-related deaths now comprise 11% of all childhood deaths and 17% for those aged 15 to 19 years, including 41% of deaths among black males of this age. Firearm-related suicides among black teenage males aged 15 to 19 years doubled from 1982 to 1987, and although the rate for white males the same age did not change substantially during this period, it was nearly twice as high. The risk of suicide among adolescents has been found to be nearly three times greater in homes where a gun is kept. Moreover, guns kept in homes as protection have been found to be several times more likely to kill a family member than an intruder. The prominent, detrimental effect of firearms on overall death rates in the U.S. is unique in comparison with other countries.

### Sexual Behavior

Unprotected sexual intercourse was accountable for approximately 30,000 deaths in 1990. Sexual behavior is associated with substantially increased risk for preventable disease and disability and is the source of some of today's most prominent social challenges. Each year, 12 million persons (two thirds of whom are under 25 years of age) are newly infected with a sexually transmitted disease. An estimated 56% of all pregnancies among U.S. women are unintended, including most of the 1 million that occur among U.S. teenagers each year. One of the most rapidly increasing causes of serious illness is hepatitis B infection, of which about a third is estimated to be sexually transmitted. Among women, pelvic inflammatory disease is a severe complication of lower genital tract infections such as gonorrhea and chlamydia. Each year, pelvic inflammatory disease affects an estimated 1 million U.S. women, of whom perhaps as many as 150,000 become sterile as a result.

The 30,000 deaths in 1990 attributed in the table to unprotected sexual intercourse include approximately 5,000 from excess infant mortality rates among those whose pregnancies were unintended, 4,000 from cervical cancer, 1,600 from sexually acquired hepatitis B infection, and 21,000 from sexually acquired HIV infection. As indicated by the nearly 20% increase over deaths in the previous year from sexually acquired HIV infection, unprotected intercourse now represents one of the most rapidly increasing causes of death in the country.

## Motor Vehicles

Motor vehicle injuries to passengers and pedestrians caused about 47,000 deaths in 1990. Nearly 40% of all deaths among those aged 15 to 24 years were caused by motor vehicles. The chances of surviving a serious motor vehicle crash are increased severalfold if an occupant is protected. Lap and shoulder belts have been shown to reduce the risk of death by about 45% to 65%, and of serious injury by about 40% to 55%. Airbags have been shown to yield a 30% reduction in fatalities and a 35% reduction in serious injury in frontal crashes. Child passenger restraints can reduce fatalities by 50% to 90%. Use of motorcycle helmets can reduce fatalities by 30% and serious head injuries by 75%. The estimate of 25,000 deaths attributed in the table to motor vehicles does not include those already recorded as relating to alcohol or drug use.

## Illicit Use of Drugs

Approximately 20,000 deaths were caused in 1990 by illicit use of drugs. It is estimated that some 3 million people in the U.S. have serious drug problems. Illicit use of drugs contributes to infant deaths and to deaths reported for such causes as overdose, suicide, homicide, motor vehicle injury, HIV infection, pneumonia, hepatitis, and endocarditis. In 1990, approximately 9,000 deaths nationwide were attributed to illicit use of drugs (both legal and illegal) by vital statistics reports. This figure, however, does not include those indirectly related, such as deaths from accidents, homicides, infections with HIV, and hepatitis. In 1990, approximately 9,000 HIV deaths resulted from intravenous drug use (20% more than 1989), as did at least another 1,300 hepatitis B–related deaths. . . . The 20,000 deaths attributed in the table to drug use represents deaths reported to the vital statistics system as drug-related, as well as those from drug-related HIV infection, automobile injuries, and hepatitis infections. It, too, is expected to increase substantially in future years as a result of HIV deaths associated with intravenous drug use.

*Other Factors*

Lack of access to a reliable source of primary care is also associated with an increased risk of death from a variety of causes, although quantifying the impact is complicated by the challenges of appropriately characterizing the various elements of access and distinguishing their effects on a given health outcome from other confounding variables. Comparisons of the health status profiles of various developed countries suggest that residents of countries that provide relatively greater access to a full range of primary care services generally fare better than residents of countries with poorer access. . . .

Poverty, too, has its own direct effect on mortality rates, although it is difficult to separate the effect of lack of access to primary care from that of social and economic status. In the United Kingdom, which guarantees universal access to services, a substantial differential remains in health status outcomes by social class despite improved access, and overall scores in health status indicators are somewhat lower than those for other more socially homogeneous Western European countries. Similarly, reports indicate that poor Canadians have a projected 11 fewer years of disability-free life than their more affluent counterparts, despite guaranteed access to medical care. Several studies that have controlled for other risk factors have shown that populations characterized by low educational or income status experience poorer health prospects. . . .

COMMENT AND CONCLUSIONS

Approximately half of all deaths that occurred among U.S. residents in 1990 could be attributed to the factors identified. Despite their approximate nature, the estimates presented here hold implications for program priorities. At the most basic level, they compel examination of the way the U.S. tracks its health status. Clearly, there is a need to improve the assessment of the contributory effects of etiologic factors on deaths among U.S. residents and to clarify the role of factors such as poverty and restricted access to health services. There is also a need to look more specifically at how these factors affect the 50% of all deaths that occur before age 75. Moreover, there is a need to assess how they affect our measures on the increasingly important dimensions of morbidity and quality of life. Our national efficiency in changing the health profile is dependent on our ability to identify and monitor trends for the major factors that give direct shape to that profile.

The most important implications of this assessment of the actual causes of death in the U.S. are found in the way the nation allocates its social resources and shapes its program emphases. In 1993, health care costs in the U.S. are expected to reach approximately $900 billion, an average of more than $14,000 annually for each family of four, if equally allocated across the population. The preponderance of this expenditure will be devoted to treatment of conditions ultimately recorded on death certificates as the nation's leading killers. Only a small fraction will go toward the control of many of the factors that the table indicates imposed a substantial public health burden. The national investment in prevention is estimated at less than 5% of the total annual health care cost.

There can be no illusions about the difficulty of the challenges in changing the impact these factors have on health status. Of those identified here, the three leading causes of death—tobacco, diet and activity patterns, and alcohol—are all rooted in behavioral choices. Behavioral change is motivated not by knowledge alone, but also by a supportive social environment and the availability of rehabilitative services. The most rapidly increasing among these causes of death— sexual behavior and illicit use of drugs—take place behind closed doors and are difficult to confront directly even in a putatively open society. Several, such as firearms, are the focal point of powerful lobbies that impede constructive exploration of the full range of social options.

Nonetheless, the central public health focus for each of these factors must be the possibility for improvement. Change can occur. In recent years, trends have been salutary on several dimensions, e.g., reductions in tobacco use, saturated fat consumption, and motor vehicle fatalities. The discouraging trends with respect to the effects of sexual behavior, firearms, and illicit use of drugs need not be inexorable. If the nation is to achieve its full potential for better health, public policy must focus directly and actively on those factors that represent the root determinants of death and disability.

## Sick Individuals and Sick Populations*
*Geoffrey Rose*

### THE DETERMINANTS OF INDIVIDUAL CASES

In teaching epidemiology to medical students, I have often encouraged them to consider a question which I first heard enunciated by Roy Acheson: "Why did *this* patient get *this* disease at *this* time?" It is an excellent starting-point, because students and doctors feel a natural concern for the problems of the individual. Indeed, the central ethos of medicine is seen as an acceptance of responsibility for sick individuals.

It is an integral part of good doctoring to ask not only, "What is the diagnosis, and what is the treatment?" but also, "Why did this happen, and could it have been prevented?" Such thinking shapes the approach to nearly all clinical and laboratory research into the causes and mechanisms of illness. Hypertension research, for example, is almost wholly preoccupied with the characteristics which distinguish individuals at the hypertensive and normotensive ends of the blood pressure distribution. Research into diabetes looks for genetic, nutritional and metabolic reasons to explain why some people get diabetes and others do not. The constant aim in such work is to answer Acheson's question: "Why did *this* patient get this disease at this time?"

The same concern has continued to shape the thinking of all of us who came to epidemiology from a background in clinical practice. The whole basis of the case-control method is to discover how sick and healthy individuals differ. Equally the basis of many cohort studies is the search for "risk factors," which identify certain individuals as being more susceptible to disease; and from this we proceed to test whether these risk factors are also causes, capable of explaining why some individuals get sick while others remain healthy, and applicable as a guide to prevention.

*Reprinted from *International Journal of Epidemiology* 14 (March 1985): 32–38 by permission of Oxford University Press.

To confine attention in this way to within-population comparisons has caused much confusion (particularly in the clinical world) in the definition of normality. Laboratory ranges of normal are based on what is common within the local population. Individuals with normal blood pressure are those who do not stand out from their local contemporaries; and so on. What is common is all right, we presume.

Applied to aetiology, the individual-centered approach leads to the use of relative risk as the basic representation of aetiological force: that is, "the risk in exposed individuals relative to risk in non-exposed individuals." Indeed, the concept of relative risk has almost excluded any other approach to quantifying causal importance. It may generally be the best measure of aetiological force, but it is no measure at all of aetiological outcome or of public health importance.

Unfortunately this approach to the search for causes, and the measuring of their potency, has to assume a heterogeneity of exposure within the study population. If everyone smoked 20 cigarettes a day, then clinical, case-control and cohort studies alike would lead us to conclude that lung cancer was a genetic disease; and in one sense that would be true, since if everyone is exposed to the necessary agent, then the distribution of cases is wholly determined by individual susceptibility. . . .

## THE DETERMINANTS OF POPULATION INCIDENCE RATE

I find it increasingly helpful to distinguish two kinds of aetiological questions. The first seeks the causes of cases, and the second seeks the causes of incidence. "Why do some individuals have hypertension?" is a quite different question from "Why do some populations have much hypertension, whilst in others it is rare?" The questions require different kinds of study, and they have different answers. . . .

To find the determinants of prevalence and incidence rates, we need to study characteristics of populations, not characteristics of individuals. . . . Within populations it has proved almost impossible to demonstrate any relation between an individual's diet and his serum cholesterol level; and the same applies to the relation of individual diet to blood pressure and to overweight. But at the level of populations it is a different story: it has proved easy to show strong associations between population mean values for saturated fat intake *versus* serum cholesterol level and coronary heart disease incidence, sodium intake *versus* blood pressure, or energy intake *versus* overweight. The determinants of incidence are not necessarily the same as the causes of cases.

## HOW DO THE CAUSES OF CASES
## RELATE TO THE CAUSES OF INCIDENCE?

This is largely a matter of whether exposure varies similarly within a population and between populations (or over a period of time within the same population). Softness of water supply may be a determinant of cardiovascular mortality, but it is unlikely to be identifiable as a risk factor for individuals, because exposure tends to be locally uniform. Dietary fat is, I believe, the main determinant of a population's incidence rate for coronary heart disease; but it quite fails to identify high-risk individuals.

In the case of cigarettes and lung cancer it so happened that the study populations contained about equal numbers of smokers and non-smokers, and in such a situation case-control and cohort studies were able to identify what was also the main determinant of population differences amid time trends.

There is a broad tendency for genetic factors to dominate individual susceptibility, but to explain rather little of population differences in incidence. Genetic heterogeneity, it seems, is mostly much greater within than between populations. This is the contrary situation to that seen for environmental factors. Thus migrants, whatever the colour of their skin, tend to acquire the disease rates of their country of adoption.

Most non-infectious diseases are still of largely unknown cause. If you take a textbook of medicine and look at the list of contents you will still find, despite all our aetiological research, that most are still of basically unknown aetiology. We know quite a lot about the personal characteristics of individuals who are susceptible to them, but for a remarkably large number of our major non-infectious diseases we still do not know the determinants of the incidence rate. . . .

There is hardly a disease whose incidence rate does not vary widely, either over time or between populations at the same time. This means that these causes of incidence rate, unknown though they are, are not inevitable. It is possible to live without them, and if we knew what they were it might be possible to control them. But to identify the causal agent by the traditional case-control and cohort methods will be unsuccessful if there are not sufficient differences in exposure within the study population at the time of the study. In those circumstances all that these traditional methods do is to find markers of individual susceptibility. The clues must be sought from differences between populations or from changes within populations over time.

PREVENTION

These two approaches to aetiology—the individual and the population-based—have their counterparts in prevention. In the first, preventive strategy seeks to identify high-risk susceptible individuals and to offer them some individual protection. In contrast, the "population strategy" seeks to control the determinants of incidence in the population as a whole.

### The "High-Risk" Strategy

This is the traditional and natural medical approach to prevention. If a doctor accepts that he is responsible for an individual who is sick today, then it is a short step to accept responsibility also for the individual who may well be sick tomorrow. Thus, screening is used to detect certain individuals who hitherto thought they were well but who must now understand that they are in effect patients. This is the process, for example, in the detection and treatment of symptomless hypertension, the transition from healthy subject to patient being ratified by the giving and receiving of tablets. (Anyone who takes medicines is by definition a patient.)

What the "high-risk" strategy seeks to achieve is something like a truncation of the risk distribution. This general concept applies to all special preventive action in high-risk individuals—in at-risk pregnancies, in small babies, or in any other particularly susceptible group. It is a strategy with some clear and important advantages.

Its first advantage is that it leads to intervention which is appropriate to the individual. A smoker who has a cough or who is found to have impaired ventilatory function has a special reason for stopping smoking. The doctor will see it as making sense to advise salt restriction in a hypertensive. In such instances the intervention makes sense because that individual already has a problem which that particular measure may possibly ameliorate. If we consider screening a population to discover those with high serum cholesterol levels and advising them on dietary change, then that intervention is appropriate to those people in particular: they have a diet-related metabolic problem.

The "high-risk" strategy produces interventions that are appropriate to the particular individuals advised to take them. Consequently, it has the advantage of enhanced subject motivation. In our randomized controlled trial of smoking cessation in London civil servants we first screened some 20,000 men and from them selected about 1,500 who were smokers with, in addition, markers of specially high risk for cardiorespiratory disease. They were recalled and a random half received anti-smoking counselling. The results, in terms of smoking cessation, were excellent because those men knew they had a special reason to stop. They had been picked out from others in their offices because, although everyone knows that smoking is a bad thing, they had a special reason why it was particularly unwise for them.

There is, of course, another and less reputable reason why screening enhances subject motivation, and that is the mystique of a scientific investigation. A ventilatory function test is a powerful enhancer of motivation to stop smoking: an instrument which the subject does not quite understand, that looks rather impressive, has produced evidence that he is a special person with a special problem. . . .

For rather similar reasons the "high-risk" approach also motivates physicians. Doctors, quite rightly, are uncomfortable about intervening in a situation where their help was not asked for. Before imposing advice on somebody who was getting on all right without them, they like to feel that there is a proper and special justification in that particular case.

The "high-risk" approach offers a more cost-effective use of limited resources. One of the things we have learned in health education at the individual level is that once-only advice is a waste of time. To see results we may need a considerable investment of counselling time and follow-up. It is costly in use of time and effort and resources, and therefore it is more effective to concentrate limited medical services and time where the need—and therefore also the benefit—is likely to be greatest.

A final advantage of the "high-risk" approach is that it offers a more favourable ratio of benefits to risks. If intervention must carry some adverse effects or costs, and if the risk and cost are much the same for everybody, then the ratio of the costs to the benefits will be more favourable where the benefits are larger.

Unfortunately the "high-risk" strategy of prevention also has some serious disadvantages and limitations. The first centers around the difficulties and costs of screening. Supposing that we were to embark, as some had advocated, on a policy of screening for high cholesterol levels and giving dietary advice to those individuals at special risk. The disease process we are trying to prevent (atherosclerosis and its complications) begins early in life, so we should have to initiate screening perhaps at the age of ten. However, the abnormality we seek to detect is not a stable lifetime characteristic, so we must advocate repeated screening at suitable intervals.

In all screening one meets problems with uptake, and the tendency for the response to be greater amongst those sections of the population who are often least at risk of the disease. Often there is an even greater problem: screening detects certain individuals who will receive special advice, but at the same time it cannot help also discovering much larger numbers of "borderliners," that is, people whose results mark them as at increased risk but for whom we do not have an appropriate treatment to reduce their risk. . . .

The second disadvantage of the "high-risk" strategy is that it is palliative and temporary, not radical. It does not seek to alter the underlying causes of the disease but to identify individuals who are particularly susceptible to those causes. Presumably in every generation there will be such susceptibles, and if prevention and control efforts were confined to these high-risk individuals, then that approach would need to be sustained year after year and generation after generation. It does not deal with the root of the problem, but seeks to protect those who are vulnerable to it; and they will always be around.

The potential for this approach is limited—sometimes more than we could have expected—both for the individual and for the population. There are two reasons for this. The first is that our power to predict future disease is usually very weak. Most individuals with risk factors will remain well, at least for some years; contrariwise, unexpected illness may happen to someone who has just received an "all clear" report from a screening examination. One of the limitations of the relative risk statistic is that it gives no idea of the absolute level of danger. . . .

Often the best predictor of future major disease is the presence of existing minor disease. A low ventilatory function today is the best predictor of its future rate of decline. A high blood pressure today is the best predictor of its future rate of rise. Early coronary heart disease is better than all the conventional risk factors as a predictor of future fatal disease. . . .

This point came home to me only recently. I have long congratulated myself on my low levels of coronary risk factors, and I joked to my friends that if I were to die suddenly, I should be very surprised. I even speculated on what other disease—perhaps colon cancer—would be the commonest cause of death for a man in the lowest group of cardiovascular risk. The painful truth is that for such an individual in a Western population the commonest cause of death—by far—is coronary heart disease! Everyone, in fact, is a high-risk individual for this uniquely mass disease. . . .

A further disadvantage of the "high-risk" strategy is that it is behaviourally inappropriate. Eating, smoking, exercise and all our other lifestyle characteristics are constrained by social norms. If we try to eat differently from our friends, it will not only be inconvenient, but we risk being regarded as cranks or hypochondriacs. If a man's work environment encourages heavy drinking, then advice that he is damaging his liver is unlikely to have any effect. No one who has attempted any sort of health education effort in individuals needs to be told that it is difficult for such people to step out of line with their peers. This is what the "high-risk" preventive strategy requires them to do.

### The Population Strategy

This is the attempt to control the determinants of incidence, to lower the mean level of risk factors, to shift the whole distribution of exposure in a favourable direction. In its traditional "public health" form it has involved mass environmental control methods; in its modern form it is attempting (less successfully) to alter some of society's norms of behaviour.

The advantages are powerful. The first is that it is radical. It attempts to remove the underlying causes that make the disease common. It has a large potential—often larger than one would have expected—for the population as a whole. . . .

The approach is behaviourally appropriate. If nonsmoking eventually becomes "normal," then it will be much less necessary to keep on persuading individuals. Once a social norm of behaviour has become accepted and (as in the case of diet) once the supply industries have adapted themselves to the new pattern, then the maintenance of that situation no longer requires effort from individuals. The health education phase aimed at changing individuals is, we hope, a temporary necessity, pending changes in the norms of what is socially acceptable.

Unfortunately the population strategy of prevention has also some weighty drawbacks. It offers only a small benefit to each individual, since most of them were going to be all right anyway, at least for many years. This leads to the *Prevention Paradox* (Rose 1981): "A preventive measure which brings much benefit to the population offers little to each participating individual." This has been the history of public health—of immunization, the wearing of seat belts and now the attempt to change various lifestyle characteristics. Of enormous potential importance to the population as a whole, these measures offer very little—particularly in the short term—to each individual; and thus there is poor motivation of the subject. We should not be surprised that health education tends to be relatively ineffective for individuals and in the short term. Most people act for substantial and immediate rewards, and the medical motivation for health education is inherently weak. Their health next year is not likely to be much better if they accept our advice or if they reject it. Much more powerful as motivators for health education are the social rewards of enhanced self-esteem and social approval. . . .

In mass prevention each individual has usually only a small expectation of benefit, and this small benefit can easily be outweighed by a small risk. This happened in the World Health Organization clofibrate trial, where a cholesterol-lowering drug seems to have killed more than it saved, even though the fatal complication rate was only about $1/1,000$/year. Such low-order risks, which can be vitally important to the balance sheet of mass preventive plans, may be hard or impossible to detect. This makes it important to distinguish two approaches. The first is the restoration of biological normality by the removal of an abnormal exposure (e.g., stopping smoking, controlling air pollution, moderating some of our recently acquired dietary deviations); here there can be some presumption of safety. This is not true for the other kind of preventive approach, which leaves intact the underlying causes of incidence and seeks instead to interpose some new, supposedly protective intervention (e.g., immunization, drugs, jogging). Here the onus is on the activists to produce adequate evidence of safety.

*   *   *   *   *

The field of public health, as we have seen, is deeply complex, riddled with contradictions, and influenced by politics, culture, and economics. It has struggled through the years to gain the attention, respect, and resources it deserves. Workers in this field are only beginning to develop a sense of professionalism, expertise, and competency comparable to that of practitioners of older disciplines such as medicine. The field of public health currently lacks the political visibility and funding needed to effectively accomplish the mission of community health. But beyond all these difficulties, the field of public health holds great promise for the future. No endeavor is more important than promoting health and preventing injury and disease among the population. As the field improves its scientific methods for measuring effectiveness and as it demonstrates its importance, the field will prosper and gain the attention and resources it deserves.

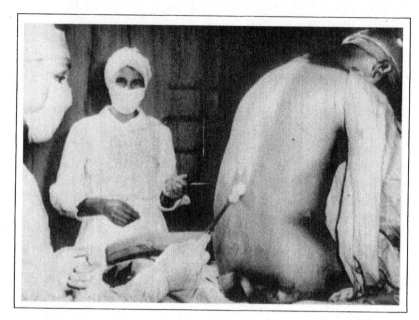

The syphilis study in Tuskegee, Alabama, is perhaps the most prominent example of unethical, government-sponsored research on human subjects in U.S. history. Spinal taps, such as this one on an unidentified man in 1933, were performed to diagnose neural syphilis. Side effects of the procedure included painful headaches and, in rare cases, paralysis or death.

# THREE

# Public Health Ethics

## The Communitarian Tradition

Bioethicists often stress the importance of individual freedoms rather than the general health and well-being of the community. There is, of course, an alternative philosophical tradition that sees individuals primarily as members of communities. This communitarian tradition views individuals as parts of social and political networks, with each individual reliant on the other for health and security. Individuals, according to this tradition, gain value from being a part of a well-regulated society that seeks to prevent risks that all members share. The three readings in this chapter introduce this important philosophical tradition.

The authors discuss several concepts that establish a moral basis for public health. Michael Walzer, an influential political philosopher at the Institute for Advanced Study at Princeton, describes the meaning of social membership, arguing that government is formed principally to meet communal needs for health and security. Dan Beauchamp, one of the pioneers of public health ethics at the State University of New York at Albany, analyzes a classic conflict between the need for population-based measures to improve the well-being of the entire community and American individualism, which, at times, seems to require only restraint from harming others. He builds on Walzer's ideas of political community, arguing that the health of populations has moral standing. In the third reading, Norman Daniels, a Tufts University philosopher who has championed the cause of social justice, and his colleagues use comparative international health data to offer a convincing argument that community wellness is dependent on the existence of democratic structures. Daniels views equal opportunity, personal liberty, and mitigation of socioeconomic inequity as essential conditions for healthier populations. In short, he argues, "justice is good for our health."

## I. POLITICAL THEORY AND PUBLIC HEALTH

With the knowledge that injury and disease can be understood and prevented on a population basis, it is important to consider the nature of social and moral obligations to those in our community. Simply because disease prevention is *possible* does not necessarily make it a desirable goal. *Why* should the government promote the public's health? Or, relatedly, why should society prefer population health to other social values? Though the following authors express distinct arguments about moral obligation, each supports an implied, shared commitment to the common good. The contribution to the common good of society is seen as an ethical imperative, even if the individual benefit is very small. Consider the underlying theories offered by Walzer and Beauchamp to support their ideal of a political commitment to the public's health.

Walzer, in the following selection, tells us that "men and women come together because they literally cannot live apart." In his writing, Walzer describes the importance of membership in a community as a vehicle for the provision for communal needs. Conversely, by providing for those needs on a community basis, individuals reaffirm and strengthen the sense of membership in society.

While Walzer offers a basic framework for understanding the provision of needs in a political community, Beauchamp describes how these communal needs are often misconstrued in American society. Beauchamp argues that communal needs are often mistakenly perceived as collections of individual needs to prevent harm to other individuals. For example, instead of perceiving pollution controls as fulfilling the societal need for clean air, regulations are often perceived as laws that prevent harm to individuals who may be affected by poor-quality air. To advance his argument, he describes the "second language" of republicanism, a language that acknowledges the community roots of the republican tradition, a language that is not drowned out by individualism and paternalism. This second language, he claims, brings the community together toward common goals and, in turn, strengthens desires to achieve public health goals (see also Beauchamp 1998).

## Security and Welfare*
*Michael Walzer*

Membership is important because of what the members of a political community owe to one another and to no one else, or to no one else in the same degree. And the first thing they owe is the communal provision of security and welfare. This claim might be reversed: communal provision is important because it teaches us the value of membership. If we did not provide for one another, if we recognized no distinction between members and strangers, we would have no reason to form and maintain political communities. "How shall men love their country?" Rousseau asked, "if it is nothing more for them than for strangers, and bestows on them only that which it can refuse to none?" Rousseau believed that citizens ought to love their country and therefore that their country ought to give them particular reasons to do so. Membership (like kinship) is a special relation. It's not enough to say, as Edmund Burke did, that "to make us love our country, our country ought to be lovely." The crucial thing is that it be lovely for us—though we always hope that it will be lovely for others (we also love its reflected loveliness).

Political community for the sake of provision, provision for the sake of community: the process works both ways, and that is perhaps its crucial feature. Philosophers and political theorists have been too quick to turn it into a simple calculation. Indeed, we are rationalists of everyday life; we come together, we sign the social contract or reiterate the signing of it, in order to provide for our needs. And we value the contract insofar as those needs are met. But one of our needs is community itself: culture, religion, and politics. It is only under the aegis of these three that all the other things we need become *socially recognized needs,* take on historical and determinate form. The social contract is an agreement to reach decisions together about what goods are necessary to our common life, and then to provide those goods for one another. The signers owe one another more than mutual aid, for that they owe or can owe to anyone. They owe mutual provision of all those things for the sake of which they have separated themselves from mankind as a whole and

*Reprinted from *Spheres of Justice: A Defense of Pluralism and Equality* by permission of Basic Books, a member of Perseus Books, L.L.C. © 1983 by Basic Books, Inc.

joined forces in a particular community. *Amour social* is one of those
things; but though it is a distributed good—often unevenly distributed—
it arises only in the course of other distributions (and of the political
choices that the other distributions require). Mutual provision breeds
mutuality. So the common life is simultaneously the prerequisite of provision and one of its products.

Men and women come together because they literally cannot live
apart. But they can live together in many different ways. Their survival
and then their well-being require a common effort: against the wrath of
the gods, the hostility of other people, the indifference and malevolence
of nature (famine, flood, fire, and disease), the brief transit of a human
life. No army camps alone, as David Hume wrote, but temples, store-
houses, irrigation works, and burial grounds are the true mothers of
cities. As the list suggests, origins are not singular in character. Cities
differ from one another, partly because of the natural environments in
which they are built and the immediate dangers their builders encounter, partly because of the conceptions of social goods that the
builders hold. They recognize but also create one another's needs and
so give a particular shape to what I will call the "sphere of security and
welfare." The sphere itself is as old as the oldest human community. Indeed, one might say that the original community is a sphere of security
and welfare, a system of communal provision, distorted, no doubt, by
gross inequalities of strength and cunning. But the system has, in any
case, no natural form. Different experiences and different conceptions
lead to different patterns of provision. Though there are some goods
that are needed absolutely, there is no good such that once we see it, we
know how it stands vis-à-vis all other goods and how much of it we
owe to one another. The nature of a need is not self-evident.

Communal provision is both general and particular. It is general
whenever public funds are spent so as to benefit all or most of the
members without any distribution to individuals. It is particular whenever goods are actually handed over to all or any of the members.
Water, for example, is one of "the bare requirements of civil life," and
the building of reservoirs is a form of general provision. But the delivery of water to one rather than to another neighborhood (where, say,
the wealthier citizens live) is particular. The securing of the food supply is general; the distribution of food to widows and orphans is particular. Public health is most often general, the care of the sick, most
often particular. . . .

Despite the inherent forcefulness of the word, needs are elusive. People don't just have needs, they have ideas about their needs; they have priorities, they have degrees of need; and these priorities and degrees are related not only to their human nature but also to their history and culture. Since resources are always scarce, hard choices have to be made. I suspect that these can only be political choices. They are subject to a certain philosophical elucidation, but the idea of need and the commitment to communal provision do not by themselves yield any clear determination of priorities or degrees. Clearly we can't meet and we don't have to meet every need to the same degree or any need to the ultimate degree. . . .

The question of degree suggests even more clearly the importance of political choice and the irrelevance of any merely philosophical stipulation. Needs are not only elusive; they are also expansive. In the phrase of the contemporary philosopher Charles Fried, needs are voracious; they eat up resources. But it would be wrong to suggest that therefore need cannot be a distributive principle. It is, rather, a principle subject to political limitation, and the limits (within limits) can be arbitrary, fixed by some temporary coalition of interests or majority of voters. Consider the case of physical security in a modern American city. We could provide absolute security, eliminate every source of violence except domestic violence, if we put a street light every ten yards and stationed a policeman every thirty yards throughout the city. But that would be very expensive, and so we settle for something less. How much less can only be decided politically. One can imagine the sorts of things that would figure in the debates. Above all, I think, there would be a certain understanding—more or less widely shared, controversial only at the margins—of what constitutes "enough" security or of what level of insecurity is simply intolerable. The decision would also be affected by other factors: alternate needs, the state of the economy, the agitation of the policemen's union, and so on. But whatever the decisions ultimately reached, for whatever reasons, security is provided because the citizens need it. And because, at some level, they all need it, the criterion of need remains a critical standard (as we shall see) even though it cannot determine priority and degree.

## COMMUNAL PROVISION

There has never been a political community that did not provide, or try to provide, or claim to provide, for the needs of its members as its members understood those needs. And there has never been a political community that did not engage its collective strength—its capacity to direct, regulate, pressure, and coerce—in this project. The modes of organization, the levels of taxation, the timing and reach of conscription: these have always been a focus of political controversy. But the use of political power has not, until very recently, been controversial. The building of fortresses, dams, and irrigation works, the mobilization of armies, the securing of the food supply and of trade generally—all these require coercion. The state is a tool that cannot be made without iron. And coercion, in turn, requires agents of coercion. Communal provision is always mediated by a set of officials (priests, soldiers, and bureaucrats) who introduce characteristic distortions into the process, siphoning off money and labor for their own purposes or using provision as a form of control. But these distortions are not my immediate concern. I want to stress instead the sense in which every political community is in principle a "welfare state." Every set of officials is at least putatively committed to the provision of security and welfare; every set of members is committed to bear the necessary burdens (and actually does bear them). The first commitment has to do with the duties of office; the second, with the dues of membership. Without some shared sense of the duty and the dues there would be no political community at all and no security or welfare—and the life of mankind "solitary, poor, nasty, brutish, and short."

## AN AMERICAN WELFARE STATE

What sort of communal provision is appropriate in a society like our own? It's not my purpose here to anticipate the outcomes of democratic debate or to stipulate in detail the extent or the forms of provision. But it can be argued, I think, that the citizens of modern industrial democracy owe a great deal to one another, and the argument will provide a useful opportunity to test the critical force of the principles I have defended up until now: that every political community must attend to the needs of its members as they collectively understand those needs; that the goods that are distributed must be distributed in proportion to need; and that the distribution must recognize and uphold the underlying equality of membership. These are very general principles; they are meant to apply to a wide range of communities—to any community, in fact, where the members are each other's equals (before God or the law), or where it can plausibly be said that, however they are treated in fact, they ought to be each other's equals. . . .

Clearly, the three principles apply to the citizens of the United States, and they have considerable force here because of the affluence of the community and the expansive understanding of individual need. On the other hand, the United States currently maintains one of the shabbier systems of communal provision in the Western world. This is so for a variety of reasons: the community of citizens is loosely organized; various ethnic and religious groups run welfare programs of their own; the ideology of self-reliance and entrepreneurial opportunity is widely accepted; and the movements of the left, particularly the labor movement, are relatively weak. Democratic decision making reflects these realities, and there is nothing in principle wrong with that. Nevertheless, the established pattern of provision doesn't measure up to the internal requirements of the sphere of security and welfare, and the common understandings of the citizens point toward a more elaborate pattern. One might also argue that American citizens should work to build a stronger and more intensely experienced political community. But this argument, though it would have distributive consequences, is not, properly speaking, an argument about distributive justice. The question is, What do the citizens owe one another, given the community they actually inhabit? . . .

## The Case of Medical Care

Until recent times, the practice of medicine was mostly a matter of free enterprise. Doctors made their diagnosis, gave their advice, healed or didn't heal their patients, for a fee. Perhaps the private character of the economic relationship was connected to the intimate character of the professional relationship. More likely, I think, it had to do with the relative marginality of medicine itself. Doctors could, in fact, do very little for their patients, and the common attitude in the face of disease (as in the face of poverty) was a stoical fatalism. Or, popular remedies were developed that were not much less effective, sometimes more effective, than those prescribed by established physicians. Folk medicine sometimes produced a kind of communal provision at the local level, but it was equally likely to generate new practitioners, charging fees in their turn. Faith healing followed a similar pattern.

Leaving these two aside, we can say that the distribution of medical care has historically rested in the hands of the medical profession, a guild of physicians that dates at least from the time of Hippocrates in the fifth century B.C. The guild has functioned to exclude unconventional practitioners and to regulate the number of physicians in any given community.

A genuinely free market has never been in the interest of its members. But it is in the interest of the members to sell their services to individual patients; and thus, by and large, the well-to-do have been well cared for (in accordance with the current understanding of good care) and the poor hardly cared for at all. . . . Most doctors, present in an emergency, still feel bound to help the victim without regard to his material status. It is a matter of professional Good Samaritanism that the call "Is there a doctor in the house?" should not go unanswered if there is a doctor to answer it. In ordinary times, however, there was little call for medical help, largely because there was little faith in its actual helpfulness. And so the bad conscience of the profession was not echoed by any political demand for the replacement of free enterprise by communal provision. . . .

Among modern citizens, longevity is a socially recognized need, and increasingly every effort is made to see that it is widely and equally distributed, that every citizen has an equal chance at a long and healthy life: hence doctors and hospitals in every district, regular check-ups, health education for the young, compulsory vaccination, and so on.

Parallel to the shift in attitudes, and following naturally from it, was a shift in institutions: from the church to the clinic and the hospital. But the shift has been gradual: a slow development of communal interest in medical care, a slow erosion of interest in religious care. The first major form of medical provision came in the area of prevention, not of treatment, probably because the former involved no interference with the prerogatives of the guild of physicians. But the beginnings of provision in the area of treatment were roughly simultaneous with the great public health campaigns of the late nineteenth century, and the two undoubtedly reflect the same sensitivity to questions of physical survival. The licensing of physicians, the establishment of state medical schools and urban clinics, the filtering of tax money into the great voluntary hospitals: these measures involved, perhaps, only marginal interference with the profession—some of them, in fact, reinforced its guild-like character; but they already represent an important public commitment. Indeed, they represent a commitment that ultimately can be formed only by turning physicians, or some substantial number of them, into public physicians (as a smaller number once turned themselves into court physicians) and by abolishing or constraining the market in medical care. But before I defend that transformation, I want to stress the unavoidability of the commitment from which it follows.

What has happened in the modern world is simply that disease itself, even when it is endemic rather than epidemic, has come to be seen as a plague. And since the plague can be dealt with, it must be dealt with. People will not endure what they no longer believe they have to endure. Dealing with tuberculosis, cancer, or heart failure, however, requires a common effort. Medical research is expensive, and the treatment of many particular diseases lies far beyond the resources of ordinary citizens. So the community must step in, and any democratic community will in fact step in, more or less vigorously, more or less effectively, depending on the outcome of particular political battles. Thus, the role of the American government (or governments, for much of the activity is at the state and local levels): subsidizing research, training doctors, providing hospitals and equipment, regulating voluntary insurance schemes, underwriting the treatment of the very old. All this represents "the contrivance of human wisdom to provide for human wants." And all that is required to make it morally necessary is the development of a "want" so widely and deeply felt that it can plausibly be said that it is the want not of this or that person alone but of the community generally, a human "want" even though culturally shaped and stressed.

But once communal provision begins, it is subject to further moral constraints: it must provide what is "wanted" equally to all the members of the community; and it must do so in ways that respect their membership. Now, even the pattern of medical provision in the United States, though it stops far short of a national health service, is intended to provide minimally decent care to all who need it. Once public funds are committed, public officials can hardly intend anything less. At the same time, however, no political decision has yet been made to challenge directly the system of free enterprise in medical care. And so long as that system exists, wealth will be dominant in (this part of) the sphere of security and welfare; individuals will be cared for in proportion to their ability to pay and not to their need for care. . . .

But any fully developed system of medical provision will require the constraint of the guild of physicians. Indeed, this is more generally true. The provision of security and welfare requires the constraint of those men and women who had previously controlled the goods in question and sold them on the market (assuming, what is by no means always true, that the market predates communal provision). For what we do when we declare this or that good to be a needed good is to block or constrain its free exchange. We also block any other distributive procedure that doesn't attend to need—popular election, meritocratic competition, personal or familial preference, and so on. But the market is, at least in the United States today, the chief rival of the sphere of security and welfare; and it is most importantly the market that is pre-empted by the welfare state. Needed goods cannot be left to the whim, or distributed in the interest, of some powerful group of owners or practitioners. . . .

This, then, is the argument for an expanded American welfare state. It follows from the three principles with which I began, and it suggests that the tendency of those principles is to free security and welfare from the prevailing patterns of dominance. Though a variety of institutional arrangements is possible, the three principles would seem to favor provision in kind; they suggest an important argument against current proposals to distribute money [e.g., the negative income tax] instead of education, legal aid, or medical care. . . .

I want to stress again that no *a priori* stipulation of what needs ought to be recognized is possible; nor is there any *a priori* way of determining appropriate levels of provision. Our attitudes toward medical care have a history; they have been different; they will be different again. The forms of communal provision have changed in the past and will continue to change. But they don't change automatically as attitudes change. The old order has its clients; there is a lethargy in institutions as in individuals. Moreover, popular attitudes are rarely so clear as they are in the case of medical care. So change is always a matter of political argument, organization, and struggle. All that the philosopher can do is to describe the basic structure of the arguments and the constraints they entail. Hence the three principles, which can be summed up in a revised version of Marx's famous maxim: From each according to his ability (or his resources); to each according to his socially recognized needs. This, I think, is the deepest meaning of the social contract. It only remains to work out the details, but in everyday life, the details are everything.

---

### Community: The Neglected Tradition of Public Health*
*Dan Beauchamp*

THE MEANING OF THE COMMON GOOD

In one version of democratic theory, the state has no legitimate role in restricting personal conduct that is substantially voluntary and that has little or no direct consequence for anyone other than the individual. This

---

*Reprinted from *Hastings Center Report* 15 (December 1985): 28–36.

strong antipaternalist position is associated with John Stuart Mill. In his essay "On Liberty," which has deeply influenced American and British thought for over one hundred years, Mill wrote: "The only purpose for which power can be rightfully exercised over any member of a civilized community, against his will, is to prevent harms to others." Mill restricts paternalism to children and the incompetent. In this view the common good consists in maximizing the freedom of each individual to pursue his or her own interests, subject to a like freedom for every other individual. In the words of Blackstone, "The public good is . . . essentially interested in the protection of every individual's private rights."

In a second version, health and safety remain private interests but some paternalism is accepted, albeit reluctantly. As Joel Feinberg argues, common sense makes us reject a thoroughgoing antipaternalism. Many restrictions on liberty are relatively minor and the savings in life and limb extremely great. Further, often voluntary choices are not completely so; many choices are impaired in some sense. But, as Dennis Thompson contends, even where choices are not impaired, as in the choice not to wear seatbelts or to take up smoking, paternalism might still be accepted, because the alternative would be a great loss of life and a society in which each citizen was, for many important decisions, left alone with the consequences of his or her choice.

This reluctant acceptance of paternalism leaves many democrats uneasy. Another alternative is to redefine voluntary risks to an individual as risks to others. Indeed, many argue that all such risks have serious consequences for others, and that the state may therefore limit such activities on the basis of the harm principle. Others challenge the category of voluntariness head on, arguing that most such risks, like cigarettes and alcohol use, have powerful social determinants.

The constitutional basis for the protection of the public health and safety has largely been ignored in this debate. This tradition, and particularly the regulatory power (often called the police power), flows from a view of democracy that sees the essential task of government as protecting and promoting both private and group interests. Government is supposed to defend both sets of interests through an evolving set of practices and institutions, and it is left to the legislatures to determine which set of interests predominate when conflicts arise.

In the constitutional tradition, the common good refers to the welfare of individuals considered as a group, the public or the people generally, the "body politic" or the "commonwealth" as it was termed in the early days of the American Republic. The public or the people were presumed to have an interest, held in common, in self-protection or preservation from threats of all kinds to their welfare. The commonwealth idea was widely influential among New England states during the first half of the nineteenth century.

The commonwealth doctrine helped shape the regulatory power in Massachusetts and throughout the U.S. The central principles underlying the police or regulatory power were the treatment of health and safety as a shared purpose and need of the community and (aside from basic constitutional rights such as due process) the subordination of the market, property, and individual liberty to protect compelling community interests.

This republican image of democracy was a blending of social contract and republican thought, as well as Judeo-Christian notions of covenant. In the republican vision of society, the individual has a dual status. On the one hand, individuals have private interests and private rights; political association serves to protect these rights. On the other hand, individuals are members of a political community—a body politic.

This common citizenship, despite diversity and divergence of interests, presumes an underlying shared set of loyalties and obligations to support the ends of the political community, among which public health and safety are central. In this scheme, public health and safety are not simply the aggregate of each private individual's interests in health and safety, interests which can be pursued more effectively through collective action. Public health and safety are community or group interests (often referred to as "state interests" in the law), interests that can transcend and take priority over private interests if the legislature so chooses.

The idea of democracy as promoting the common or group interest is captured in Joseph Tussman's classic work on political obligation: "Familiar as it is, there is something fundamentally misleading about the slogan that the aim of government is 'welfare of the individual.' . . . [T]he government's concern for the individual is not to be understood as a special concern for *this* or *that* individual but rather a concern for all individuals. Government, that is to say, serves the welfare of the community.". . .

## THE LANGUAGE OF PUBLIC HEALTH

What are we to make of this constitutional tradition surrounding the development of the regulatory power for health and safety? What relevance does it have for the policy disputes of today, particularly those concerning the limitation of lifestyle risks?

The constitutional tradition for public health constitutes one of those "second languages" of republicanism that Robert Bellah and his coauthors (1985) speak of in their book *Habits of the Heart*. In their book, the first language (or tradition of moral discourse) of American politics is political individualism. But there are "second languages" of community rooted in the republican and biblical tradition that limit and qualify the scope and consequences of political individualism. Public health as a second language reminds us that we are not only individuals, we are also a community and a body politic, and that we have shared commitments to one another and promises to keep. . . .

The danger is that we can come to discuss public health exclusively within the dominant discourse of political individualism, relying either on the harm principle or a narrow paternalism justified on grounds of self-protection alone. By ignoring the communitarian language of public health, we risk shrinking its claims. We also risk undermining the sense in which health and safety are a signal commitment of the common life—a central *practice* by which the body-politic defines itself and affirms its values. . . .

Public health belongs to the realm of the political and the ethical. Public health belongs to the ethical because it is concerned not only with explaining the occurrence of illness and disease in society, but also with ameliorating them. Beyond instrumental goals, public health is concerned with integrative goals expressing the commitment of the whole people to face the threat of death and disease in solidarity.

Public health is also a practical science. Spanning the world of science and practical action, it seeks reasonable and practical means of altering property arrangements or limiting liberty to promote the health of the public generally.

These two ideas, the ideas of second languages and of social practices, shed light on why paternalism—at least public health paternalism—plays an affirmative role in the republican tradition. In the constitutional categories for protecting the public health, the regulatory power is to protect not individual citizens, but rather citizens considered as a group, the public health. In this tradition, the public, as well as the community itself, has a reality apart from the citizens who comprise it. Fundamental constituents of the community and the common life are its practices and institutions.

Practices are communal in nature and concerned with the well-being of the community as a whole and not just the well-being of any particular person. Policy, and here public health paternalism, operates at the level of practices and not at the level of individual behavior. . . .

This distinction between practices and behavior should help us see the difference between public health paternalism aimed at the group and the "personal paternalism" of the doctor-patient, lawyer-client relationship. While there are public elements of these professional relationships—and while the state can (rightly or wrongly) structure these relationships in a paternalistic fashion—their essence is based on a personal encounter between a professional and a client. This is not the case with public health paternalism. Public health paternalism should also be kept separate from the legal doctrine of *parens patriae*, where the state assumes the role of parent in instances where parental supervision is absent or deemed deficient.

This suggests that public health paternalism and the language of community on which it is based fit the parent-child analogy very poorly. To Mill, all paternalism was wrong because the individual is best placed to know his own good: "He is the person most interested in his own well-being—the interest which any other person, except in cases of strong personal attachment, can have in it, is trifling. . . ."

But precisely because public health paternalism is aimed at the group and its practices, and not the specific individual, Mill's point is wrong. The good of the particular person is not the aim of health policy in a democracy which defends both the community and the individual. In fact, Mill is wrong twice—because particular individuals are often very poorly placed to judge the effects that market arrangements and practices have on the population as a whole. This is the task for legislatures, for organized groups of citizens, and for other agents of the public, including the citizen as voter.

Mill's dichotomy of either the harm principle or self-protection is too limited; the world of harms is not exhausted by self-imposed and other-imposed injuries. There is a third and very large set of problems that afflicts the community as a whole and that results primarily from inadequate safeguards over the practices of the common life. Economists and others often refer to this class of harms as "summing up problems" or "choice-in-the-small versus choice-in-the-large."

Creating, extending, or strengthening the practices of public health—and the collective goods principle that underlies [them]—ought to be the primary justification for our health and safety policy. Instead we usually base these regulations on the harm principle. We usually justify regulating the steel or coal industry on the grounds that workers and the general public have the risks of pollution or black lung visited on them, but consumers are not obliged to drink alcohol or smoke cigarettes. While this may be true, in the communitarian language and categories of public health, fixing blame is not the main point. We regulate the steel or coal industry because market competition undervalues collective goods like a clean environment or workers' safety. Using social organization to secure collective goods like public health, not preventing harms to others, is the proper rationale for health and safety regulations imposed on the steel or coal industry, or the alcohol or cigarette industry. . . .

The main lesson to learn from public health paternalism as it has developed in the constitutional tradition may well be that the second language of community and the virtues of cooperation and beneficence still exist, albeit precariously, alongside a tradition of political individualism. Strengthening the public health includes not only the practical task of improving aggregate welfare, it also involves the task of reacquainting the American public with its republican and communitarian heritage, and encouraging citizens to share in reasonable and practical group schemes to promote a wider welfare of which their own welfare is only a part. In political individualism, seatbelt legislation or signs on the beach restricting swimming when a lifeguard is not present restrict the individual's liberty for his or her own good. In this circumstance the appropriate slogan is: "The life you save may be your own." But in the second language of public health these restrictions define a common practice which shapes our life together, for the general or the common good. In the language of public health, the motto for such paternalistic legislation might be: "The lives we save together might include your own."

---

## II. SOCIAL AND ECONOMIC INEQUALITIES

Norman Daniels and his colleagues present a different framework for community membership and public health. Using the Rawlsian concept of justice, he describes the political institutions necessary for a healthy population. Essentially, John Rawls embraced the idea that a social contract designed to be fair to free and equal people would lead to equal basic liberties and equal opportunity. Rawls, Daniels argues, did not incorporate premature illness into his account of justice. By correcting Rawls's model to account for health disparities, Daniels predicts the political conditions necessary to achieve health equity (see further, Daniels, Kennedy, and Kawachi 2000b; Daniels 1985; and Evans, Barer, and Marmor 1994).

## Justice Is Good for Our Health*
*Norman Daniels, Bruce Kennedy, and Ichiro Kawachi*

We have long known that the more affluent and better-educated members of a society tend to live longer and healthier lives: Rene Louis Villerme made this point as early as 1840, and it has been shown to hold for just about every human society. Recent research suggests that the correlations between income and health do not end there. We now know, for example, that countries with a greater degree of socioeconomic inequality show greater inequality in health status; also, that middle-income groups in relatively unequal societies have worse health than comparable, or even poorer, groups in more equal societies. Inequality, in short, seems to be bad for our health.

Moreover, and perhaps more surprisingly, universal access to health care does not necessarily break the link between social status and health. Our health is affected not simply by the ease with which we can see a doctor—though that surely matters—but also by our social position and the underlying inequality of our society. We cannot, of course, infer causation from these correlations between social inequality and health inequality (though we will explore some ideas about how the one might lead to the other). Suffice to say that, while the exact processes are not fully understood, the evidence suggests that there are *social determinants of health.*

These social determinants offer a distinctive angle on how to think about justice, public health, and reform of the health care system. If social factors play a large role in determining our health, then efforts to ensure greater justice in health care should not focus simply on the traditional health sector. Health is produced not merely by having access to medical prevention and treatment, but also, to a measurably greater extent, by the cumulative experience of social conditions over the course of one's life. By the time a sixty-year-old heart attack victim arrives at the emergency room, bodily insults have accumulated over a lifetime. For such a person, medical care is, figuratively speaking, "the ambulance waiting at the bottom of the cliff." Much contemporary discussion about reducing health inequalities by increasing access to medical care misses this point. We should be looking as well to improve social conditions—such as access to basic education, levels of material

*Reprinted from *The Boston Review* (February/March 2000): 6–15.

deprivation, a healthy workplace environment, and equality of political participation—that help to determine the health of societies.

These conditions have unfortunately been virtually ignored within the academic field of bioethics, and in public discussions about health care reform. Academic bioethics is quick to focus on exotic new technologies and the vexing questions they raise for doctors and health administrators, who must make decisions about patient care and the allocation of scarce medical resources. And we all worry about the doctor-patient relationship under managed care, as insurance companies have taken a newly aggressive role in making medical decisions. But with some significant exceptions neither academic nor popular discussion has looked "upstream," past the new technologies, managed care, and the organization of health insurance, to the social arrangements that determine the health achievement of societies.

We hope to fill this gap by exploring some broader issues about health and social justice. To avoid vague generalities about justice, we shall advance a line of argument inspired principally by the theory of "justice as fairness" put forth by the philosopher John Rawls. We find Rawls's theory compelling as an account of justice quite apart from its usefulness as an approach to the health care issue. But even those who do not share our ideas about justice may find our argument a helpful first step in thinking about social justice and public health.

Rawls's theory of justice as fairness was not designed to address issues of health care. He assumed a completely healthy population, and argued that a just society must assure people equal basic liberties, guarantee that the right of political participation has roughly equal value for all, provide a robust form of equal opportunity, and limit inequalities to those that benefit the least advantaged. When these requirements of justice are met, Rawls argued, we can have reasonable confidence that others are showing us the respect that is essential to our sense of self-worth.

Recent empirical literature about the social determinants of health suggests that the failure to meet Rawlsian criteria for a just society is closely related to health inequality. The conjecture we propose to explore, then, is that by establishing equal liberties, robustly equal opportunity, a fair distribution of resources, and support for our self-respect—the basics of Rawlsian justice—we would go a long way to eliminating the most important injustices in health outcomes. To be sure, social justice is valuable for reasons other than its effects on health. And social reform in the direction of greater justice would not eliminate the need to think hard about fair allocation of resources within the health care system. Still, acting to promote social justice may be a key step toward improving our health.

## SOCIAL DETERMINANTS OF HEALTH

### Cross-National Inequalities

A country's prosperity is related to its health, as measured, for example, by life expectancy: in richer countries people tend to live longer. This well-established finding suggests a natural ordering of societies along some fixed path of economic development: as a country or region develops economically average health improves. But the evidence suggests that things are more complicated. Figure 5 shows the relationship between the wealth of nations, as measured by per capita gross domestic product (GDPpc), and the health of nations, as measured by life expectancy. Clearly, GDPpc and life expectancy are closely associated, but only up to a point. The relationship levels off when GDPpc reaches $8,000 to $10,000; beyond this threshold, further economic advance buys virtually no further gains in life expectancy. This leveling effect is most apparent among the advanced industrial economies (see Figure 6), which largely account for the upper tail of the curve in Figure 5. Closer inspection of these two figures shows some startling discrepancies.

Though Cuba and Iraq are equally poor (each has a GDPpc of about $3,100), life expectancy in Cuba exceeds that in Iraq by 17.2 years. The difference between the GDPpc for Costa Rica and the United States is enormous (about $21,000), yet Costa Rica's life expectancy exceeds that of the United States (76.6 to 76.4). In fact, despite being the richest nation on the globe, the United States performs rather poorly on major health indicators.

Taken together, these observations show that the health of nations may depend, in part, on factors other than wealth. Culture, social organization, and government policies also help determine population health, and variations in these factors may explain many of the differences in health outcomes among nations.

### Relative Income

One especially important factor in explaining the health of a society is the distribution of income: the health of a population depends not just on the size of the economic pie, but on how the pie is shared. Differences in health outcomes among developed nations cannot be explained simply by the absolute deprivation associated with low economic development—lack of access to the basic material conditions

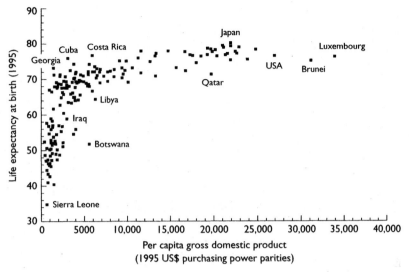

Figure 5. Life expectancy and per capita GDP. (*Source:* United Nations Human Development Report Statistics 1998.)

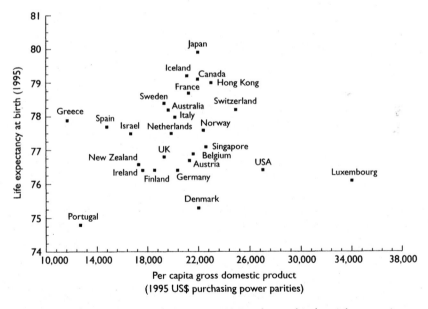

Figure 6. Life expectancy and per capita GDP: advanced industrial economies. (*Source:* United Nations Human Development Report Statistics 1998.)

necessary for health such as clean water, adequate nutrition and housing, and general sanitary living conditions. The degree of relative deprivation within a society also matters.

Numerous studies have provided support for this *relative-income hypothesis,* which states, more precisely, that inequality is strongly associated with population mortality and life expectancy across nations. To be sure, wealthier countries generally have higher average life expectancy. But rich countries, too, vary in life expectancy (see the tail of Figure 5), and that variation dovetails with income distribution. Wealthy countries with more equal income distributions, such as Sweden and Japan, have higher life expectancies than does the United States, despite their having lower per capita GDP. Likewise, countries with low GDPpc but remarkably high life expectancy, such as Costa Rica, tend to have a more equitable distribution of income. . . .

## Individual SES [socioeconomic status]

Finally, when we move from comparing whole societies to comparing their individual members, we find, once more, that inequality is important. At the individual level, numerous studies have documented what has come to be known as the *socioeconomic gradient:* at each step along the socioeconomic ladder, we see improved health outcomes over the rung below. This suggests that differences in health outcomes are not confined to the extremes of rich and poor, but are observed across all levels of socioeconomic status.

Moreover, the SES gradient does not appear to be explained by differences in access to health care. Steep gradients have been observed even among groups of individuals, such as British civil servants, who all have adequate access to health care, housing, and transport. The slope of the gradient varies substantially across societies. Some societies show a relatively shallow gradient in mortality rates: being better off confers a health advantage, but not so large an advantage as elsewhere. Others, with comparable or even higher levels of economic development, show much steeper gradients.

The slope of the gradient appears to be fixed by the level of income inequality in a society: the more unequal a society is in economic terms, the more unequal it is in health terms. Moreover, middle income groups in a country with high income inequality typically do worse in terms of health than comparable or even poorer groups in a society with less income inequality. We find the same pattern within the United States when we examine state and metropolitan area variations in inequality and health outcomes.

## Pathways

Earlier, we cautioned that correlations between inequality and health do not necessarily imply causation. Still, there are plausible and identifiable pathways through which social inequalities appear to produce health inequalities. In the United States, the states with the most unequal income distributions invest less in public education, have larger uninsured populations, and spend less on social safety nets. The facts on educational spending and educational outcomes are especially striking: controlling for median income, income inequality explains about 40 percent of the variation between states in the percentage of children in the fourth grade who are below the basic reading level. Similarly strong associations are seen for high school drop-out rates. It is evident from these data that educational opportunities for children in high-income-inequality states are quite different from those in states with more egalitarian distributions. These effects on education have an immediate impact on health, increasing the likelihood of premature death during childhood and adolescence (as evidenced by the much higher death rates for infants and children in the high inequality states). Later in life, they appear in the SES gradient in health.

When we compare countries, we also find that differential investment in human capital—in particular, education—is a strong predictor of health. Indeed, one of the strongest predictors of life expectancy among developing countries is adult literacy, particularly the disparity between male and female adult literacy, which explains much of the variation in health achievement among these countries after accounting for GDPpc. For example, among the 125 developing countries with GDPpcs less than $10,000, the difference between male and female literacy accounts for 40 percent of the variation in life expectancy after factoring out the effect of GDPpc. The fact that gender disparities in access to basic education drives the level of health achievement further emphasizes the role of broader social inequalities in patterning health inequalities. Indeed, in the United States, differences between the states in women's status—measured in terms of their economic autonomy and political participation—are strongly correlated with higher female mortality rates.

These societal mechanisms—for example, income inequality leading to educational inequality leading to health inequality—are tightly linked to the political processes that influence government policy. For example, income inequality appears to affect health by undermining civil society. Income inequality erodes social cohesion, as measured by higher levels of social mistrust and reduced participation in civic organizations. Lack of social cohesion leads to lower participation in political activity (such as voting, serving in local government, volunteering for political campaigns). And lower participation, in turn, undermines the responsiveness of government institutions in addressing the needs of the worst off. States with the highest income inequality, and thus lowest levels of social capital and political participation, are less likely to invest in human capital and provide far less generous social safety nets.

In short, the case for social determinants of health is strong. What are the implications of this fact for ideas of justice?

## INEQUALITIES AND INEQUITIES

When is a health inequality between two groups "inequitable"? Margaret Whitehead and Goran Dahlgren have suggested a useful and influential answer: health inequalities count as inequities when they are avoidable, unnecessary, and unfair.

The Whitehead/Dahlgren analysis is deliberately broad. Age, gender, race, and ethnic differences in health status exist independent of the socioeconomic differences we have been discussing, and they raise distinct questions about equity. For example, should we view the lower life expectancy of men compared to women in developed countries as an inequity? If it is rooted in biological differences that we do not know how to overcome, then it is unavoidable (and therefore not an inequity). This is not an idle controversy: taking average, rather than gender-differentiated, life expectancy in developed countries as a benchmark will yield different estimates of the degree of inequity women face in some developing countries. In any case, the analysis of inequity is only as good as our understanding of what is avoidable or unnecessary.

The same point applies to judgments about fairness. Is the poorer health status of groups whose members smoke and drink heavily unfair? We may be inclined to say it is not unfair, provided that participation in such risky behaviors is truly voluntary. But if many people in a cultural group or class behave similarly, then the behavior might acquire the qualities of a social norm—in which case we might wonder just how voluntary the behavior is (and therefore how much responsibility we should ascribe to them for it). Whitehead's and Dahlgren's terms leave us with an unresolved complexity of judgments about responsibility, and, as a result, with disagreements about fairness and avoidability.

The poor in many countries lack access to clean water, sanitation, adequate shelter, basic education, vaccinations, and prenatal and maternal care. As a result of some, or all, of these factors, infant mortality rates for the poor exceed those of the rich. Since social policies could supply the missing determinants of infant health, these inequalities are avoidable.

Are these inequalities also unfair? Most of us would think they are, perhaps because we believe that policies that create and sustain poverty are unjust, and perhaps also because we object to social policies that compound economic poverty with lack of access to the determinants of health. The problem of justice in health care becomes more complicated, however, when we remember one of the basic findings from the literature on social determinants: we cannot eliminate health inequalities simply by eliminating poverty. Health inequalities persist even in societies that provide the poor with access to all standard public health and medical services, as well as basic income and education health, and they persist as a gradient of health throughout the social hierarchy, not just between the very poorest groups and those above them.

What, then, are we to think of the health inequalities that would persist, even if poverty were eliminated? To eliminate health inequalities, should we eliminate all socioeconomic inequalities? We might believe that all socioeconomic inequalities, or at least all inequalities we did not freely choose, are unjust—but very few embrace such a radical egalitarian view. Indeed, we may well believe that some degree of socioeconomic inequality is unavoidable, or even necessary, and therefore not unjust. On issues of this kind, we should take guidance from a well-articulated account of social justice—the one put forth by John Rawls.

## JUSTICE AS FAIRNESS

In *A Theory of Justice*, Rawls sought to show that a social contract designed to be fair to free and equal people would lead to equal basic liberties and equal opportunity, and would permit inequalities only when they work to make the worst-off groups fare as well as possible. Though Rawls's account was devised for the most general questions of social justice, it also provides a set of principles for the just distribution of the social determinants of health.

Rawls did not talk about disease or health in his original account. To simplify the construction of his theory, he assumed that his contractors were fully functional over a normal life span—no one becomes ill or dies prematurely. This idealization provides a clue about how to extend this theory to the real world of illness and premature death. The goal of public health and medicine is to keep people as close to the idealization of normal functioning as possible under reasonable resource constraints. Maintaining normal functioning, in turn, makes a limited but significant contribution to protecting the range of opportunities open to individuals. So one might see the distribution of health care as governed by a norm of fair equality of opportunity. We can now say more directly why justice, as described by Rawls's principles, is good for our health.

Let us start by considering what a just society would require with regard to the distribution of the social determinants of health. In such an ideal society, everyone is guaranteed equal basic liberties, including the right to participate in politics. In addition, there are safeguards aimed at assuring for all, whether richer or poorer, the worth or value of those rights. Since, as we argued above, there is evidence that political participation is a social determinant of health, the Rawlsian ideal assures institutional protections that counter the usual effects of socioeconomic inequalities on participation—and thus on health.

Moreover, according to Rawls, justice requires fair equality of opportunity. This principle condemns discriminatory barriers and requires robust measures aimed at mitigating the effects of socioeconomic inequalities and other contingencies on opportunity. In addition to equitable public education, such measures would include the provision of developmentally appropriate day care and early childhood interventions intended to promote the development of capabilities independently of the advantages of family background. Such measures match, or go beyond, the best models of such interventions currently in place, such as European efforts at day care and early childhood education. We also note that the strategic importance of education for protecting equal opportunity has implications for all levels of education, including access to graduate and professional education.

The equal opportunity principle also requires extensive public health, medical, and social support services aimed at promoting normal functioning for all. It even provides a rationale for the social costs of reasonable accommodation to incurable disabilities, as required by the Americans with Disabilities Act. Because the equal opportunity principle aims at promoting normal functioning for all as a way of protecting opportunity for all, it at once aims at improving population health and the reduction of health inequalities. Obviously, this focus requires provision of universal access to comprehensive health care, including public health, primary health care, and medical and social support services.

To act justly in health policy, we must have knowledge about the causal pathways through which socioeconomic (and other) inequalities work to produce differential health outcomes. Suppose we learn, for example, that workplace organization induces stress and a loss of control, and that these tend, in turn, to promote health inequalities. We should then think of modifying those features of workplace organization in order to mitigate their negative effects on health as a public health requirement of the equal opportunity approach.

Finally, a just society restricts allowable inequalities in income and wealth to those that benefit the least advantaged. The inequalities allowed by this principle—in conjunction with the principles assuring equal opportunity and the value of political participation—are probably more constrained than those we observe in even the most industrialized societies. If so, just inequalities would produce a flatter gradient of health inequality than we currently observe in even the more extensive welfare systems of Northern Europe.

In short, Rawlsian justice—though not devised for the case of health—regulates the distribution of the key social determinants of health, including the social bases of self-respect. There is nothing about the theory that should make us focus narrowly on medical services. Properly understood, justice as fairness tells us what justice requires in the distribution of all socially controllable determinants of health. . . .

Suppose we reduce socioeconomic inequalities, and thereby reduce health inequalities—but the result is that the health of all is worsened because productivity is reduced so much that important institutions are undermined. That is not acceptable. Our commitment to reducing health inequality should not require steps that threaten to make health worse off for those with less-than-equal health status. So the theoretical issue reduces to this: would it ever be reasonable to allow some health inequality in order to produce some non-health benefits for those with the worst health prospects?

We know that in real life people routinely trade health risks for other benefits. They do so when they commute longer distances for a better job or take a ski vacation. Trades of this kind raise questions of fairness. For example, when is hazard pay a benefit workers gain only because their opportunities are unfairly restricted? When is it an appropriate exercise of their autonomy? Some such trades are unfair; others will only be restricted by paternalists.

Rawls gave priority to the principle of protecting equal basic liberties because he believed that once people achieve some threshold level of material well-being, they will not trade away the fundamental importance of liberty for other goods. Making such a trade might deny them the liberty to pursue their most cherished ideals, including their religious beliefs, whatever they turn out to be. Can we make the same argument about trading health for other goods?

There is some plausibility to the claim that rational people should refrain from trading their health for other goods. Loss of health may preclude us from pursuing what we most value in life. We do, after all, see people willing to trade almost anything to regain health once they lose it.

Nevertheless, there is also strong reason to think this priority is not clear-cut, especially where the trade is between a risk to health and other goods that people highly value. Refusing to allow any (*ex ante*) trades of health risks for other goods, even when the background conditions on choice are otherwise fair, may seem unjustifiably paternalistic, perhaps in a way that refusal to allow trades of basic liberties is not.

We propose a pragmatic route around this problem. Fair equality of opportunity is only approximated even in an ideally just system, because we can only mitigate, not eliminate, the effects of family and other social contingencies. For example, only if we were willing to violate widely respected parental liberties could we intrude into family life and "rescue" children from parental values that arguably interfere with equal opportunity. Similarly, though we give a general priority to equal opportunity over the Difference Principle, we cannot achieve complete equality in health any more than we can achieve completely equal opportunity. Justice is always rough around the edges.

Suppose, then, that the decision about trade-offs is made by the legislature in a democratic society where everyone has a fair chance to participate. Because those principles require effective political participation across all socioeconomic groups, we can suppose that groups most directly affected by any trade-off decision have a voice in the decision. Since there is a residual health gradient, groups affected by the trade-off include not only the worst off, but those in the middle as well. A democratic process that involved deliberation about the trade-off and its effects might be the best we could do to provide a resolution of the unanswered theoretical question.

In contrast, where the fair value of political participation is not adequately assured—and we doubt it is so assured in even our most democratic societies—we have much less confidence in the fairness of a democratic decision about how to trade health against other goods. It is much more likely under actual conditions that those who benefit most from the inequalities—that is, those who are better off—also wield disproportionate political power and will influence decisions about trade-offs to serve their interests. It may still be that the use of a democratic process in non-ideal conditions is the fairest resolution we can practically achieve, but it still falls well short of what an ideally just democratic process involves.

If we were to achieve a just distribution of resources, then, with the least well-off being as well off as possible, there would still be health inequalities. But decisions about whether to reduce those inequalities even more are matters for democratic process. Justice itself does not command their reduction.

---

*     *     *     *     *

This chapter has explored a different tradition in modern philosophy—one that sees people not as independent "rights-bearing" individuals, but as members of a community. Under this conception, people's primary claims are not to autonomy, privacy, and liberty, but to mutual security and well-being. Rather than stressing individual entitlements, this tradition stresses the duties all members of society owe, one to another. Rather than seeing government's role as defending personal interests and avoiding taxation and regulation, this tradition examines the affirmative powers and obligations of the state to safeguard the common weal. This is the philosophic tradition of public health: it maximizes health and security and minimizes social and economic inequalities.

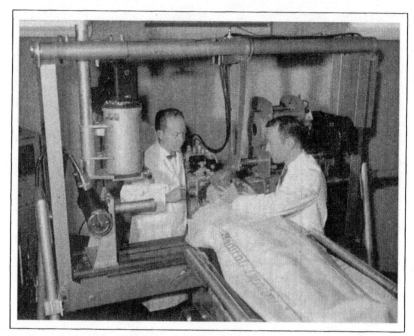

This photo, taken in 1958 at the Lawrence Radiation Laboratory at Berkeley, shows Dr. Richard A. Carlson and Hal O. Anger, an electronics engineer, preparing a patient for irradiation using a 184-inch cyclotron (a particle accelerator). Although the cyclotron enabled physicians to detect tumors, it exposed individuals to unhealthy doses of radiation. (Courtesy of Lawrence Berkeley National Laboratory.)

# FOUR

# Human Rights
# and Public Health

It is not necessary to recount the numerous charters and
declarations . . . to understand human rights. . . . All persons
are born free and equal in dignity and rights. Everyone . . . is
entitled to all the rights and freedoms set forth in the
international human rights instruments without discrimination,
such as the rights to life, liberty, security of the person, privacy,
health, education, work, social security, and to marry and
found a family. Yet, violations of human rights are a reality to
be found in every corner of the globe.

> *Jose Ayala Lasso (UN High Commissioner for*
> *Human Rights) and Peter Piot (Executive*
> *Director of UNAIDS) (1997)*

In recent years, human rights have profoundly influenced the field of
public health (Mann, Gruskin, Grodin, and Annas 1999). Historians
may reasonably inquire why a body of international law dating back to
the mid-twentieth century would suddenly become part of public health
discourse. The emphasis on individual rights and liberties that became
fashionable in the AIDS pandemic later in the century provides a partial explanation. Civil libertarians turned to the language of human
rights to defend persons living with HIV/AIDS from stigma and discrimination (Gostin and Lazzarini 1997).

Scholars and practitioners came to see human rights as essential
tools in the work of public health. They reasoned that persons who fear
government coercion or private discrimination would not come forward for testing, treatment, and partner notification. Individuals who
lacked social status and economic power, moreover, would be more vulnerable to infection. Women, for example, may understand that unprotected sex or needle sharing transmits HIV infection, and they may
even have the means of protection available (e.g., condoms and sterile
injection equipment). But if these women remain powerless in abusive

relationships or economically dependent on their partners, they cannot resist unwanted sex or needle sharing, which places them at risk.

There are other possible historical explanations for the current use of human rights discourse in public health. During the Clinton administration's effort to achieve universal access to medical insurance, advocates began to claim that health care is a human right. This rhetorical device elevated health care from a market commodity to a basic entitlement.

The first reading in this chapter discusses human rights and health in commemoration of the fiftieth anniversary of the Universal Declaration of Human Rights (UDHR), which took place in 1998. George Annas, a well-known scholar in health law from Boston University, explains the legal basis for human rights and applies international human rights law to contemporary health issues. He describes why human rights law has inspired international activism and scholarship in public health.

The second reading is coauthored by perhaps the most prominent figure in public health and human rights. The late Jonathan M. Mann, as the first head of the World Health Organization's Global Programme on AIDS (which has evolved into the United Nations Joint Programme on AIDS [UNAIDS]), drew inspiration from his work on the pandemic. Mann later became the first François-Xavier Bagnoud Professor of Health and Human Rights at Harvard University. He theorized that human rights and public health are complementary fields motivated by the paramount value of human well-being. He felt that people could not be healthy if governments did not respect their rights and dignity. Nor could people maintain their rights and dignity if they were not healthy. Mann and his colleagues argue that public health and human rights are integrally connected: human rights violations adversely affect the community's health, coercive public health policies violate human rights, and advancement of human rights and public health reinforce one another. This synergy between human rights and public health is illustrated in Figure 7.

When reading Mann's article, consider whether human rights and public health are indeed complementary pursuits. Do public health and human rights share the goal of improving human well-being? Can the individualistic thinking inherent in human rights sometimes impede public health goals? Human rights characteristically defend individual interests and civil liberties. Is this approach always consistent with public health's focus on collective well-being?

The third article in this chapter is also written by Mann. Later in his career, Mann came to have an interest in the relationships between public health, human rights, and bioethics. In this article, he offers suggestions for the development of a code of ethics for public health. Should

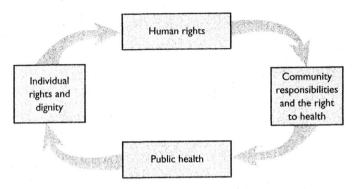

Figure 7.  Synergy between public health and human rights.

public health professionals be guided by a code of ethical practice or at least a well-articulated set of ethical principles? Are the multiple professions engaged in the enterprise of public health sufficiently similar to justify a single set of ethical guidelines?

Thus far, most of the discussion of human rights has assumed that the field is devoted principally to individual rights and liberties. Civil and political rights are characteristically negative or defensive in character, requiring government to refrain from abuse and overreaching. Put another way, human rights advocates argue that individuals have a right to be free from government interference.

Although this view of human rights certainly is correct, there is another important human rights tradition. Many human rights scholars stress the equal importance of economic, social, and cultural rights, which are characteristically "positive" in nature, placing obligations on government to act for the communal good. Unfortunately, the international community has not rigorously defined the parameters of positive rights (Gostin 2000d). When does a country violate an economic, social, or cultural right, such as the right to health? Should the right apply in different ways depending on the wealth of a country? How can the right be enforced, and by whom? The international community has only begun to explore these kinds of difficult and challenging questions (Jamar 1994; Kinney 2001).

The final article in this chapter examines the most important economic, social, and cultural right—the right to health. Human rights scholar Brigit Toebes surveys the various international instruments supporting a right to health. She also discusses the significant problems of definition, scope, and enforcement (see further Toebes [1999b] and Leary [1994]). Toebes' article was written before the publication of the United Nations Committee on Economic, Social,

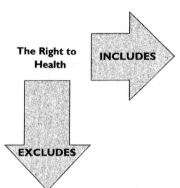

- The right to the highest attainable standard of health
- The right to basic, essential health services
- The right to affordable, quality health care
- The right to equality of access to health services
- The right to conditions needed to protect health (e.g., clean water, housing, sanitation)
- The right to be free from serious environmental threats
- The right to occupational health
- The right to some level of health education
- The right to enhanced health measures for vulnerable populations

- The right to be healthy
- The right to health care no matter the cost
- The right to premium quality health care
- The right to unlimited access to health care services
- The right not to be injured at work
- The right to regular health education in schools
- The right to prohibit experimental medical or scientific procedures or research

Figure 8.   The human right to health.

and Cultural Rights *General Comment No. 14: The Right to the Highest Attainable Standard of Health,* 22nd Session, April 25–May 12, 2000. The General Comment represents the most authoritative statement of the United Nations on the meaning of the right to health. It can be found on the *Reader* web site. Figure 8 lists the various elements of the right to health—services that are included and excluded from the entitlement according to Toebes and the General Comment.

## I. THE RELATIONSHIPS BETWEEN PUBLIC HEALTH, HUMAN RIGHTS, AND ETHICS

### Human Rights and Health— The Universal Declaration of Human Rights at 50*

*George J. Annas*

War, famine, pestilence, and poverty have had obvious and devastating effects on health throughout human history. In recent times, human

*Reprinted from *New England Journal of Medicine* 339 (1998): 1777–81.

rights have come to be viewed as essential to freedom and individual development. But it is only since the end of World War II that the link between human rights and these causes of disease and death has been recognized. The 50th anniversary of the UDHR—signed on December 10, 1948—provides an opportunity to review its genesis, to explore the contemporary link between health and human rights, and to develop effective human-rights strategies in order to promote health and prevent and treat disease.

## WAR AND HUMAN RIGHTS

The modern human-rights movement was born from the devastation of World War II. Nonetheless, appeals to universal human rights are at least as old as government. When Jean Anouilh staged Sophocles' *Antigone* in Nazi-occupied Paris in early 1944, the French audience applauded the performance, identifying Antigone with the French resistance. Antigone was sentenced to be buried alive for defying King Creon's order not to bury her dead brother (whom the king considered a traitor) but to leave his body to rot in public. The Nazis in the audience also applauded the performance, apparently because they identified with Creon and his difficulty in maintaining law and order in the face of seemingly fanatical resistance. *Antigone,* which was written more than 2400 years ago, focuses on a central moral question: Is there a higher, universal law to which all humans must answer, or is simply obeying the written law of one's country sufficient? Antigone justified her defiance of the king on the basis of an unwritten, higher law: "Nor did I think your edict had such force that you, a mere mortal, could override the gods, the great unwritten, unshakable traditions" (Knox 1984, 82).

The source of higher law has varied throughout human history and has included the mythical gods of Olympus, the God of the Old Testament, the God of the New Testament, human reason, and respect for human dignity. The multinational trial of the Nazi war criminals at Nuremberg after World War II was held on the premise that there is a higher law of humanity (derived from rules of "natural law" that are based on an understanding of the essential nature of humans) and that persons may be properly tried for violating this law. Universal criminal law concerns crimes against humanity, such as state-sanctioned genocide, torture, and slavery. Obeying the orders of superiors is no defense: the state cannot shield its agents from prosecution for crimes against humanity. Another major step toward incorporating human rights into international law was taken when the UDHR was signed in a liberated Paris.

## THE UNITED NATIONS

The United Nations (UN) was formed at the end of World War II as a permanent peace-keeping organization. The charter of the UN, signed by the 50 original member nations in San Francisco on June 26, 1945, spells out the organization's goals. The first two goals are "to save succeeding generations from the scourge of war . . . and to reaffirm faith in fundamental human rights, in the dignity and worth of the human person, in the equal rights of men and women and of nations large and small." After the charter was signed, the adoption of an international bill of rights with legal authority proceeded in three steps: a declaration, a treaty-based covenant, and implementation measures.

## THE UNIVERSAL DECLARATION OF HUMAN RIGHTS

The UDHR was adopted by the United Nations General Assembly in 1948, with 48 member states voting in favor of adoption and 8 (Saudi Arabia, South Africa, and the Soviet Union together with 5 other countries whose votes it controlled) abstaining. The declaration was adopted as a "common standard for all people and nations" (Steiner and Alston 2000). As Steiner (1998) notes, "No other document has so caught the historical moment, achieved the same moral and rhetorical force, or exerted so much influence on the human rights movement as a whole." The rights enumerated in the declaration "stem from the cardinal axiom that all human beings are born free and equal, in dignity and rights, and are endowed with reason and conscience. All the rights and freedoms belong to everybody" (Kunz 1949, 319). These points are spelled out in Articles 1 and 2. Nondiscrimination is the overarching principle. Article 7, for example, is explicit: "All are equal before the law and are entitled without any discrimination to equal protection of the law." Other articles prohibit slavery, torture, and arbitrary detention and protect freedom of expression, assembly, and religion, the right to own property, and the right to work and receive an education. Of special importance to health care professionals is Article 25, which states, in part, "Everyone has the right to a standard of living adequate for the health and well-being of himself and his family, including food, clothing, housing and medical care and necessary social services."

Human rights are primarily rights individuals have in relation to governments. Human rights require governments to refrain from doing certain things, such as torturing persons or limiting freedom of religion, and also require that they take actions to make people's lives better, such as providing education and nutrition programs. The UN adopted the UDHR as a statement of aspirations. The legal obligations of governments were to derive from formal treaties that member nations would individually sign and incorporate into domestic law.

## THE TREATIES

Because of the Cold War, with its conflicting ideologies, it took almost 20 years to reach an agreement on the texts of the two human-rights treaties. On December 16, 1966, both the International Covenant on Civil and Political Rights (ICCPR) and the International Covenant on Economic, Social, and Cultural Rights (ICESCR) were adopted by the General Assembly and offered for signature and ratification by the member nations. The United States ratified the ICCPR in 1992, but not surprisingly, given our capitalist economic system with its emphasis on private property, we have yet to act on the ICESCR. The division of human rights into two separate treaties illustrates the tension between liberal states founded on civil and political rights and socialist and communist welfare states founded on solidarity and the government's obligation to meet basic economic and social needs.

The rights spelled out in the ICCPR include equality, the right to liberty and security of person, and freedom of movement, religion, expression, and association. The ICESCR focuses on well-being, including the right to work, the right to receive fair wages, the right to make a decent living, the right to work under safe and healthy conditions, the right to be free from hunger, the right to education, and "the right of everyone to the enjoyment of the highest attainable standard of physical and mental health."

Given the horrors of poverty, disease, and civil wars over the past 50 years, it is easy to dismiss the rights enunciated in these documents as empty gestures. Indeed, Amnesty International, in marking the 50th anniversary of the UDHR, has labeled the rights it articulates "little more than a paper promise for most people in the world" (Palmer 1998, 1940). It is certainly true that unadulterated celebration is not in order, but as Kunz (1949) noted almost 50 years ago in writing about the birth of the declaration, "In the field of human rights as in other actual problems of international law it is necessary to avoid the Scylla of a pessimistic cynicism and the Charybdis of mere wishful thinking and superficial optimism."

## HUMAN RIGHTS AND HEALTH

The UDHR and the two subsequent treaties form a global human-rights framework for action and have a special relevance for global health. In recent years, the relation between health and human rights has been most persuasively articulated and tirelessly championed by Dr. Jonathan Mann, the first director of the World Health Organization's Global Programme on AIDS, whose life was tragically cut short in the September 1998 crash of Swissair flight 111. The strongest predictor of health is income—that is, poverty is strongly correlated with disease and disability—and one way to attack disease and improve health internationally is to redistribute income. This seems a hopeless goal to most people in developing nations. Reliance on income redistribution as a single or primary strategy can lead to pessimism about the possibility that anything can be done or cynicism about the likelihood that anything will be done. Equality of income may be unattainable. But it is not unreasonable to expect the rich to share their wealth with the poor, and thereby help create the conditions necessary for good health for all. The UN has noted, for example, that the cost of universal access to basic education, health care, food, and clean water is only $40 billion a year—less than 4 percent of the combined wealth of the 225 richest people in the world. This figure seems too low (if 2 billion people needed additional resources, it would provide only $20 for each); nonetheless, it focuses on proper global goals and suggests that not much redistribution is required to have a major impact on the lives of most people in the world.

Multinational corporations should be actively involved in promoting human rights as well, because they control much of the wealth of the world. This has become evident in the global environmental movement in the areas of pollution, resource conservation, and global warming, and should be evident in the area of health care as well. Much of the agenda for research on drugs and vaccines, for example, is controlled by large multinational corporations, not by governments.

By broadening our perspective, the language of human rights highlights basic needs, such as equality, education, nutrition, and sanitation. Improvement in each of these areas can have a major role in improving health. Over the past decade, the World Bank has become involved in international health. In 1993, the World Bank issued a report entitled *Investing in Health*. Although not stated in the language of human rights, the report's agenda for action implicitly acknowledged that only the recognition of basic human rights could improve the health status of most of the world's population. In low-income countries, for example, the World Bank's two primary recommendations for improvement of health were "increased investment in schooling for girls" and the financing and delivery of a basic package of public health programs, including AIDS prevention. The other major recommendations included increasing the income of the poor, promoting the rights and status of women through "political and economic empowerment and legal protection against abuse," and delivering essential clinical services to the poor. These recommendations directly address the human-rights issues of access to education, access to health care, and discrimination against women.

## HUMAN RIGHTS AND PUBLIC HEALTH

World War II, arguably the first truly global war, led many nations to acknowledge the universality of human rights and the responsibility of governments to promote them. Mann perceptively noted that the AIDS epidemic can be viewed as the first global epidemic, because it is taking place at a time when all countries are linked both electronically and by easy transportation. Like World War II, this tragedy requires us to think in new ways and to develop effective methods to prevent and treat disease on a global level. Globalization is a mercantile and ecologic fact; it is also a reality in health care. The challenge facing medicine and health care is to develop a global language and strategy to improve the health of all the world's citizens.

Clinical medicine is practiced one patient at a time. The language of medical ethics is the language of self-determination and beneficence: doing what is in the best interests of the patient with the patient's informed consent. This language is powerful, but often has little application in countries where physicians are scarce and medical resources very limited.

Public health deals with populations and prevention of disease—the necessary frame of reference in the global context. In the context of clinical practice, the treatment of human immunodeficiency virus infection with a combination of antiviral medicines makes sense. In the context of worldwide public health, however, such treatment may be available to less than 5 percent of people with AIDS. To control AIDS, it has become necessary to deal directly with discrimination, immigration status, and the rights of women, as well as with the rights of privacy, informed consent, education, and access to health care. It is clear that population-based prevention is required to address the AIDS epidemic effectively on a global level (as well as, for example, tuberculosis, malaria, and tobacco-related illness). Nonetheless, it has been much harder to articulate a global public health ethic. The field of public health itself has had an extraordinarily difficult time developing its own ethical language. This problem of language has two basic causes: the incredibly large array of factors that influence health at the population level, and the emphasis by contemporary public health professionals on individualism and market forces rather than on the collective responsibility for social welfare. Because of its universality and its emphasis on equality and dignity, the language of human rights is well suited to public health.

On the 50th anniversary of the UDHR, I suggest that the declaration itself sets forth the ethics of public health, since its goal is to provide the conditions under which people can flourish. This is also the goal of public health. The unification of public health and human-rights efforts throughout the world could be a powerful force to improve the lives of every person. In my view, the declaration is a much more powerful public health document in 1998 than it was in 1948, because global interdependence and human equality are better recognized today.

## HUMAN RIGHTS AND PHYSICIANS

Both medical ethics and human rights represent aspirations that are difficult to enforce. Over the past two decades, medical ethics has been transformed into medical law, with more litigation and regulation. In the United States, for example, medical organizations, hospitals, and health plans often emphasize avoiding legal liability rather than doing the best or right thing. The domain of medical ethics is shrinking.

The domain of human rights, on the other hand, is growing. Not only are human rights being taken more seriously by governments, but they are also becoming a major driving force in private, nongovernmental organizations. Of course, there are different kinds of rights and different ways to enforce them, some of which are more effective than others. Earlier this year [1998], for example, at a meeting in Rome held under the auspices of the UN, the countries in attendance voted overwhelmingly (120 to 7) to propose the establishment of a permanent International Criminal Court with jurisdiction over war crimes, crimes against humanity, genocide, and aggression. The United States refused to support the establishment of the court unless it could, among other things, veto trials of Americans, especially American troops acting abroad. But this condition, of course, is incompatible with the entire purpose of the court: to punish violations of basic human rights regardless of the perpetrator. The court will be established without U.S. involvement if it is ratified by 60 nations by the end of the year 2000. [Ed.: Forty-three nations ratified as of October 2001.]

Individuals and nongovernmental organizations can use the language and concepts of human rights to energize their own activities. Many groups of physicians have taken the lead in promoting human rights, including International Physicians for the Prevention of Nuclear War and its U.S. affiliate, Physicians for Social Responsibility, Physicians for Human Rights, Medecins sans Frontieres (Doctors without Borders), and Medecins du Monde (Physicians of the World). Global Lawyers and Physicians (of which I am a cofounder) broadens the base by providing an opportunity for physicians and lawyers to work together to promote human rights in health care. The Consortium for Health and Human Rights has provided a new forum for cooperative action among health-related nongovernmental organizations. Other groups, such as Amnesty International and the National Academy of Sciences Committee on Human Rights, have developed very effective letter-writing campaigns on behalf of persons who have been arbitrarily detained and imprisoned. Physicians interested in promoting human rights thus have many organizations they can support. Most of these organizations have concentrated on the medical consequences of wars, torture, abuses of prisoners, and arbitrary detention, as well as the threats to health posed by nuclear, chemical, and biologic weapons, landmines, and other means of killing and maiming.

The fact that the UDHR is a declaration, not a treaty, need not limit its reach to human rights violations involving crimes against humanity any more than the reach of the Declaration of Independence has been limited by this fact. Although the Declaration of Independence started a war and the UDHR was drafted to prevent war, it is the power of the concepts and language that matters most. As Maier (1997, 214) has noted, the Declaration of Independence "rests less in law than in the minds and hearts of the people, and its meaning changes as new groups and new causes claim its mantle." Lincoln, for example, claimed to be upholding the "all men are created equal" pronouncement of the declaration both when he spoke at Gettysburg and when he issued the Emancipation Proclamation. And a century later, Martin Luther King, Jr., stood at the site of the Lincoln Memorial and invoked the words of the Declaration of Independence in calling for a new birth of the freedom

Lincoln had promised, by which he meant "an end to the poverty, discrimination, and segregation that left black citizens 'languishing in the corners of American society,' exiles in their own land" (Maier 1997, 214). The meaning of the UDHR will also be invoked and reinterpreted to meet the changing challenges of the times. The agenda for human rights should be broad; it should include efforts to make basic health care available to everyone and to prevent disease and injury and promote health worldwide. Fifty years after the signing of the UDHR, the language of human rights pervades international politics, law, and morality. The challenge now is to make the promise of the UDHR a reality.

## Health and Human Rights*
*Jonathan M. Mann, Lawrence O. Gostin, Sofia Gruskin, Troyen Brennan, Zita Lazzarini, and Harvey Fineberg.*

Health and human rights have rarely been linked in an explicit manner. With few exceptions, notably involving access to health care, discussions about health have not included human rights considerations. Similarly, except when obvious damage to health is the primary manifestation of a human rights abuse, such as with torture, health perspectives have been generally absent from human rights discourse.

Explanations for the dearth of communication between the fields of health and human rights include differing philosophical perspectives, vocabularies, professional recruitment and training, societal roles, and methods of work. In addition, modern concepts of both health and human rights are complex and steadily evolving. On a practical level, health workers may wonder about the applicability or utility ("added value"), let alone necessity, of incorporating human rights perspectives into their work, and vice versa. In addition, despite pioneering work seeking to bridge this gap in bioethics, jurisprudence, and public health law, a history of conflictual relationships between medicine and law, or between public health officials and civil liberties advocates, may contribute to anxiety and doubt about the potential for mutually beneficial collaboration.

---

*Reprinted from "Health and Human Rights," *Health and Human Rights* 1994, 1(1): 6–23, by permission of the François-Xavier Bagnoud Center for Health and Human Rights and the President and Fellows of Harvard College.

Yet health and human rights are both powerful, modern approaches to defining and advancing human well-being. Attention to the intersection of health and human rights may provide practical benefits to those engaged in health or human rights work, may help reorient thinking about major global health challenges, and may contribute to broadening human rights thinking and practice. However, meaningful dialogue about interactions between health and human rights requires a common ground. To this end, following a brief overview of selected features of modern health and human rights, this article proposes a provisional, mutually accessible framework for structuring discussions about research, promoting cross-disciplinary education, and exploring the potential for health and human rights collaboration. . . .

## A PROVISIONAL FRAMEWORK:
## LINKAGES BETWEEN HEALTH AND HUMAN RIGHTS

The goal of linking health and human rights is to contribute to advancing human well-being beyond what could be achieved through an isolated health or human rights–based approach. This [article] proposes a three-part framework for considering linkages between health and human rights; all are interconnected, and each has substantial practical consequences. . . .

First, the impact (positive and negative) of health policies, programs, and practices on human rights will be considered. This linkage will be illustrated by focusing on the use of state power in the context of public health.

### The First Relationship: The Impact of
### Health Policies, Programs, and Practices on Human Rights

Around the world, health care is provided through many diverse public and private mechanisms. However, the responsibilities of public health are carried out in large measure through policies and programs promulgated, implemented, and enforced by, or with support from, the state. Therefore, this first linkage may be best explored by considering the impact of public health policies, programs, and practices on human rights.

The three central functions of public health are: assessing health needs and problems; developing policies designed to address priority health issues; and assuring programs to implement strategic health goals. Potential benefits to and burdens on human rights may occur in the pursuit of each of these major areas of public health responsibility.

For example, assessment involves collection of data on important health problems in a population. However, data are not collected on all possible health problems, nor does the selection of which issues to assess occur in a societal vacuum. Thus, a state's failure to recognize or acknowledge health problems that preferentially affect a marginalized or stigmatized group may violate the right to nondiscrimination by leading to neglect of necessary services, and in so doing, may adversely affect the realization of other rights, including the right to "security in the event of . . . sickness [or] disability" or to the "special care and assistance" to which mothers and children are entitled (UDHR, Art. 25).

Once decisions about which problems to assess have been made, the methodology of data collection may create additional human rights burdens. Collecting information from individuals, such as whether they are infected with HIV, have breast cancer, or are genetically predisposed to heart disease, can clearly burden rights to security of person (associated with the concept of informed consent) and of arbitrary interference with privacy. In addition, the right of nondiscrimination may be threatened even by an apparently simple information-gathering exercise. For example, a health survey conducted via telephone, by excluding households without telephones (usually associated with lower socioeconomic status), may result in a biased assessment, which may in turn lead to policies or programs that fail to recognize or meet needs of the entire population. Also, personal health status or health behavior information (such as sexual orientation or history of drug use) has the potential for misuse by the state, whether directly or if it is made available to others, resulting in grievous harm to individuals and violations of many rights. Thus, misuse of information about HIV infection status has led to: restrictions of the right to work and to education; violations of the right to marry and found a family; attacks upon honor and reputation; limitations of freedom of movement; arbitrary detention or exile; and even cruel, inhuman, or degrading treatment.

The second major task of public health is to develop policies to prevent and control priority health problems. Important burdens on human rights may arise in the policy development process. For example, if a government refuses to disclose the scientific basis of health policy or permit debate on its merits, or in other ways refuses to inform and involve the public in policy development, the rights to "seek, receive and impart information and ideas . . . regardless of frontiers" (UDHR, Art. 19) and "to take part in the government . . . directly or through freely chosen representatives" (UDHR, Art. 21) may be violated. Then, prioritization of health issues may result in discrimination against individuals, as when the major health problems of a population of a specific sex, race, religion, or language are systematically given lower priority (e.g., sickle-cell disease in the United States, which affects primarily the African-American population; or, more globally, maternal mortality, breast cancer, and other health problems of women).

The third core function of public health, to assure services capable of realizing policy goals, is also closely linked with the right to nondiscrimination. When health and social services do not take logistic, financial, and sociocultural barriers to their access and enjoyment into account, intentional or unintentional discrimination may readily occur. For example, in clinics for maternal and child health, details such as hours of service, accessibility via public transportation, and availability of day care may strongly and adversely influence service utilization.

It is essential to recognize that in seeking to fulfill each of its core functions and responsibilities, public health may burden human rights. In the past, when restrictions on human rights were recognized, they were often simply justified as necessary to protect public health. Indeed, public health has a long tradition, anchored in the history of infectious disease control, of limiting the "rights of the few" for the "good of the many." . . .

Unfortunately, public health decisions to restrict human rights have frequently been made in an uncritical, unsystematic, and unscientific manner. Therefore, the prevailing assumption that public health, as articulated through specific policies and programs, is an unalloyed public good that does not require consideration of human rights norms must be challenged. For the present, it may be useful to adopt the maxim that health policies and programs should be considered discriminatory and burdensome on human rights until proven otherwise. . . .

The idea that human rights and public health must inevitably conflict is increasingly tempered with awareness of their complementarity. . . . Recently, in the context of HIV/AIDS, new approaches have been developed, seeking to maximize realization of public health goals while simultaneously protecting and promoting human rights. Yet HIV/AIDS is not unique; efforts to harmonize health and human rights goals are clearly possible in other areas. At present, an effort to identify human rights burdens created by public health policies, programs, and practices, followed by negotiation toward an optimal balance whenever public health and human rights goals appear to conflict, is a necessary minimum. An approach to realizing health objectives that simultaneously promotes—or at least respects—rights and dignity is clearly desirable.

### The Second Relationship: Health Impacts
### Resulting from Violations of Human Rights

Health impacts are obvious and inherent in the popular understanding of certain severe human rights violations, such as torture, imprisonment under inhumane conditions, summary execution, and "disappearances." For this reason, health experts concerned about human rights have increasingly made their expertise available to help document such abuses. Examples of this type of medical–human rights collaboration include: exhumation of mass graves to examine allegations of executions; examination of torture victims; and entry of health personnel into prisons to assess health status.

However, health impacts of rights violations go beyond these issues in at least two ways. First, the duration and extent of health impacts resulting from severe abuses of rights and dignity remain generally underappreciated. Torture, imprisonment under inhumane conditions, or trauma associated with witnessing summary executions, torture, rape, or mistreatment of others have been shown to lead to severe, probably lifelong effects on physical, mental, and social well-being. In addition, a more complete understanding of the negative health effects of torture must also include its broad influence on mental and social well-being; torture is often used as a political tool to discourage people from meaningful participation in or resistance to government.

Second, and beyond these serious problems, it is increasingly evident that violations of many more, if not all, human rights have negative effects on health. For example, the right to information may be violated when cigarettes are marketed without governmental assurance that information regarding the harmful health effects of tobacco smoking will also be available. . . . Other violations of the right to information, with substantial health impacts, include governmental withholding of valid scientific health information about contraception or measures (e.g., condoms) to prevent infection with a fatal virus (HIV). . . .

A related, yet even more complex problem involves the potential health impact associated with violating individual and collective dignity. The UDHR considers dignity, along with rights, to be inherent, inalienable, and universal. While important dignity-related health impacts may include such problems as the poor health status of many indigenous peoples, a coherent vocabulary and framework to characterize dignity and different forms of dignity violations are lacking. A taxonomy and an epidemiology of violations of dignity may uncover an enormous field of previously suspected, yet thus far unnamed and therefore undocumented damage to physical, mental, and social well-being.

Assessment of rights violations' health impacts is in its infancy. Progress will require: a more sophisticated capacity to document and assess rights violations; the application of medical, social science, and public health methodologies to identify and assess effects on physical, mental, and social well-being; and research to establish valid associations between rights violations and health impacts.

### The Third Relationship: Health and
### Human Rights—Exploring an Inextricable Linkage

The proposal that promoting and protecting human rights is inextricably linked to the challenge of promoting and protecting health derives in part from recognition that health and human rights are complementary approaches to the central problem of defining and advancing human well-being. This fundamental connection leads beyond the single, albeit broad mention of health in the UDHR (Art. 25) and the specific health-related responsibilities of states listed in Article 12 of the ICESCR, including: reducing stillbirth and infant mortality and promoting healthy child development; improving environmental and industrial hygiene; preventing, treating, and controlling epidemic, endemic, occupational, and other diseases; and assuring medical care.

Modern concepts of health recognize that underlying "conditions" establish the foundation for realizing physical, mental, and social well-being. Given the importance of these conditions, it is remarkable how little priority has been given within health research to their precise identification and understanding of their modes of action, relative importance, and possible interactions.

The most widely accepted analysis focuses on socioeconomic status; the positive relationship between higher socioeconomic status and better health status is well documented. Yet this analysis has at least three important limitations. First, it cannot adequately account for a growing number of discordant observations, such as: the increased longevity of married Canadian men and women compared with their single (widowed, divorced, never married) counterparts; health status differences between minority and majority populations which persist even when traditional measures of socioeconomic status are considered; or reports of differential marital, economic, and educational outcomes among obese women, compared with non-obese women.

A second problem lies in the definition of poverty and its relationship to health status. Clearly, poverty may have different health meanings; for example, distinctions between the health-related meaning of absolute poverty and relative poverty have been proposed.

A third, practical difficulty is that the socioeconomic paradigm creates an overwhelming challenge with which health workers are neither trained nor equipped to deal. Therefore, the identification of socioeconomic status as the "essential conditions" for good health paradoxically may encourage complacency, apathy, and even policy and programmatic paralysis. . . .

Experience with the global epidemic of HIV/AIDS suggests a further analytic approach, using a rights analysis. For example, married, monogamous women in East Africa have been documented to be infected with HIV. Although these women know about HIV and condoms are accessible in the marketplace, their risk factor is their inability to control their husbands' sexual behavior or to refuse unprotected or unwanted sexual intercourse. Refusal may result in physical harm, or in divorce, the equivalent of social and economic death for the woman. Therefore, women's vulnerability to HIV is now recognized to be integrally connected with discrimination and unequal rights, involving property, marriage, divorce, and inheritance. The success of condom promotion for HIV prevention in this population is inherently limited in the absence of legal and societal changes which, by promoting and protecting women's rights, would strengthen their ability to negotiate sexual practice and protect themselves from HIV infection.

More broadly, the evolving HIV/AIDS pandemic has shown a consistent pattern through which discrimination, marginalization, stigmatization, and, more generally, a lack of respect for the human rights and dignity of individuals and groups heighten their vulnerability to becoming exposed to HIV. In this regard, HIV/AIDS may be illustrative of a more general phenomenon in which individual and population vulnerability to disease, disability, and premature death is linked to the status of respect for human rights and dignity. . . .

The hypothesis that promotion and protection of rights and health are inextricably linked requires much creative exploration and rigorous evaluation. The concept of an inextricable relationship between health and human rights also has enormous potential practical consequences. For example, health professionals could consider using the International Bill of Human Rights as a coherent guide for assessing health status of individuals or populations; the extent to which human rights are realized may represent a better and more comprehensive index of well-being than traditional health status indicators. Health professionals would also have to consider their responsibility not only to respect human rights in developing policies, programs, and practices, but to contribute actively from their position as health workers to improving societal realization of rights. Health workers have long acknowledged the societal roots of health status; the human rights linkage may help health professionals engage in specific and concrete ways with the full range of those working to promote and protect human rights and dignity in each society.

From the perspective of human rights, health experts and expertise may contribute usefully to societal recognition of the benefits and costs associated with realizing, or failing to respect, human rights and dignity. This can be accomplished without seeking to justify human rights and dignity on health grounds (or for any pragmatic purposes). Rather, collaboration with health experts can help give voice to the pervasive and serious impact on health associated with lack of respect for rights and dignity. In addition, the right to health can be developed and made meaningful only through dialogue between health and human rights disciplines. Finally, the importance of health as a precondition for the capacity to realize and enjoy human rights and dignity must be appreciated. For example, poor nutritional status of children can contribute subtly yet importantly to limiting realization of the right to education; in general, people who are healthy may be best equipped to participate fully and benefit optimally from the protections and opportunities inherent in the International Bill of Human Rights.

## Medicine and Public Health, Ethics and Human Rights*
*Jonathan M. Mann*

Where are the ethics of public health? In contrast to the important declarations of medical ethics such as the International Code of Medical Ethics of the World Medical Association and the Nuremberg Principles,

---

*Reprinted from *Hastings Center Report* 27 (May–June 1997): 6–13.

the world of public health does not have a reasonably explicit set of ethical guidelines. [The Public Health Leadership Society issued ethical guidelines in 2002, posted on the *Reader* web site.] In part, this deficiency may stem from the broad diversity of professional identities within public health. Yet, curiously, many of the occupational groups central to public health (epidemiologists, policy analysts, social scientists, biostatisticians, nutritionists, health system managers) have not yet developed, or are only now developing, widely accepted ethical guidelines or statements of principle for their work in the public health context. Thus, while a public health physician may draw upon medical ethics for guidance, the ethics of a public health physician have yet to be clearly articulated.

The central problem is one of coherence and identity: public health cannot develop an ethics until it has achieved clarity about its own identity; technical expertise and methodology are not substitutes for conceptual coherence. Or, as one student remarked a few years ago, public health spends too much time on the "p" values of biostatistics and not enough time on values.

To have an ethic, a profession needs clarity about central issues, including its major role and responsibilities. Two steps will be essential for public health to reach toward this analytic and definitional clarity.

First, public health must divest itself of its biomedical conceptual foundation. The language of disease, disability, and death is not the language of well-being; the vocabulary of diseases may detract from analysis and response to underlying societal conditions, of which traditional morbidity and mortality are expressions. It is clear that we do not yet know all about the universe of human suffering. Just as in the microbial world, in which new discoveries have become the norm—Ebola virus, hantavirus, toxic shock syndrome, Legionnaires' disease, AIDS—we are explorers in the larger world of human suffering and well-being. And our current maps of this universe, like world maps from sixteenth century Europe, have some very well-defined, familiar coastlines and territories and also contain large blank spaces, which beckon the explorer.

The language of biomedicine is cumbersome and ultimately perhaps of little usefulness in exploring the impacts of violations of dignity on physical, mental, and social well-being. The definition of dignity itself is complex and thus far elusive and unsatisfying. While the UDHR starts by placing dignity first, "all people are born equal in dignity and rights," we do not yet have a vocabulary, or taxonomy, let alone an epidemiology of dignity violations.

Yet it seems we all know when our dignity is violated or impugned. Perform the following experiment: recall, in detail, an incident from your own life in which your dignity was violated, for whatever reason. If you will immerse yourself in the memory, powerful feelings will likely arise—of anger, shame, powerlessness, despair. When you connect with the power of these feelings, it seems intuitively obvious that such feelings, particularly if evoked repetitively, could have deleterious impacts on health. Yet most of us are relatively privileged; we live in a generally dignity-affirming environment, and suffer only the occasional lapse of indignity. However, many people live constantly in a dignity-impugning environment, in which affirmations of dignity may be the exceptional occurrence. An exploration of the meanings of dignity and the forms of its violation—and the impact on physical, mental, and social well-being—may help uncover a new universe of human suffering, for which the biomedical language may be inapt and even inept. After all, the power of naming, describing, and then measuring is truly enormous—child abuse did not exist in meaningful societal terms until it was named and then measured; nor did domestic violence.

A second precondition for developing an ethics of public health is the adoption and application of a human rights framework for analyzing and responding to the societal determinants of health. The human rights framework can provide the coherence and clarity required for public health to identify and work with conscious attention to its roles and responsibilities. At that point, an ethics of public health, rather than the ethics of individual constituent disciplines within public health, can emerge.

Issues of respect for autonomy, beneficence, nonmaleficence, and justice can then be articulated from within the set of goals and responsibilities called for by seeking to improve public health through the combination of traditional approaches and those that strive concretely to promote realization of human rights. This is not to replace health education, information, and clinical service-based activities of public health with an exclusive focus on human rights and dignity. Both are necessary.

For example, the challenges for public health officials in balancing the goals of promoting and protecting public health and ensuring that human rights and dignity are not violated call urgently for ethical analysis. The official nature of much public health work places public health practitioners in a complex environment, in which work to promote rights inevitably challenges the state system within which the official is employed. Ethical dimensions are highly relevant to collecting, disseminating, and acting on information about the health impacts of the entire range of human rights violations. And as public health seeks to "ensure the conditions in which people can be healthy" (IOM 1988, 19) and as those conditions are societal, to be engaged in public health necessarily involves a commitment to societal transformation. The difficulties in assessing human rights status and in developing useful and appropriate ways to promote human rights and dignity necessarily engage ethical considerations. . . . [P]ublic health must engage difficult issues even when no cure or effective instruments are yet available, and public health also must accompany, remain with, and not abandon vulnerable populations.

That this work—added to, not substituted for, the current approach of public health—will require major changes in public health reflection, analysis, action, and education, is clear. That it is urgently required, in order to confront the major health challenges of the modern world, is equally clear.

## II. THE HUMAN RIGHT TO HEALTH

### Towards an Improved Understanding of the International Human Right to Health*
*Brigit Toebes*

In the context of international human rights, economic, social, and cultural rights are generally distinguished from civil and political rights. Although it is often asserted that both sets of rights are interdependent, interrelated, and of equal importance, in practice, Western states and NGOs [nongovernmental organizations], in particular, have tended to treat economic, social, and cultural rights as if they were less important than civil and political rights. Civil and political rights, for example, are frequently invoked in national judicial proceedings, and several complaint mechanisms are designed to protect these rights at the international level. In contrast, economic, social, and cultural rights are often considered nonjusticiable and are regarded as general directives for states rather than rights.

Another serious obstacle to the implementation of economic, social, and cultural rights is their lack of conceptual clarity. An economic and social right that is characterized by particular vagueness is the interna-

*Reprinted from *Human Rights Quarterly* 21:3 (1999), 661–679. © The John Hopkins University Press.

tional human right to health. It is by no means clear precisely what individuals are entitled to under the right to health, nor is it clear what the resulting obligations are on the part of states. . . .

## THE PROBLEM OF DEFINITION

When it comes to health as a human right, there is an initial problem with regard to its definition. Specifically, there is confusion and disagreement over what is the most appropriate term to use to address health as a human right. Due to this disagreement, different terms are used by various authors. The terms that most commonly appear in human rights and health law literature are: the "right to health," the "right to healthcare" or to "medical care," and to a lesser extent, the "right to health protection."

It has been argued that the term "right to health" is awkward because it suggests that people have a right to something that cannot be guaranteed, namely perfect health or to be healthy. It has also been noted that health is a highly subjective matter, varying from person to person and from country to country. It is argued, therefore, that the terms "right to healthcare" and "right to health protection" are more realistic.

At the international level, however, the term "right to health" is most commonly used. This term best matches the international human rights treaty provisions that formulate health as a human right. These provisions not only proclaim a right to healthcare but also a right to other health services such as environmental health protection and occupational health services. The term "healthcare" would accordingly not cover this broader understanding of health as a human right. Thus, in practice the term "right to health" is generally used as a shorthand expression for the more elaborate treaty texts. Using such shorthand expressions is rather common in human rights discourse; terms such as the rights to life, privacy, a fair trial, and housing have all obtained a very specific practical connotation, as has the right to health.

## INTERNATIONAL CODIFICATION OF THE RIGHT TO HEALTH

The right to health is firmly embedded in a considerable number of international human rights instruments. The right to health as laid down in the preamble to the Constitution of the World Health Organization (WHO) constitutes the point of departure on which most of the provisions in these instruments are based. The preamble formulates the "highest attainable standard of health" as a fundamental right of everyone and defines health as a "state of complete physical, mental, and social well-being and not merely the absence of disease or infirmity." In the same vein, most treaty provisions stipulate a right to the highest attainable standard of (physical and mental) health and include a number of government obligations as well. These government undertakings usually include commitments regarding healthcare and also mention a number of underlying preconditions for health, such as occupational health, environmental health, clean drinking water, and adequate sanitation.

In addition to specific treaty provisions addressing the right to health, there are a number of general treaty provisions that stipulate that there is a universal right to health. The most well-known and influential of these provisions is Article 12 of the ICESCR. In addition to Article 12 of the ICESCR, there are a number of other treaty provisions that stipulate a right to health for particular vulnerable groups, such as women, children, racial minorities, prisoners, migrant workers, and indigenous populations. . . .

Finally, a great number of national constitutions include a right to health (care) or stipulate states' duties with regard to the health of their people. Some of these provisions existed before the international human right to health was formulated.

## IMPLEMENTATION PRACTICE OF THE RIGHT TO HEALTH

In view of the above, it becomes clear that the problem with the right to health is not so much a lack of codification but rather an absence of a consistent implementation practice through reporting procedures and before judicial and quasi-judicial bodies, as well as a lack of conceptual clarity. These problems are interrelated: a lack of understanding of the meaning and scope of a right makes it difficult to implement, and the absence of a frequent practice of implementation in turn hampers the possibility of obtaining a greater understanding of its meaning and scope.

### Reporting Procedures

International treaty monitoring bodies do not have a very clear understanding of how they should implement the right to health. Under the heading of the "right to health," these bodies deal with a great number of health-related issues in a somewhat haphazard fashion. The treaty monitoring body of the ICESCR, the Committee on Economic, Social, and Cultural Rights ("the Committee"), for example, addresses the following broad range of topics within the framework of the right to health: the national health policies adopted, issues related to healthcare, issues related to environmental health, accessibility of clean drinking water and adequate sanitation, availability of health-related information, occupational health, and the accessibility of health services for various vulnerable groups. . . .

### General Issues

Included within the category of general issues is the overall requirement that state parties make certain commitments in the area of public health. First, state parties are required to devote a sufficient percentage of their GNP [gross national product] to health. If, for example, military spending is high as compared to health expenditure, the Committee assumes that the country concerned should have spent its budget otherwise. Second, this health commitment entails an obligation to adopt a national health policy, including the adoption of the Primary Health Care strategy (PHC) of WHO. Also, state parties have to ensure that no disparities exist between the standard of health services offered in the private and public sectors. The Committee opines that, although the right to health may be satisfied through whatever mix of public and private sector services is appropriate in the national context, state parties are responsible for the equality of access to healthcare services, whether privately or publicly provided. Plans to privatize and decentralize healthcare services do not in any way relieve state parties of their obligation to use all available means to promote adequate access to healthcare services, particularly for the poorer segments of the population. The health legislation adopted by states is discussed; however, the type of legislation state parties must adopt is not further spelled out by the Committee.

### Healthcare

As far as the provision of healthcare services is concerned, a distinction between availability, accessibility, affordability, and quality of healthcare services proves useful in order to scrutinize the Committee's approach. With regard to the *availability* of healthcare services, the Committee assesses the aggregate of hospital beds and the population per nurse and per doctor. In order to guarantee the availability of healthcare facilities, the Committee notes that state parties should encourage health personnel to stay and practice in the country. Regarding the *accessibility* of healthcare services, the Committee focuses on the most vulnerable groups, who are generally minority and indigenous populations, women, children, the elderly, disabled persons, and persons with HIV/AIDS. In addition, the Committee expresses its concern about the accessibility of healthcare facilities in remote, rural areas. State parties are to make efforts to institute rural health sub-centers and to stimulate doctors and nurses to set up practice in rural areas. An important aspect of the accessibility of healthcare facilities is the *affordability* of the available services. State parties are to ensure that healthcare services are affordable for the economically underprivileged in general and for the elderly and low-income women in particular. As part of the affordability requirement, state parties must make sure that privatization does not constitute a threat to the affordability of healthcare services. Finally, state parties must ensure that the available healthcare services are of good *quality*. This requires that doctors and nurses are skilled and that equipment and drugs are adequate.

### Underlying Preconditions for Health

When it comes to the underlying preconditions for health there is some overlap with other rights. In particular, there is overlap with those rights contained in Article 11 of the ICESCR: food, housing, and clothing. Of these, the most explicitly health related are food-related issues. Additional preconditions for health that are not covered by other rights but are discussed within the framework of Article 12 are access to safe water and the provision of adequate sanitary facilities, environmental hygiene, occupational hygiene, and health education. State parties have to make sure that their population has sufficient access to safe water and adequate sanitation. In particular, they have to ensure that people living in remote, rural areas have sufficient access to these facilities.

The Committee is also interested in environmental policies. However, it seeks to address environmental issues only in as far as they affect, or may affect, human health. For example, state parties have to take safety measures for the protection against radioactive radiation. The area of occupational health requires the implementation and monitoring of health and safety measures in the workplace. Finally, health education requires that measures be taken to provide education concerning prevailing health problems, as well as the measures that are necessary for preventing and controlling them.

### Vulnerable Groups and Health-Specific Subjects

With regard to vulnerable groups and health-specific subjects, multiple topics have emerged in the reporting procedure. When the inhabitants of remote, rural areas are concerned, state parties must ensure that there is not an imbalance between rural and urban areas when it comes to access to health services. With regard to indigenous populations, state parties are required to both guarantee respect for the cultural identity of those populations (for example, their use of traditional medicine) and to improve their health status. State parties are also required to improve poor sanitary and hygiene conditions prevailing in penal institutions. With respect to women, state parties are expected to combat maternal mortality, to provide medical assistance to low-income women, and to combat "traditional practices," including female circumcision. Moreover, state parties are to reduce infant mortality and to ensure that the rising costs of healthcare do not disadvantage the elderly.

. . . [The Committee urges State parties] to take measures to reduce the spread of HIV/AIDS, to set up information campaigns, . . . and . . . to avoid measures that discriminate against people with HIV/AIDS. These measures are in response to some states' adoption of coercive measures, including transit restrictions to minimize the risk of the spread of AIDS, mandatory testing, and control of prostitution. . . .

[In July 2000, the Committee on Economic, Social and Cultural Rights adopted General Comment 14 on the right to health in Article 12 ICESCR (UN Doc. E/C.12/2000/4). This General Comment provides an authoritative interpretation of the meaning and significance of the right to health in the ICESCR. General comment is posted on the *Reader* web site.]

### Justiciability of the Right to Health

At the UN, as well as the regional and national levels, very few examples exist where courts have reviewed the right to health; however, there are some sources of inspiration for judicial review of the right to health. At the UN level there are no specific complaint procedures in force to make health rights and other economic, social, and cultural rights justiciable. . . .

At the regional level the situation is somewhat more encouraging. For example, the development of complaint procedures for economic, social, and cultural rights has proceeded somewhat further at the regional levels than at the UN. In principle, the right to health as contained in the African Charter is susceptible to invocation before and review by the African Commission, although this procedure has not often been used. The Organization of American States has adopted a limited complaints procedure; however, it has yet to come into force. However, given the limited scope of the Inter-American Protocol of San Salvador, the right to health would not be susceptible to judicial review. Nevertheless, it is possible to submit complaints to the Inter-American Commission on Human Rights (IACHR) on the basis of the right to health as provided for in the American Declaration. This, in fact, was tried in the case of the Yanomami Indians, where the IACHR declared that the right to health in Article XI of the American Declaration was violated. The Government of Brazil was held to have failed to protect the Yanomami against the exploitation of the rainforest and the detrimental health effects that could be caused. Finally, with the adoption of a complaint procedure under the European Social Charter (ESC) of the Council of Europe, the right to protection of health in the ESC will become susceptible to (quasi-) judicial review. This procedure will, however, only allow specific organizations to submit complaints, not individuals.

Inspiration for the justiciability of the right to health can be derived from the national level. In some countries either the constitutional or the international right to health has been given effect before domestic courts. Whereas some of these cases involve a right to certain healthcare facilities, others concern a right to environmental health. With regard to healthcare, a 1992 Colombian case that concerned the terminal illness of an AIDS patient is worth mentioning. In that case the Colombian Supreme Court ruled that the state was required, by the right to health in Article 13 of the Colombian constitution, to provide special protection when the lack of economic resources "prevents a person from decreasing the suffering, discrimination, and social risk involved in being afflicted by a terminal, transmissible, and incurable illness." (Constitutional Court, Judgment No. T-505 of 28 August 1992). To this end, the Court decided that the hospital was required to provide the AIDS patient the necessary services. With regard to environmental health, the well-known 1993 Philippine *Minors Oposa* case is significant. (Minors Oposa v. Factoran, Supreme Court of Philippines, 33 I.L.M. 173 (1994)). In that case the Philippine Supreme Court ruled that the state should stop providing logging licenses in order to protect the health of present and future generations. The decision was based on Article II of the Declaration of Principles and State Policies of the 1987 Philippine constitution, which sets forth the rights to health and ecology.

Finally, one may derive inspiration from the justiciability of civil and political rights. On some occasions, civil and political rights have offered protections similar to that of the right to health. Again, such protections may concern access to a certain healthcare facility or protection against environmental health threats. A case indirectly involving a right to access to healthcare services has been brought before the Human Rights Committee (HRC). This body has adopted the practice of considering ICCPR Article 26 (nondiscrimination) as an autonomous provision that may include the prohibition of discriminatory actions with relation to social rights. In *Hendrika S. Vos v. the Netherlands* (Communication No. 218/1986, adopted 29 Mar. 1989, U.N. GAOR, Hum. Rts. Comm., 44th

Sess., Supp. No. 40, at 232, U.N. Doc. A/44/40 (1989)), the HRC considered whether the denial of a disability benefit constituted a violation of Article 26 of the ICCPR. Although the HRC held that there was no violation of the nondiscrimination clause in Article 26, the fact that the HRC tested the denial of the sickness benefit against Article 26 shows its willingness to read social rights into the nondiscrimination clause. . . .

Regarding environmental health, a case on point is *López Ostra v. Spain* (303 Eur. Ct. H.R. (ser. A) at 47 (1995)), which concerned the nuisance caused by a waste treatment plant and its effects on the applicant's daughter's health in the town of Lorca, Spain. The Spanish court opined that "severe environmental pollution may affect individuals' well-being and prevent them from enjoying their homes in such a way as to affect their private and family life adversely. . . . " 303 Eur. Ct. H.R. (ser. A) at 54. It concluded that the municipality of Lorca had failed to take steps to respect the applicant's right to respect for her home and for her private life under Article 8 of the European Convention on Human Rights and that Article 8 had accordingly been violated.

## THE CREATION OF CONCEPTUAL CLARITY WITH REGARD TO THE RIGHT TO HEALTH

### In Search of Its Scope and Core Content

On the basis of the above findings, one can clarify further the meaning of the right to health and delineate its scope and core content. Whereas the scope constitutes the general content of the right to health, the core content consists of those elements that a state has to guarantee under any circumstances, irrespective of its available resources.

Regarding the scope, it is important to recognize the broad character of the right to health and not recognize a right to "healthcare" only. The right to health can be said to embrace two larger parts: (1) elements related to "healthcare" and (2) elements concerning the "underlying preconditions for health" (these may include a healthy environment, safe drinking water and adequate sanitation, occupational health, and health-related information). Simultaneously, it is important to demarcate limits on the right to health and not allow it to include everything that might involve health. For example, with a few minor exceptions, the right to health does not include a prohibition against torture or inhuman and degrading treatment, nor does it include protection against arbitrary killing or medical or scientific experimentation. The right to health also does not include regular education at schools or a right to adequate housing. It offers protection against environmental pollution only if there are clear health risks, and it is related to the right to work only if it concerns the safeguarding of industrial hygiene and the prevention, treatment, and control of occupational diseases. On the other hand, it is important to recognize that there is a certain overlap with several civil and political as well as other economic, social, and cultural rights, in that on some occasions the right to health may offer protection similar to that of other rights. For example, the right to health may overlap with other human rights where it concerns prevention of infant mortality (right to life), the safeguarding of adequate prison conditions, measures to combat "traditional practices" (prohibition of torture and inhuman and degrading treatment), and access to healthy foodstuffs (right to food).

Secondly, there is a trend among scholars and activists towards delineating a certain core in the right to health. This so-called core content consists of a set of elements that states have to guarantee immediately, irrespective of their available resources. The core content stands in contrast to some elements of the right to health that are to be realized "progressively." This core content . . . refers to those elements that encompass the essence of the right. For the definition of the core content of the right to health, one may derive inspiration from the PHC of WHO. The core content of the right to health accordingly consists of a number of basic health services. Irrespective of their available resources, states are to provide access to: maternal and child healthcare (including family planning), immunization against the major infectious diseases, appropriate treatment for common diseases and injuries, essential drugs, and an adequate supply of safe water and basic sanitation. In addition, they should ensure freedom from serious environmental health threats.

Finally, in addition to the scope and core content, a number of guiding principles constitute the framework of the right to health. States should safeguard the availability, equality, accessibility (financial, geographic, and cultural), and quality of the above mentioned health services.

### Obligations Resulting from the Right to Health

For further clarification of the normative content of the right to health, it is helpful to approach it from the angle of (state) obligations. A useful concept in this regard is the tripartite typology of duties, which assumes that obligations to respect, protect, and fulfill can be derived from each human right. An analysis of the right to health on the basis of this typology demonstrates that the right to health not only gives rise to positive obligations to protect and to fulfill but also embraces negative obligations to respect. Obligations to respect the right to health include, for example, the obligation to respect equal access to health services and to refrain from health-harming activities, as in the sphere of environmental health. The fact that an economic and social right embraces negative obligations underlines the interdependence and interrelatedness of civil and political rights with economic, social, and cultural rights. In effect, both sets of rights—civil and political, and economic, social, and cultural—require state abstention. . . .

## CONCLUSION

It will take a long time for economic, social, and cultural rights to obtain the same status and impact as civil and political rights. States will continue to fear the financial commitments of guaranteeing such rights. A conceptual clarification of the separate economic, social, and cultural rights may nevertheless contribute to their recognition and implementation. In addition, this clarification reveals that economic, social, and cultural rights, equal to civil and political rights, may require state abstention, a commitment that requires no financial resources on the part of states. Simultaneously, the fact that civil and political rights may embrace positive obligations underlines the interdependence and interrelatedness of both sets of rights. If positive obligations are derived from civil and political rights, why not recognize similar obligations with regard to economic, social, and cultural rights?

*     *     *     *     *

In this chapter human rights are viewed as necessary tools for the work of public health. The authors argue that public health and human rights are interrelated: citizens cannot be healthy unless governments recognize their rights and dignity, and citizens cannot enjoy human rights unless they are healthy.

Critics of human rights instruments (e.g., the UDHR and the ICESCR) point to their ineffectiveness in improving the health of citizens, particularly in resource-poor countries. They argue that social and economic rights, such as the right to health, are vague and unenforceable. Human rights advocates, however, believe that although ensuring the right to health may be a distant goal, its recognition in international law is a crucial step toward securing healthier populations. Advocates also see the right to health as an important rhetorical device that can be inspiring.

The right to the highest attainable standard of health for all citizens requires governments to develop and implement law and policy that will best serve the public's health. The ensuing chapters closely examine public health law and policy, as well as methods of reasoning in public health.

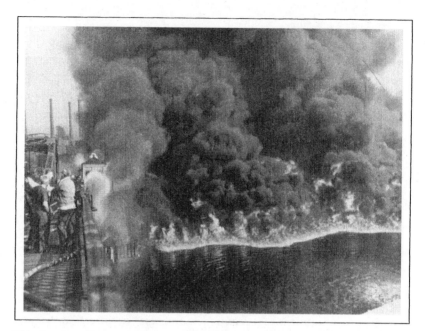

The Cuyahoga River in flames on November 3, 1952. This river in Cleveland, Ohio, caught fire several times during the twentieth century when oil and other contaminants on the water's surface were ignited. The 1969 river fire prompted outrage nationwide and galvanized the environmental movement. (James Thomas, 11/3/52.)

# FIVE

# Reasoning in Public Health

*Philosophy, Risk, and Cost*

Government regulates to prevent injury and disease and to promote the population's health and safety. The mere fact that the government's intentions are benevolent does not necessarily mean that regulation is warranted. Public health regulation needs to be justified because it intrudes on individual interests in liberty and property. But when is a public health intervention justified? The most thoughtful approach is to seek general principles and objective criteria to assess the worth of public health interventions. Scholars and practitioners use various forms of reasoning to accomplish this difficult task—e.g., philosophical inquiry, risk assessment, and cost-effectiveness analysis. See Figure 9.

Philosophers seek general ethical principles in justifying public health regulation. For example, University of Arizona political philosopher Joel Feinberg (1987–1990) examines the types of conduct the state may appropriately proscribe. Among the "liberty-limiting" principles he discusses are harm to others (the "harm principle") and offense to others (the "offense principle"). The "liberal position" holds that the harm and offense principles exhaust the class of good reasons for legal prohibitions. Liberal thinkers exclude harm to oneself (paternalism) as a sufficient justification for legal prohibitions.

The liberal position is not universally accepted (see Kuczewski 2001). Some ethicists believe that the state is warranted in coercing

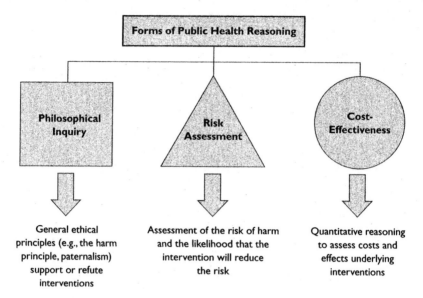

Figure 9.   Justifying public health regulation.

competent individuals to act in their own best interests (Pope 2000). Under this view, government may coerce individuals to refrain from behavior that poses a risk primarily to the person herself and not to others. Classic illustrations of "self-regarding" behavior include the use of seatbelts and motorcycle helmets as well as gambling and fluoridation of water.

Risk assessment is another widely used form of reasoning in public health regulation (Graham and Wiener 1995). According to this form of thinking, it is important to understand the risk posed to the community's health. Risk is a highly complex concept, and a great deal of literature exists about the analysis, perception, characterization, communication, and management of risk. Risk assessors struggle with the divergent conceptions of risk in society (National Research Council 1996). Scientists understand risk according to probabilistic assessments relating to the chance that a dangerous event will occur and, if it does, the severity of its effects. The lay public's understanding of risk, however, includes personal, social, and cultural values. People seem interested in whether the risk is imposed or voluntarily assumed, naturally occurring or introduced by novel technologies, or fairly distributed among the population.

Risk, of course, is a multidimensional concept. Public health regulations intended to reduce one kind of risk may increase another. Public health agencies have to confront these kinds of risk-risk trade-offs every day. For example, chemical disinfection of drinking water may reduce the short-term risk of waterborne infectious disease but increase the long-term risk of cancer (Gostin, Lazzarini, Neslund, and Osterholm 2000).

Finally, economists use quantitative reasoning in evaluating public health regulation. Economists want to understand both the costs of an intervention and its effects. Public health regulations impose economic costs—for example, agency resources to devise and implement the regulation, costs to individuals and businesses subject to the regulation, and lost opportunities to intervene with different, potentially more effective techniques (opportunity costs). Similarly, economists want to understand the effects of regulation—the effectiveness of the intervention in the real world and the societal benefits. Under standard economic accounts, government should favor regulatory responses that maximize health benefits (e.g., saving the most years of life or quality-adjusted years of life) at the least cost. Using this "cost-effectiveness" analysis, health economists estimate the net health effects of a regulatory program or intervention.

Needless to say, not everyone believes that sterile estimates of costs and benefits represent a fair way of evaluating policies (Powers and Faden 2000). Many argue that market exchanges should not be the principal measure of the value of human lives. In particular, critics argue that public health policies cannot be compressed, through ever more complex economic methods, into a single aggregate number, such as costs per quality-adjusted life saved (Heinzerling 1998a,b).

Many additional forms of reasoning about public health regulation exist, notably constitutional law and other legal reasoning (see Part Two of the *Reader*). This chapter, however, concentrates on philosophy, risk, and economics.

## I. PHILOSOPHICAL JUSTIFICATIONS

In the following reading, Philip Cole, from the University of Alabama at Birmingham, elaborates on the importance of providing ethical justifications for public health interventions. He provides a structured review of public health interventions and the moral claims used to justify each.

## The Moral Bases for Public Health Interventions*
*Philip Cole*

> Man is born free, but is everywhere in chains.
>
> Rousseau, *Du Contrat Social*

Members of the public health professions, practitioners and academi-
cians alike, traditionally hold as their primary goals the development and
dissemination of practices that will prevent disease and disability. Other
aspects of public health, such as those relating to medical care access and
costs, wax and wane in importance but remain secondary to disease prevention. This paper is focused on the traditional goals of public health.
My principal purpose is to suggest the need for examining the moral underpinnings of the public health interventions that we endorse. . . .

There are three major reasons why most activities intended to prevent disease require an explicit moral justification: they are enforceable
by the police power of the state; they are supported by taxes; and they
are meddlesome or intrusive. Therefore, I suggest that a preventive intervention should be endorsed only by a person who can justify it to
himself, or herself, in explicit moral terms.

I describe the four major types of prevention activities: education,
policy advocacy, legislation, and research. The potential moral justifications for programs of these types are also presented and evaluated.
The enhancement of the will of the individual, used to justify health education, is a highly moral justification when it is adhered to. Paternalism and doing the greatest good for the greatest number of people are
also moral justifications in most instances. Other justifications, such as
conserving government resources and "doing good" with funds raised
through taxes, have a limited moral basis. . . .

### BASIC ISSUES

There are two major contexts in which to consider fundamental rationales in public health. The first is that of the unofficial agency and the
individual public health worker. In this context an acceptable justification is one that is moral. Here, moral means "that which is recognized
as correct or good by the great majority of competent persons." The

*Reprinted from *Epidemiology* (January 1995): 78–83 with permission from the BMG
Publishing Group.

second context for a fundamental rationale is that of the official or governmental agency. In this context the important criterion for a justification to meet is legitimacy. Here, legitimate means "in compliance with the social contract that validates the existence of a government."

Morality and legitimacy are complex abstractions that are difficult to define and that differ from one another. Nonetheless, for brevity, I use the word moral to mean either moral or legitimate, depending on the context. These two meanings of the word are congruent because a legitimate government nearly always does that, and only that, which most of its citizens consider moral. . . .

There are several aspects of many preventive interventions that require a close examination of their moral bases. The first is that most interventions are enforceable by governmental authority. The passage of a public health law or regulation means that a non-compliant individual may suffer the consequences of the police power of the state. . . .

The second aspect of many preventive interventions that necessitates their moral justification is that they are supported by tax funds. Taxes are extracted from everyone under the threat of severe penalty for failure to pay. Each citizen must support a public health program whether or not he endorses it and whether or not he benefits from it.

The third aspect that requires a moral basis is that prevention activities are often meddlesome and sometimes quite intrusive. Consider, for example, the law that requires a person to have his physiology altered as the result of an immunization. Or consider the law that would compel a person seeking treatment for a venereal disease to identify sexual partners.

Intrusive, paid for with public funds, and backed by the police power of the state. Clearly, activities with such attributes may readily violate the contract that each of us has with our government. Yet, in our complex society, the considerations that underlie that contract have been lost sight of. I reaffirm them: The individual human being is the fundamental unit of society. . . .

It is the inalienable right to liberty (and closely related, autonomy) that requires particular consideration, since meddlesome preventive programs often infringe upon it. For example, a motorist is required in some jurisdictions to restrain himself with a seatbelt. A seatbelt law reduces the liberty of a person, while failure to use a belt poses no threat to anyone other than the person himself. Seatbelt laws are justified currently by the "common resource" rationale. But this rationale (explained below) relates to a minor function of government; it cannot be used legitimately to abrogate an inalienable right the protection of which is fundamental to the existence of government. . . .

## INTERVENTIONS

Legislating and regulating, the regimentation of individual and corporate behavior by law and by the enabling authority of a law, are used in public health to criminalize behavior. Criminalizing may be in the form of requiring or forbidding certain behaviors or of levying a tax. The criminalizing of behavior is the adoption of laws or regulations that make illegal an activity that previously was acceptable and legal (and that often remains so in similar jurisdictions). Criminalizing must have a compelling moral basis since its purpose is to change the moral code of the individual. For example, a seatbelt law is intended to cause a responsible citizen to break the law (that is, to feel immoral) if he fails to use his seatbelt. Levying a tax is also done through legislation and, while subtly different from mandating or forbidding behavior, has the same need for a moral basis, since the tax evader is deemed a criminal. All behaviors can be criminalized and de-criminalized by the state, but few can be rendered immoral or moral. . . . A law that may reasonably be seen as arbitrary or quite transitory must draw its moral basis from its compliance with the social contract, for it has no inherent or God-given moral basis. . . .

## JUSTIFICATIONS

Many moral bases have been offered for public health interventions. Almost all of these fall into one of the following categories: (1) informed people make healthful choices; (2) we professionals know what is best; (3) we must bring about the greatest good for the greatest number of people; (4) common resources must be conserved and government services maintained; (5) the funds generated will be used for a good purpose.

The "informed people" rationale is used to support education and, to some extent, research. Educating is highly moral when it is intended to enhance the will of the individual and no penalty is imposed on persons who do not accept the educational message. In fact, education is almost always the ideal preventative since it honors the social contract and no inalienable right is threatened. Moreover, education is valuable in its scope: people may respond to education with healthful behavior in many areas of their lives. However, when this does not occur, and unhealthful behavior persists, education may be supplemented, or replaced, by a law that criminalizes that behavior. From this perspective, most public health laws that dictate personal actions (for example, a seatbelt law) are testimony to the state's failure as an educator. . . .

We professionals know what is best, or "paternalism," is the second rationale. Paternalism has its place, of course, and can be moral in dealing with children and with adults who are unable to make an informed judgment. But paternalism is immoral as a basis for attempting to dictate the behavior of a competent adult. . . . It is sometimes contended that technical issues in public health render most adults unable to make an informed judgment. This contention is usually an excuse for the failure of education and propaganda to bring about behavior change and is a rationalization for criminalizing the undesirable behavior. In reality, nearly all public health issues can be explained satisfactorily to almost every adult. Paternalism is most odious when used as a justification for limiting the choices that adults make in their everyday lives. Nonetheless, paternalism is a common rationale behind much life style propaganda that is passed off as education. It has been suggested that paternalism can be defended because it is efficient and because it works. Then, a cudgel should be even better. No, the criterion of morality is not efficiency and not even success, but compliance with the social contract.

To bring about the greatest good for the greatest number, the "commonweal" rationale, is a third justification that can be moral. The morality of commonweal lies in the reality that the protection of the rights of a larger number of people sometimes requires the abrogation of the rights of a smaller number. It is the most common rationale and, in fact, along with paternalism, is the only rationale seemingly widely recognized. Commonweal is at the core of most public health laws and regulations. It is used, for example, to enact and to enforce standards of hygiene for the control of infectious diseases. It is also used as a basis for setting standards relating to health and safety in the work place and in residences and with regard to matters such as the purity of foods. We acknowledge that a society as technologically advanced as ours poses many hidden threats to its citizens. It is not reasonable to expect each citizen to be aware of all of these; thus standards-setting is justified even when the standard alienates the rights of the people who own the productive resources that are regulated. . . .

Despite its usual morality, the commonweal justification is potentially dangerous and must be used carefully. The danger lies in its inappropriate use to infringe upon the rights of a minority group, even of a large minority group. For example, commonweal was a major justification, with paternalism, for criminalizing the drinking of alcohol. Prohibition failed as social engineering primarily because it infringed upon the rights of many. . . .

The conserving of "common resources" and the maintenance of ancillary government services is a rationale that underlies many public health laws in socialist states. It is gaining in popularity in the USA. The reasoning behind this justification is that there is a pool of common resources (usually money) held by the government to meet claims that may be made by individuals. Now, since any individual may (under certain conditions) make a claim on these funds, and since resources must be conserved, the government can require people to behave in a way that reduces the prospect that they will, in fact, make any such claim. An example may clarify this. The common resources justification is used to defend the rather extreme law requiring a helmet to be worn by motorcyclists. The reasoning is that if you have a motorcycle accident, the state may be responsible for paying for your medical care. These costs will be lower if you wear a helmet and so suffer a less severe injury. Therefore, so goes the reasoning, you must wear a helmet. Here, an ancillary government service (a welfare function) is used to deny the individual the inalienable right to choose whether to wear a helmet. The issue is more obvious when based on the state's serving not as a welfare provider but rather as the universal medical insurer or guarantor. However, there is a major implication in having a governmental universal medical guarantor involve itself in preventive activities. Why should the universal medical guarantor stop at requiring a helmet (or a seatbelt, or whatever)? No, the universal medical guarantor should penalize all unhealthful behaviors. For example, obesity could be fined. Or the state might try to enforce a law requiring regular exercise. There could be no end to it. Parenthetically, an interesting aspect of the common resources rationale as a defense for the helmet law is that the underlying premise is probably false. While there is evidence that helmets reduce the severity of injuries, there is none that they lower medical care costs. This seeming paradox is explained by recognizing that helmets may cause persons who otherwise would have been injured fatally to survive and require considerable medical care.

The "funds for good purpose" rationale is used, of course, to justify levying a tax and has a moral basis in only a few circumstances. A major good purpose for which taxes are levied is to support research.

The authority of the state to deprive individuals of their assets in order to support research on communicable diseases is not questioned. In addition, a reasonable defense can be put forward for the use of taxes to support research on very common diseases. But what can be the moral basis for using taxes to support research into the causes, or means of control, of an uncommon noncommunicable disease? The customary response to that inquiry is: It is the will of the majority that such research be done. In reality, this response is unsubstantiated, and it is unlikely to be correct for much of this type of research. But more important, if the justification is "the will of the majority," then there is no need to support such research with taxes. Let that majority whose will this is pay the full cost, through donations to private agencies. Government need not be involved. . . .

The funds for good purpose rationale has a second major application. It is often combined with other rationales to justify the so-called sin taxes. These are the relatively exorbitant levies placed on alcohol and tobacco products. The endorsement of sin taxes is increasing, especially among public health professionals, who, I expect, are a rather abstemious group. Therefore, this approach to disease prevention warrants a detailed consideration of its moral underpinnings.

Three purposes are commonly put forward to justify a sin tax: to discourage use of the taxed product (actually, paternalism); to cause users to pay in advance for their future medical care (a variation of the common resources rationale); and to provide funds for a good purpose. The use of law to discourage the use of a product that harms only the user is not moral. A competent adult is entitled to decide for himself whether he will accept the risk of harm attendant upon the use of such a product. On the other hand, if the goal of discouraging use is to protect non-users from the effects of a harmful product, a commonweal rationale might be sustainable. For example, knowledge of the health effects of environmental tobacco smoke might justify cigarette taxes. (However, since smoking in public places is now effectively banned, this particular commonwealth rationale loses much of its force.) . . .

Finally, we come to the funds for "good purpose" rationale. This is quite popular among persons who believe that they, or their work, will receive some of the funds raised. Thus, cancer researchers, especially institute directors, will endorse a tobacco tax if some of the proceeds are earmarked for cancer research. I do not imply that these people are selfish or self-serving. They are well intentioned in their belief that their work warrants support and that taxing a disease-causing product is a good way to raise funds. The error comes from thinking that because the funds will be used for a good purpose, the police power of the state should be marshaled to extract them from unwilling contributors.

In the final analysis, taxes cannot enhance the will of the individual and may not reduce the spread of a disease-causing agent; they will therefore prove difficult or impossible to defend in moral terms.

\*      \*      \*      \*      \*

Cole defends the liberal position and exhibits suspicion of coercive public health interventions. Compare this approach with the vigorous defense of regulation for the common good offered by two prominent ethicists working on a Hastings Center project on health promotion (Bayer and Moreno 1986, 84):

> For two decades advocates of aggressive government intervention in this arena [e.g., cigarette, alcohol, and motor vehicle regulation] have had to bear the burden of proof. Politics, economics, and ethics have all been relied upon to provide arguments against anything but the most modest of efforts. The sheer toll in morbidity and mortality associated with such behavior provides ample justification for shifting the burden of proof. Those who oppose government health promotion efforts, including the use of fiscal measures and even carefully designed restrictions and prohibitions, ought to be compelled to provide arguments against proceeding more aggressively.

Paternalism represents the most controversial justification for public health regulation. Gerald Dworkin (2000, 271) defines paternalism as "the interference with a person's liberty of action justified by reasons referring exclusively to the welfare, good, happiness, needs, interests, or values of the person being coerced" (e.g., laws relating to seatbelts, drugs, gambling, and licensing of professionals). Dworkin (2000, 278) offers a spirited defense of paternalism: "It is reasonable to suppose that there are 'goods' such as health which any person would want to have in order to pursue his own good—no matter how that good is conceived."

Many courts uphold government regulation of self-regarding behavior. Some courts do so based on a belief in paternalism, whereas most others focus on the harms to family and society that inevitably occur when people cause harm to themselves—as in the case of *Benning v. Vermont*.

## Benning v. Vermont*

*Supreme Court of Vermont*
*Decided January 28, 1994*

Justice DOOLEY delivered the opinion of the court.

[Plaintiffs bring a state constitutional challenge against Vermont's motorcycle law, § 1256, which requires motorcyclists to wear reflective helmets with neck or chin straps when on highways. The challenge is based on the language in the first amendment of the Vermont Constitution guaranteeing citizens the right of "enjoying and defending . . . liberty" and "pursuing and obtaining . . . safety."]

At the center of plaintiffs' argument is the assertion that Vermont values personal liberty interests so highly that the analysis under the federal constitution or the constitutions of other states is simply inapplicable here. In support of this contention, plaintiffs rely on political theorists, sociological materials, and incidents in Vermont's history. Without detailing this argument, we find it unpersuasive not because it overvalues Vermont's devotion to personal liberty and autonomy, but because it undervalues the commitment of other governments to those values. . . . Certainly, if there was a heightened concern for personal liberty, there is no evidence of it in the text of the Constitution. . . .

As a result, we reject the notion that this case can be resolved on the basis of a broad right to be let alone without government interference. We accept the federal analysis of such a claim in the context of a public safety restriction applicable to motorists using public roads. We agree with Justice Powell, recently sitting by designation with the Court of Appeals for the Eleventh Circuit, who stated:

> There is no broad legal or constitutional "right to be let alone" by government. In the complex society in which we live, the action and notation of citizens are subject to countless local, state, and federal laws and regulations. Bare invocation of a right to be let alone is an appealing rhetorical device, but it seldom advances legal inquiry, as the "right" —to the extent it exists—has no meaning outside its application to specific activities. The [federal] Constitution does protect citizens from government interference in many areas— speech, religion, the security of the home. But the unconstrained right asserted by appellant has no discernible bounds, and bears little resemblance to the important but limited privacy rights recognized by our highest Court.
>
> Picou v. Gillum, 874 F.2d 1519, 1521 (11th Cir. 1989)

---

*641 A.2d 757 (Vt. 1994).

We are left then with the familiar standard for evaluating police power regulations—essentially, that expressed in *State v. Solomon*, 260 A.2d 377, 379 (Vt. 1969) [holding that § 1256 did not exceed the state's police power or violate due process of law and was "directly related to highway safety" because without a helmet, a motorcyclist could be affected by highway hazards, lose control, and injure other motorists]. Plaintiffs urge us to overrule *Solomon* because it was based on an analysis of the safety risk to other users of the roadway that is incredible. In support of their position, they offered evidence from motorcycle operators that the possibility of an operator losing control of a motorcycle and becoming a menace to others is remote. On the other hand, these operators assert that helmets make a motorcycle operator dangerous. Plaintiffs also emphasize that even supporters of helmet laws agree that their purpose is to protect the motorcycle operator, not other highway users.

We are not willing to abandon the primary rationale of *Solomon* because of plaintiffs' evidence. The statute is entitled to a presumption of constitutionality. Plaintiffs are not entitled to have the courts act as a super-legislature and retry legislative judgments based on evidence presented to the court. Thus, the question before us is whether the link between safety for highway users and the helmet law is rational, not whether we agree that the statute actually leads to safer highways. The *Solomon* reasoning has been widely adopted in the many courts that have considered the constitutionality of motorcycle helmet laws. We still believe it supports the constitutionality of § 1256.

There are at least two additional reasons why we conclude § 1256 is constitutional. . . . Although plaintiffs argue that the only person affected by the failure to wear a helmet is the operator of the motorcycle, the impact of that decision would be felt well beyond that individual. Such a decision imposes great costs on the public. As Professor Laurence Tribe (1988, 1372) has commented, ours is "a society unwilling to abandon bleeding bodies on the highway, [and] the motorcyclist or driver who endangers himself plainly imposes costs on others." This concern has been echoed in a number of opinions upholding motorcycle helmet laws. . . . This rationale is particularly apparent as the nation as a whole, and this state in particular, debate reform of a health care system that has become too costly although many do not have access to it. Whether in taxes or insurance rates, our costs are linked to the actions of others and are driven up when others fail to take preventive steps that would minimize health care consumption. We see no constitutional barrier to legislation that requires preventive measures to minimize health care costs that are inevitably imposed on society.

A second rationale supports this type of a safety requirement on a public highway. Our decisions show that in numerous circumstances the liability for injuries that occur on our public roads may be imposed on the state, or other governmental units, and their employees. It is rational for the state to act to minimize the extent of the injuries for which it or other governmental units may be financially responsible. The burden placed on plaintiffs who receive the benefit of the liability system is reasonable. . . .

As a result, we reiterate our conclusion that § 1256 "in no way violates any of the provisions of our state and federal constitutions." *Solomon*, 260 A.2d at 380.

---

## II. UNDERSTANDING RISK

Not every threat to self or others merits intervention. Risks should rise to a certain threshold before they warrant a regulatory response. Of course, it is difficult to know what level of risk ought to trigger regulation. In *School Board of Nassau County, Florida v. Arline*, 480 U.S. 273 (1987) (see *Reader* web site), Justice William Brennan reasons that risks should be weighed based on their nature, the probability of their occurrence, and the severity of the harm should the risk materialize. Although Brennan's arguments are written in the context of disability discrimination law, they say something important about the weighing of risk.

The risk assessment formula proposed in *Arline* represents a scientific approach to assessing health risks. The current regulatory system purports to use scientific methods to measure risk, but policy in the real world is confounded by scientific uncertainties, human values, and political compromises. The result appears to be a combination of "over-regulated risk," such as the removal of apples treated with the pesticide Alar from supermarkets, and "underregulated risk," such as the regulation of personal handguns.

Justice Stephen Breyer's book *Breaking the Vicious Circle* sharply criticizes existing public health regulation, particularly in the environmental area. In the following reading, Breyer discusses one of the most important factors contributing to what he sees as inefficient risk regulation—public risk perception. He outlines the cognitive attributions and schemata the public uses to inaccurately assess risk. Poor public perception of risk, together with politics and the technical uncertainties of the regulatory process, create what Breyer terms the "vicious circle" of risk regulation. The vicious circle, argues Breyer, leads agencies to overregulate tiny health risks while ignoring larger, more pressing health concerns.

---

### Breaking the Vicious Circle:
### Toward Effective Risk Regulation*
*Stephen Breyer*

PUBLIC PERCEPTIONS

Study after study shows that the public's evaluation of risk problems differs radically from any consensus of experts in the field. Risks associated with toxic waste dumps and nuclear power appear near the bottom of most expert lists; they appear near the top of the public's list of concerns, which more directly influences regulatory agendas. To some extent, these differences may reflect that the public fears certain risks more than others with the same probability of harm. . . . [O]f two equal risks, one could rationally dislike or fear more the risk that is involuntarily suffered, new, unobservable, uncontrollable, catastrophic, delayed, a threat to future generations, or likely accompanied by pain or dread.

Still, these differences in the source, quality, or nature of a risk may not account for the different ranking by the public and the experts. A typical member of the public would like to minimize risks of death to himself, to his family, to his neighbors; he would normally prefer that regulation buy more safety for a given expenditure or the same amount of safety for less. Not many of us would like to shift resources to increase overall risks of death significantly in order to increase the likelihood that death will occur on a bicycle or in a fire, rather than through disease. There is a far simpler explanation for the public's aversion to toxic waste dumps than an enormous desire for supersafety, or a strong aversion to the tiniest risk of harm—namely, the public does not *believe* that the risks are tiny. The public's "nonexpert" reactions reflect not

---

different values but different understandings about the underlying risk-related facts.

My assumption that the public assigns "rational" values to risks, however, does not entail rational public reactions to risk. Psychologists have found several examples of thinking that impede rational understanding, but may have helped us survive as we lived throughout much of prehistory, in small groups of hunter-gatherers, depending upon grain, honey, and animals for sustenance. The following, rather well-documented aspects of risk perception are probably familiar.

*Rules of thumb.* In daily life most of us do not weigh all the pros and cons of feasible alternatives. We use rules of thumb, more formally called "heuristic devices." We simplify radically; we reason with the help of a few readily understandable examples; we categorize (events and other people) in simple ways that tend to create binary choices— yes/no, friend/foe, eat/abstain, safe/dangerous, act/don't act—and may reflect deeply rooted aversions, such as fear of poisons. The resulting categorizations do not always accurately describe another person of circumstance, but they help us make quick decisions, most of which prove helpful. This kind of quick decision-making may help cut a swath through the modern information jungle, but it oversimplifies dramatically and thereby inhibits an understanding of risks, particularly small risks.

*Prominence.* People react more strongly, and give greater importance, to events that stand out from the background. Unusual events are striking. We more likely notice the (low-risk) nuclear waste disposal truck driving past the school than the (much higher-risk) gasoline delivery trucks on their way to local service stations. Journalists, whose job is to write interesting stories, know this psychological fact well. The American Medical Association examined how the press treated two similar stories, one finding increased leukemia rates among nuclear workers, the other finding no increased cancer rates among those living near nuclear plants. More than half of the newspapers in the study mentioned the first story but not the second; and more than half of those that mentioned both emphasized the first.

*Ethics.* The strength of our feelings of ethical obligation seems to diminish with distance. That is to say, feelings of obligation are stronger (or we have different, more time-consuming obligations) toward family, neighbors, friends, community, and those with whom we have direct contact, those whom we see, than toward those who live in distant places, whom we do not see but only read or hear about.

*Trust in experts.* People cannot easily judge between experts when those experts disagree with each other. The public, since the mid-1960s, has shown increasing distrust of experts and the institutions, private, academic, or governmental, that employ them.

*Fixed decisions.* A person who has made up his or her mind about something is very reluctant to change it.

*Mathematics.* Most people have considerable difficulty understanding the mathematical probabilities involved in assessing risk. People consistently overestimate small probabilities. What is the likelihood of death by botulism? (One in two million.) They underestimate large ones. What is the likelihood of death by diabetes? (One in fifty thousand.) People cannot detect inconsistencies in their own risk-related choices. . . .

These few, near-commonsense propositions, with strong statistical support in the technical literature, verify Oliver Wendell Holmes's own observation that "most people think dramatically, not quantitatively." They also have important consequences. Consider the public reaction to toxic waste dumps. Start with the mathematical facts about the probability of various occurrences: In 1985 a New Jersey woman won the state lottery twice. What are the odds against this, billions to one? Given the vast number of lotteries in the world, the odds come close to favoring someone somewhere winning a lottery twice. Given the population of the world, and the number of dreams each night, the odds favor someone somewhere dreaming he marries a girl who looks very much like the girl he meets the next day and marries. Given the number of toxic waste dumps in the United States (26,000) and the number of places with above-average cancer rates (half of all places), obviously many cities, towns, and rural areas near toxic waste dumps must also have seriously elevated cancer rates ("mathematics").

Add what sells newspapers—interesting stories—and you can be fairly certain the press will write about the double lottery-winner, perhaps the dreamer, and, if the mathematical evidence is somewhat less crude than my example, the toxic waste dump ("prominence"). Will it be easy to convince the cancer victim that the waste dump (water that is "pure" or "not pure") had nothing to do with the disease ("rules of thumb")? And how will the public react to the image of the angry family member on nightly television ("ethics"), particularly if experts disagree ("trust in experts") as they might, for the relation between the disease and the toxic site may not be strictly chance (the lottery, too, might be fixed). If further study exonerates the dump, will the viewing public change its mind ("fixed decision")?

When we think about nuclear power controversies, we should take account of the fact that hearing about an accident is what psychologists tell us is a heuristic "tip-off" of danger, whether or not anyone is hurt. We have "seen" Chernobyl and Three Mile Island, and we may therefore doubt nuclear power's safety, whether or not experts tell us that the reactor at Chernobyl was not properly designed, that the accident at Three Mile Island hurt no one, that military weapons, not electric power generators, are responsible for 99 percent of all nuclear waste, that nuclear power's risks are minuscule compared to the risks of coal-generated power. Add a few disagreements among experts and the fact that most members of the public made up their minds long ago, and one can understand nuclear power's position on the public perception risk charts.

These few propositions suggest that better "risk communications," such as efforts to explain risks to the public at open meetings, may not suffice to alleviate risk regulation problems. It is not surprising that, after the EPA Administrator William Ruckelshaus spent days at such meetings in Tacoma, Washington, explaining why an ASARCO chemical plant that was leaking small amounts of arsenic could remain open, he was misunderstood, criticized, and accused of trying to drive a wedge between environmentalists and blue collar workers. The plant eventually closed, although perhaps for other reasons. Nor is it surprising that after special public discussions of nuclear power plants were held in Sweden, surveys of the eighty thousand Swedes who participated showed no consensus, but increased confusion.

There is little reason to hope for better risk communication over time. To the contrary, as science improves, scientists may more easily detect and identify ever tinier risks—the risks associated, for example, with the migration of a single molecule of plastic from a container into a soft drink; they may more easily identify geographical areas near toxic waste dumps with higher than average cancer rates. As international communications improve, the press will have an ever larger pool of unusual, and therefore more interesting, accident stories to write about. Why should we not expect an outcry from a public that reads about Love Canal, Times Beach, Alar, Chilean grapes laced with cyanide, and the leaflet of Villejuif, whether or not such examples reflect meaningful danger? (At the same time, how can one expect public reaction to potentially greater but more mundane problems, of which it is unaware?)

It is hard to make the normal human mind grapple with this inhuman type of problem. To change public reaction, one would either have to institute widespread public education in risk analysis or generate greater public trust in some particular group of experts or the institutions that employ them. The first alternative seems unlikely. The second, over the past thirty years, has not occurred. Ordinary, human, public perception, then, forms one element of the vicious circle.

---

*     *     *     *     *

Shortly before *Breaking the Vicious Circle* was published, Breyer delivered the opinion in *United States v. Ottati & Goss,* 900 F.2d 429 (1st Cir. 1990) (posted on the *Reader* web site). In *Ottati,* a famous case involving the "Superfund" toxic cleanup law, a federal court of appeals rejected the Environmental Protection Agency's claim that the International Minerals and Chemical Corporation did not clean up a toxic waste site sufficiently. Breyer expressed frustration at the cost and complexity of adjudicating a case involving nearly a fifty thousand–page record:

> Why . . . has this case taken ten years to litigate? The issues are complex, but not unfathomable. Why has the government not found a way to express its technical problems in English (e.g., "small children will eat tiny amounts of dirt when they play in a yard"), instead of relying upon maze-like patterns of cross-references among regulations, statutes, and "expert jargon?". . . Has the government, in fact, spent enormous administrative (and judicial) resources in an effort to force improvement from "quite clean" . . . to "extremely clean," at three to four times the "quite clean" costs?

Determining appropriate levels of toxicity in *Ottati* turned on seemingly trivial questions such as "Will a child playing in the dirt consume contaminated soil on 70 or 245 days out of the year?"

Breyer was also influenced by the Supreme Court's decision in *Industrial Union Department, AFL-CIO v. American Petroleum Institute,* 448 U.S. 607 (1980) (posted on the *Reader* web site). This case, known as the "Benzene case," illustrates an equally challenging problem in risk regulation: determining how much exposure to a harmful chemical is "safe." If exposure to benzene at a certain level is associated with an increased rate of leukemia, does *any* exposure increase the risk of leukemia? Alternatively, is there a "safe" level at which benzene exposure will have no physical effects? The Occupational Safety and Health Administration (OSHA) decided that in the absence of scientific data, there is no "safe" level of benzene exposure. The Supreme Court disagreed, holding that OSHA had the burden of proving, on the basis of substantial evidence, that long-term exposure to benzene at low levels presents a "significant risk of material health impairment."

Breyer is only one of several respected jurists and scholars who have questioned the policy of regulating exceedingly low risks while failing to regulate more serious health threats. Much of this scholarship relies on a classic empirical study by John F. Morrall III purporting to show that government often spends exorbitant sums to avert very small risks. However, Lisa Heinzerling, an environmental law scholar at Georgetown University Law Center, offers a powerful critique of Morrall's methods and thereby calls into question some of the risk scholarship that relies on his findings (Heinzerling and Ackerman 2001).

Heinzerling points out that the work by Morrall and others systematically downgrades the importance of regulation aimed at preventing long-latency diseases and long-term ecological harm. Heinzerling (1998a, 39) observes that "this is precisely the purpose of the rules that have fared so poorly in analyses of costs per life saved." She also suggests that Morrall's estimates are inflated because they reflect only one regulatory benefit (cancer sickness and death) but do not count other regulatory benefits, such as preventing respiratory illness and ecological harms. "Given all the benefits, some quantifiable, some not, most of the regulatory programs that have been portrayed as clunkers are not just barely cost-justified. They are bargains."

Risk is often expressed in absolute terms. The regulatory question asked is whether government should spend a certain amount of money to avert a particular risk. Of course, risk is a relative concept—a risk can be measured only against other health threats faced by society. Moreover, when government acts to avert a given risk, it may exacerbate another risk. In an important article, Cass R. Sunstein, a professor of law and political science at the University of Chicago, writes about "health-health" trade-offs in public health regulation.

## Health-Health Tradeoffs*
*Cass R. Sunstein*

My purpose in this essay is to discuss a pervasive problem in risk regulation, one that helps account for regulatory failure, that is an intriguing part of cost-benefit assessment, and that is only now receiving

*Reprinted from *University of Chicago Law Review* 63 (Fall 1996): 1533–71.

public attention. The problem occurs when the diminution of one health risk simultaneously increases another health risk. Thus, for example, fuel economy standards, designed to reduce environmental risks, may make automobiles less safe, and in that way increase risks to life and health. Regulations designed to control the spread of AIDS and hepatitis among health care providers may increase the costs of health care, and thus make health care less widely available, and thus cost lives. If government bans the manufacture and use of asbestos, it may lead companies to use more dangerous substitutes. Regulation of nuclear power may make nuclear power safer; but by increasing the cost of nuclear power, such regulation will ensure reliance on other energy sources, such as coal-fired power plants, which carry risks of their own. When government requires reformulated gasoline as a substitute for ordinary gasoline, it may reduce carbon monoxide emissions but produce new pollution problems from hydrocarbons and smog. When government regulates air pollution, it may encourage industry to increase the volume of solid waste, and in that sense aggravate another environmental problem. A ban on carcinogens in food additives may lead consumers to use noncarcinogenic products that carry greater risks in terms of diseases other than cancer.

The general problem is ubiquitous. It stems from the fact that government officials, like individual citizens and the public as a whole, suffer from both limited information and (even more importantly) selective attention. A large current priority is to develop mechanisms that overcome the problems posed by the fact that people—both citizens and regulators—tend to focus on problems that are parts of complex wholes. . . . Risks to life and health are qualitatively diverse, and because of their origins and nature, some risks warrant greater attention than others. . . .

## A POLEMICAL NOTE AND CONCEPTUAL MAP

### Why Does It Matter?

We have now seen enough to know that an impressive body of work attempts to measure health gains from regulation against health risks from regulation. But why should we focus on this particular question? Would it not be better to attend to the overall gains from regulation and to the overall losses from regulation? Cost-benefit analysis is receiving considerable attention in both agencies and Congress, and cost-benefit analysis, properly conceived, takes account of all of the health-related effects of regulation. [See reading by Kenneth J. Arrow et al. later in this chapter.] Health-health assessments focus on a subset of effects, and refuse to translate those effects into dollars. Such assessments ignore all costs unrelated to mortality and morbidity. But what is special about health-health tradeoffs? Why should analysis focus on such tradeoffs rather than on all relevant effects?

Part of the answer lies in existing public judgments, taken as simple brute facts. People seem to think that regulation is bad if it causes more deaths than it prevents; a demonstration that a particular regulation has this effect would count strongly against its adoption. But people do not always know how to compare health gains (fifteen lives gained, for example) with monetary losses (an expenditure of $15 million, for example). This uncertainty stems partly from the fact that lives and dollars are not easily made commensurable, and partly from the fact that the appropriate amount to spend on protection of a (statistical) life depends very much on context.

A deliberative judgment about how to assess net health tradeoffs is easier to reach than a deliberative judgment about how to assess cost-benefit tradeoffs. It may thus be possible to obtain an incompletely theorized agreement—incompletely theorized in the sense that people from diverse theoretical perspectives can agree—that a net mortality loss is bad. Incompletely theorized agreements on particular results are an important part of democratic deliberation; they are a distinctive solution to the problems of social pluralism and disagreement.

It would, however, be inadequate for present purposes to rely on existing public judgments, which may be irrational or confused. Perhaps public uncertainty about cost-benefit judgments depends on an obstinate and counterproductive unwillingness to acknowledge that even [risk to] life has its price and that risks are matters of degree rather than "dangerous or not."

But part of the answer can be found in information costs. The comparative defect of health-health assessment is also its virtue: it involves only a subset of the consequences of regulating. Fewer facts need to be compiled. The assessment may economize on the costs of inquiry into speculative issues about regulatory consequences.

Another part of the answer may lie in attending more closely to problems of incommensurability. We might understand incommensurability to arise when no single metric is available by which to assess the variables at stake in a social decision. In the area of risk regulation, a single metric is troublesome simply because it blurs qualitative distinctions.

The vice and virtue of cost-benefit analysis is that it attempts to provide such a metric. If all effects are reduced to the metric of dollars, it may be possible to make simple assessments, in the sense that comparisons and hence tradeoffs can become easier. But the reduction of mortality and morbidity effects to dollars can erase important qualitative distinctions among diverse risks. These qualitative distinctions matter, and hence it is important for officials to understand them when they make decisions.

It is in the face of qualitative distinctions—distinctions in how, not simply how much, things are valued—that participants in democratic deliberation often resist a metric of dollars. To say this is not is to say that there is a problem of incomparability or that tradeoffs do not have to be made among qualitatively diverse goods. But perhaps people can make choices more easily when the tradeoffs involve things that may seem qualitatively indistinguishable, like lives, rather than qualitatively diverse things, like lives and dollars. Most simply, when it is hard to trade off lives against dollars, the burdens of judgment might be eased when we are trading off lives against lives. A judgment of this kind undoubtedly underlies the interest in health-health analysis. . . .

What solutions are possible? It may be possible to reduce these problems by looking not at total lives lost or gained, but at the effects of regulation on the number of quality-adjusted life years. A regulation that saves thirteen children while jeopardizing fifteen elderly people may well be worthwhile, at least if the thirteen children are likely to have decent life prospects. Government might thus focus on statistical years rather than statistical lives. Through attending to years rather than lives saved, and also by making judgments about the nature of years saved, problems of incommensurability can be reduced though certainly not eliminated.

## INCORPORATING HEALTH-HEALTH COMPARISONS

### First Approximation

Let us try, in a simple, intuitive way, to identify the factors that should enter into deliberative judgments about health-health tradeoffs. Begin with a simple case in which the costs of information and inquiry are zero. If this is so, all agencies should investigate all risks potentially at stake. Agencies should always take account of ancillary risks and always try to limit overall or aggregate risks.

Of course the costs of investigation and inquiry are never zero; to the contrary, they are often very high. We can readily imagine that agencies could spend all their time investigating ancillary risks and never do anything else—a disaster for regulatory policy. (This is a potential problem with cost-benefit analysis: cost-benefit analysis may itself fail cost-benefit analysis—if the costs of undertaking cost-benefit analysis are high and the benefits lower.) When the costs of inquiry are not zero, the obligation to inquire into ancillary risks might be a function of several factors. First is the cost of delay, understood as the cost of not controlling the regulated risk until more information has been compiled. To assess this cost, it is necessary to explore the seriousness of the regulated risk and the length of time necessary to investigate the ancillary risk. Second is the cost of investigating the ancillary risk, where this cost is understood as a product of the cost of compiling and evaluating the relevant information. Third is the benefit of investigating the ancillary risk, with the benefit understood as the likelihood of uncovering information that might help to produce a different and better result.

Under this view, it is of course (and unfortunately) important to know at least something about the possible extent of the ancillary risk and the costs of discovering it. Hence there is a problem of circularity: it is impossible to know whether to undertake health-health analysis without first doing a bit of health-health analysis, at least by making some initial judgments about the ancillary risk—a risk that, by hypothesis, the agency has not yet explored. Before the actual investigation has occurred, there will be a good deal of intuition and guesswork; the full facts cannot be known until inquiries have been completed, and the real question is whether it is worthwhile to complete the inquiries or even to embark on them. . . .

### Incorporating Complexities

If aggravating and mitigating factors are taken into account, it might well be the case that people would find, say, 300 cases of cancer less acceptable than 350 cases of heart disease, given certain assumptions about what causes each. In contingent valuation studies, people purport to be willing to pay far more to prevent cancer deaths (from $1.5 million to $9.5 million) than they would to prevent unforeseen instant deaths (from $1 million to $5 million). It is similarly possible that people might therefore accept a regulated risk involving 100 annual fatalities even if the ancillary risk involves 110 annual fatalities; perhaps the ancillary risk is less severe because it is voluntarily run, not especially dreaded, and well understood. The democratic decision to look at something other than quantity is easy to defend. It is fully rational.

---

## III. COST-EFFECTIVENESS

"Cost-effectiveness" is a highly fashionable method of assessment in health care. Health economists try to ascertain how much medical interventions cost and then compare this cost with the number of lives saved. Economists prefer those interventions that save the most lives at the lowest possible cost. To compare different interventions, economists arrive at a figure that represents the "cost per life saved." Health economists have sought more sophisticated measures of the number of lives saved by factoring in the number of years the person would be expected to live (saving younger persons is "worth" more than saving older persons) and the quality of that life (a high quality of life is "worth" more than a life with pain and disability). This method of assessment is often called "cost per quality-adjusted life years saved."

Researchers have also advocated using cost-effectiveness as a tool to evaluate public health interventions (Handler, Issel, and Turnock 2001; IOM 1997). Here, economists estimate the money spent on a regulation (e.g., agency costs to devise and implement the regulation as well business costs to comply with the regulation) and compare it with the number of lives likely to be saved (Becker, Principe, Adams, and Teutsch 1998; U.S. Public Health Service 1994).

Regulated industries often argue that public health regulators must take costs into account. Consider a challenge by industry arguing that the words "public health" in § 109(b)(1) of the Clean Air Act (CAA) required the Environmental Protection Agency (EPA) to assess implementation costs in setting national ambient air quality standards. The Supreme Court in *Whitman v. American Trucking Associations, Inc.,* 121 S. Ct. 903, 908–09 (2001) held that § 109(b)(1) bars EPA from considering implementation costs. In his opinion, Justice Scalia makes some interesting observations about the use of cost-effectiveness analysis in regulation for the public's health:

> Against this most natural of readings [that EPA must identify the maximum airborne concentration of a pollutant that the public health can tolerate], respondents make a lengthy, spirited, but ultimately unsuccessful attack. They begin with the object of § 109(b)(1)'s focus, "the public health." When the

term first appeared in federal clean air legislation—in the Act of July 14, 1955 (1955 Act), 69 Stat. 322, which expressed "recognition of the dangers to the public health" from air pollution—its ordinary meaning was "the health of the community." *Webster's New International Dictionary* 2005 (2d ed. 1950). Respondents argue, however, that . . . many more factors than air pollution affect public health. In particular, the economic cost of implementing a very stringent standard might produce health losses sufficient to offset the health gains achieved in cleaning the air—for example, by closing down whole industries and thereby impoverishing the workers and consumers dependent upon those industries. That is unquestionably true, and Congress was unquestionably aware of it. [Congress specifically required cost-effectiveness analysis in other parts of the CAA, but not in § 109(b)(1).] . . . We have therefore refused to find implicit in ambiguous sections of the CAA an authorization to consider costs that has elsewhere, and so often, been expressly granted.

The two readings that follow examine cost-effectiveness analysis. Louise B. Russell, a Rutgers University researcher who has thought a great deal about measuring the costs of health care services, briefly explains the basics of cost-effectiveness analysis (see Russell et al. 1996). In the final reading in this chapter, Nobel Prize–winning economist Kenneth J. Arrow and his colleagues explain why this form of reasoning would be useful in environmental, health, and safety regulation.

---

## Cost-Effectiveness Analysis*
*Louise B. Russell*

The methodology of cost-effectiveness analysis (CEA) derives from its fundamental objective: to identify those interventions, and ways of using them, that produce the greatest improvement in health for a given quantity of resources ("budget"). The interventions that produce the greatest improvement in health also have the smallest opportunity cost, that is, the fewest health benefits lost. The services not funded would have produced less good health than those selected.

In a cost-effectiveness analysis, the intervention of interest is compared with one or more alternatives. . . . The difference in health effects between an intervention and an alternative is the net gain in

---

*Unpublished paper prepared for the Committee on Health and Behavior: Research, Practice, and Policy, Institute of Medicine, Washington, D.C., 1999.

health from the intervention. The difference in costs is its net cost (resource use). The feature that distinguishes CEA from cost-benefit analysis (CBA), an older methodology which has a similar objective and which has provided much of the theoretical basis for CEA, is that resource use is valued in monetary terms, while health is valued as cases of disease, years of life, or some other measure specific to health. CBA values both costs and health effects in monetary terms. CEA results are customarily presented as the net cost per unit of health gained, the cost-effectiveness ratio.

CEA can only serve its purpose, getting the most health possible from a given quantity of resources, if an analysis reflects everything about an intervention that is of importance to the people affected by it. On the health side, longer life is important, but so are improvements in the quality of life (fewer symptoms, better function, less pain) and adverse effects (pain from a procedure, side effects of medication, anxiety). On the cost side, services paid for by insurers and public programs are important, but so are services paid for out-of-pocket by the patient, or provided without payment by family and friends. The concept of opportunity cost emphasizes that these costs are important because they represent benefits forgone, health (or even non-health) benefits that could have been achieved if the resources had been put to other use.

## OBJECTIONS TO CEA

The most common objection to cost-effectiveness analysis is to raising the issue of cost at all. This objection is often persuasively phrased as "It is unethical to put a price on human life and health." The difficulty with this line of thinking is that if no price is put on human life, or group of human lives, then, when resources are limited, a lower price is put on some other life or lives. That is, if everything is done for some people, less can be done for others. Thus the real-world issue is one of tradeoffs and the ethical question is whether it is acceptable to favor some people without regard to others in the allocation of medical resources.

The tradeoff issue does not go away if costs are ignored. Instead resources can be badly misallocated; interventions that would bring a great deal of good health can be missed, or receive too little funding, while much less effective interventions are funded. . . . Ignoring costs and cost-effectiveness is equivalent to saying that it is unimportant how much health is lost by spending resources one way rather than another. . . .

Comprehensive as it is, however, CEA does not include everything that might be relevant to a particular decision. While CEA provides information crucial for good decisions, it should never be used mechanically. Decision makers may choose to emphasize certain groups, benefits, or costs more heavily than others in a particular decision for very legitimate reasons. In addition, they may need to consider elements that cannot be captured in CEA such as the impact of an intervention on individual privacy or liberty.

The current emphasis on presenting results in the form of cost-effectiveness ratios does not help decision makers consider the trade-offs among costs and health effects. To be more useful, CEAs need to present data on the elements that go into the cost-effectiveness ratios in addition to the ratios themselves, both so that decision makers can understand the ratios better, and so that they can consider whether some elements deserve additional thought or greater weight. Every CEA is also a cost-consequence and should be presented accordingly.

Cost-effectiveness analysis is an analytical framework that arises from asking the question "Which ways of promoting good health—procedures, tests, medications, educational programs, regulations, taxes or subsidies, or combinations and variations of these—are the most effective use of resources?" Specific recommendations about interventions will contribute the most to good health if they are set in this larger context and based on information that demonstrates that they are in the public interest.

## Is There a Role for Benefit-Cost Analysis in Environmental, Health, and Safety Regulation?*

*Kenneth J. Arrow, Maureen L. Cropper, George C. Eads, et al.*

The growing impact of regulations on the economy has led both Congress and the Administration to search for new ways of reforming the regulatory process. Many of these initiatives call for greater reliance on the use of economic analysis in the development and evaluation of

*Reprinted from *Science* 272 (April 12, 1996): 221–22 with permission. © 1996 American Association for the Advancement of Science.

regulations. One specific approach being advocated is benefit-cost analysis, an economic tool for comparing the desirable and undesirable impacts of proposed policies.

For environmental, health, and safety regulation, benefits are typically defined in terms of the value of having a cleaner environment or a safer workplace. Ideally, costs should be measured in the same terms: the losses implied by the increased prices that result from the costs of meeting a regulatory objective. In practice, the costs tend to be measured on the basis of direct compliance costs, with secondary consideration given to indirect costs, such as the value of time spent waiting in a motor vehicle inspection line.

The direct costs of federal environmental, health, and safety regulation appear to be on the order of $200 billion annually, or about the size of all domestic non-defense discretionary spending. The benefits of the regulations are less certain, but evidence suggests that some but not all recent regulations would pass a benefit-cost test. Moreover, a reallocation of expenditures on environmental, health, and safety regulations has the potential to save significant numbers of lives while using fewer resources. The estimated cost per statistical life saved has varied across regulations by a factor of more than $10 million, ranging from an estimated cost of $200,000 per statistical life saved with the Environmental Protection Agency's (EPA's) 1979 trihalomethane drinking water standard to more than $6.3 trillion with EPA's 1990 hazardous waste listing for wood-preserving chemicals. Thus, a reallocation of priorities among these same regulations could save many more lives at the given cost, or alternatively, save the same number of lives at a much lower cost.

Most economists would argue that economic efficiency, measured as the difference between benefits and costs, ought to be one of the fundamental criteria for evaluating proposed environmental, health, and safety regulations. Because society has limited resources to spend on regulation, benefit-cost analysis can help illuminate the trade-offs involved in making different kinds of social investments. In this regard, it seems almost irresponsible to not conduct such analyses, because they can inform decisions about how scarce resources can be put to the greatest social good. Benefit-cost analysis can also help answer the question of how much regulation is enough. From an efficiency standpoint, the answer to this question is simple: regulate until the incremental benefits from regulation are just offset by the incremental costs.

In practice, however, the problem is much more difficult, in large part because of inherent problems in measuring marginal benefits and costs. In addition, concerns about fairness and process may be important non-economic factors that merit consideration. Regulatory policies inevitably involve winners and losers, even when aggregate benefits exceed aggregate costs.

Over the years, policy-makers have sent mixed signals regarding the use of benefit-cost analysis in policy evaluation. Congress has passed several statutes to protect health, safety, and the environment that effectively preclude the consideration of benefits and costs in the development of certain regulations, even though other statutes actually require the use of benefit-cost analysis. Meanwhile, former presidents Carter, Reagan, and Bush and President Clinton have all introduced formal processes for reviewing economic implications of major environmental, health, and safety regulations. Apparently the Executive Branch, charged with designing and implementing regulations, has seen a need to develop a yardstick against which the efficiency of regulatory proposals can be assessed. Benefit-cost analysis has been the yardstick of choice.

We suggest that benefit-cost analysis has a potentially important role to play in helping inform regulatory decision-making, although it should not be the sole basis for such decision-making. We offer the following eight principles on the appropriate use of benefit-cost analysis.

*Benefit-cost analysis is useful for comparing the favorable and unfavorable effects of policies.* Benefit-cost analysis can help decision-makers better understand the implications of decisions by identifying and, where appropriate, quantifying the favorable and unfavorable consequences of a proposed policy change, even when information on benefits and costs is highly uncertain. In some cases, however, benefit-cost analysis cannot be used to conclude that the economic benefits of a decision will exceed or fall short of its costs, because there is simply too much uncertainty.

*Decision-makers should not be precluded from considering the economic costs and benefits of different policies in the development of regulations. Agencies should be allowed to use economic analysis to help set regulatory priorities.* Removing statutory prohibitions on the balancing of benefits and costs can help promote more efficient and effective regulation. Congress could further promote more effective use of resources by explicitly asking agencies to consider benefits and costs in formulating their regulatory priorities.

*Benefit-cost analysis should be required for all major regulatory decisions.* Although the precise definition of "major" requires judgment, this general requirement should be applied to all government agencies. The scale of a benefit-cost analysis should depend on both the stakes involved and the likelihood that the resulting information will affect the ultimate decision. For example, benefit-cost analyses of policies intended to retard or halt depletion of stratospheric ozone were worthwhile because of the large stakes involved and the potential for influencing public policy.

*Although agencies should be required to conduct benefit-cost analyses for major decisions and to explain why they have selected actions for which reliable evidence indicates that expected benefits are significantly less than expected costs, those agencies should not be bound by strict benefit-cost tests.* Factors other than aggregate economic benefits and costs, such as equity within and across generations, may be important in some decisions.

*Benefits and costs of proposed policies should be quantified wherever possible. Best estimates should be presented along with a description of the uncertainties.* In most instances, it should be possible to describe the effects of proposed policy changes in quantitative terms; however, not all impacts can be quantified, let alone be given a monetary value. Therefore, care should be taken to assure that quantitative factors do not dominate important qualitative factors in decision-making. If an agency wishes to introduce a "margin of safety" into a decision, it should do so explicitly.

Whenever possible, values used to quantify benefits and costs in monetary terms should be based on trade-offs that individuals would make, either directly or, as is often the case, indirectly in labor, housing, or other markets. Benefit-cost analysis is premised on the notion that the values to be assigned to program effects—favorable or unfavorable— should be those of the affected individuals, not the values held by economists, moral philosophers, environmentalists, or others.

*The more external review that regulatory analyses receive, the better they are likely to be.* Historically, the U.S. Office of Management and Budget has played a key role in reviewing selected major regulations, particularly those aimed at protecting the environment, health, and safety. Peer review of economic analyses should be used for regulations with potentially large economic impacts. Retrospective assessments of selected regulatory impact analyses should be carried out periodically.

*A core set of economic assumptions should be used in calculating benefits and costs. Key variables include the social discount rate, the value of reducing risks of premature death and accidents, and the values associated with other improvements in health.* It is important to be able to compare results across analyses, and a common set of economic assumptions increases the feasibility of such comparisons. In addition, a common set of appropriate economic assumptions can improve the quality of individual analyses. A single agency should establish a set of default values for typical benefits and costs and should develop a standard format for presenting results.

*Although benefit-cost analysis should focus primarily on the overall relation between benefits and costs, a good analysis will also identify important distributional consequences.* Available data often permit reliable estimation of major policy impacts on important subgroups of the population. On the other hand, environmental, health, and safety regulations are neither effective nor efficient tools for achieving redistributional goals.

*Conclusion.* Benefit-cost analysis can play an important role in legislative and regulatory policy debates on protecting and improving health, safety, and the natural environment. Although formal benefit-cost analysis should not be viewed as either necessary or sufficient for designing sensible public policy, it can provide an exceptionally useful framework for consistently organizing disparate information, and in this way, it can greatly improve the process and, hence, the outcome of policy analysis.

* * * * *

Whenever government regulates to promote health and prevent injury and disease, it almost inevitably interferes with personal liberty and economic freedom. There are various methods to assess whether the collective goods to be achieved are worth the burdens and costs, and various forms of reasoning, including philosophical inquiry, risk assessment, and cost-effectiveness analysis, may be employed.

Having examined public health, ethics, human rights, and various forms of reasoning in Part One, Part Two turns to a careful examination of public health law. One can examine the field of public health through a number of legal lenses. Part Two uses the lens of the Constitution, which covers public health powers, duties, and limits; administrative law, which covers direct regulation of persons and property by public health agencies; and tort law, which covers indirect regulation of individuals and businesses through the court system.

# The Law and the Public's Health

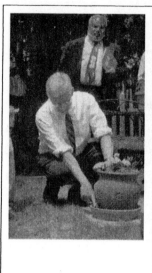
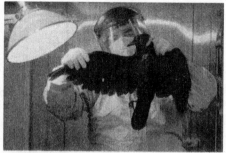
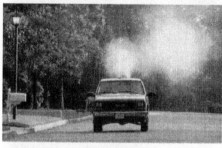
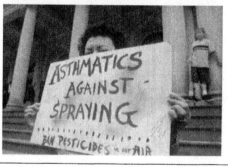

*Left:* During a press conference on preventing West Nile virus on June 21, 2000, Maryland Governor Parris Glendening points to a flowerpot that has collected stagnant water. He recommends that people empty containers filled with standing water to lower the mosquito count and reduce the risk of contracting the virus. (Mary Carty, AP/Wide World Photos, 6/21/00.) *Top right:* Ward B. Stone, a New York state wildlife pathologist, examines a dead crow for signs of West Nile encephalitis virus at his lab in Delmar, New York, on November 13, 1999. Stone received boxes of dead crows from veterinarians around the region. (David Jennings, AP/Wide World Photos, 11/13/99.) *Center right:* A Suffolk County Department of Vector Control truck sprays mosquito insecticide in Shirley, New York, on July 17, 2000, to prevent the spread of West Nile virus. (Ed Betz, AP/Wide World Photos, 7/17/00.) *Bottom right:* On the steps of New York City Hall on July 27, 2000, Tullia Limarzi, of Staten Island, protests the spraying of insecticide to kill mosquitoes carrying West Nile virus. (Kathy Willens, AP/Wide World Photos, 7/27/00.)

# SIX

# Public Health
# Duties and Powers

The United States Constitution provides the framework for the distribution of governmental power. It divides power between the federal government and the states (federalism), separates power among the three branches of government ("separation of powers"), and limits governmental power over individuals to protect a sphere of liberty (see Figure 10). Federal and state public health agencies carry out public health functions within these constitutional boundaries. Governmental actors must use their power to protect and promote public health according to the constitutional design and within the scope of legislative mandates. When disputes regarding governmental powers arise, courts often determine the lawfulness of particular public health interventions.

In thinking about government intervention to promote the common good, at least three important questions should be asked: (1) Does government have a *duty* to protect the public's health and safety? (2) What *power* does government have to regulate in the name of public health? (3) What *limits* exist in the exercise of public health powers? These three issues—governmental duties, powers, and limits—are central to understanding the role of public health authorities in the constitutional design. The readings in this chapter examine government's duty and power and also explore a corollary question: Which government—federal or state—may act to avert a health threat? The next chapter evaluates constitutional restraints on the exercise of public health power.

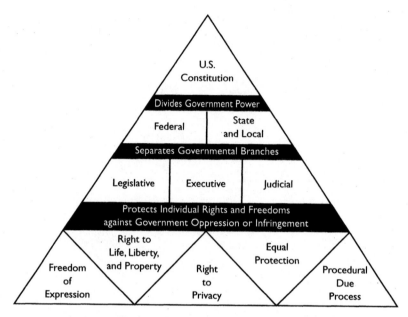

Figure 10.   Constitutional triangle.

First, the readings in this chapter offer historical and modern-day perspectives on the duties of government to safeguard the public's health. Second, the readings explore federal public health powers, principally the authority to tax and spend and to regulate interstate commerce. Third, the readings examine state public health powers, principally the police power to defend the public's health, safety, and morals. The chapter concludes with cases and materials that discuss the balance of power between the federal government and the states in our federalist system. The case holdings contain important implications for the limits on public health powers exercisable by the federal government—a concept known as "new federalism."

## I. GOVERNMENT'S DUTY
## TO PROMOTE THE PUBLIC'S HEALTH

Conventional wisdom holds that the Constitution places no affirmative duty on the government to protect individuals from harm or to promote the common good. Under this view, the Constitution is purely "negative" or "defensive" in character, protecting individuals against government's overreaching; it provides no positive obligation on government to act. Wendy Parmet, an influential public health law scholar at Northeastern University, questions this conventional position. She looks back to colonial times for a view of the state's affirmative duty to protect the public's health. Parmet provides a theory of the responsibility that government assumed for public health at the time of the framing of the Constitution and applies that theory to modern public health practice. She suggests that protection from infectious diseases was so important to our ancestors that government's duty to prevent epidemics was virtually assumed. It will become clear when reading the *DeShaney* case, which follows the Parmet article, that the Supreme Court has a very different understanding of the Constitution.

## Health Care and the Constitution: Public Health and the Role of the State in the Framing Era*
*Wendy Parmet*

### HEALTH AND GOVERNMENTS: BACKGROUND UNDERSTANDINGS

Current legal analysis assumes that the relationship between individual and state is primarily negative. The Constitution imposes no obligation upon government to protect the public health. Instead, the Constitution's role is to empower government while, at the same time, limiting its ability to impinge upon individual interests. Under constitutional theory, public goals play a role only indirectly in determining whether governmental restraints upon individuals are justified by the weight of the public interest at stake. Public goals do not form the basis of public duties. Under this view, the dilemma for judicial review is how to justify limits placed upon majoritarian policies for the protection of individual rights.

This conventional view presupposes that the role of law and legal rights is to restrain governmental action. It also assumes that individual liberty is prior to law. Whatever the general merit of this conceptualization of rights and law, in the context of health care it overlooks two fundamental facts. First, if liberty is prior to states, so is mortality. Disease, injury, and threats to health constrain freedom without the

*Reprinted from *Hastings Constitutional Law Quarterly* (Winter 1992): 267–335.

help of any state, although states can surely exacerbate such dangers. Thus, there is no ideal state of nature in which the only threat to freedom is the one libertarians identify: aggression towards property. Rather, any hypothetical state of nature would have to include dangers and threats to liberty posed by the inevitability of disease. Second, whatever the theoretical role of the law, it has always had to deal with the constraints imposed by disease and mortality. Law has always had to respond to the constraints imposed by disease. Governments typically have assumed an active role with respect to health care, acting as if their role were obligatory. . . .

## PUBLIC HEALTH LAW AND
## THE POLITICAL THEORY OF THE FRAMERS

### Public Health as a Common Good

The eighteenth century belief in government's compact obligation to fulfill the common good is consistent with the pattern of regulation and provision evident in colonial and early federalist public health regulations. More fundamentally, it suggests that the framing generation may have seen the duty to protect health as stemming from the social or governmental contract in which individual and state were related by mutual obligations.

Although social contract theorists, and the framing generation in general, spoke often about the public good, the common weal, and the general welfare, they provided remarkably little elucidation of those phrases. . . . While everyone might have agreed about the government's obligation to protect the public good, they often disagreed about exactly what that meant. To Locke (1690), the concept was ultimately individualistic. Individuals agree to leave the state of nature "for the mutual Preservation of their Lives, Liberties and Estates, which I call by the general Name Property." Jefferson, echoing that language, saw preservation of "life, liberty and the pursuit of happiness" as the goal of government. Madison saw the preservation of property as among the primary reasons for having government. He may have seen that goal as largely instrumental, however, since he believed that the preservation of property was essential to maintaining the ability of government to achieve the common good.

Despite the disagreement and uncertainty over the actual meaning of "the common good," it seems likely that the preservation of public health, as exemplified by protection against epidemics, was one meaning that all would share. Tradition and practice pointed to it. Theorists such as Montesquieu supported it. So did popular political discourse. According to historian Ronald Peters (1978), "the answer of the literature is unequivocal on this point: the only end of civil society is the common good. And the sine qua non of the common good is public safety—*salus populi suprem lex est.*" In an era of frequent epidemics, safety meant more than protection from foes—it likely included, or was often associated with, preservation of health.

The equation of public health with safety, and thereby with the common good, did not necessarily derive from any heightened sense of altruism. To say that the framing generation believed that the social contract obligated government to protect the public's health and to provide care to the ill is not to say that they were utopians or even humanitarians. Many in the framing generation supported slavery. They also held negative views about the indigent. . . . It was, therefore, not altruism that caused public health to be part of the common good, but a tradition motivated by the pragmatism and pessimism derived from the insecurity of life in a preindustrial age.

In an era of frequent epidemics, when an increasing number of physicians thought disease stemmed either from accumulated filth in public places or from contagion, . . . public health protection constituted a core element of the common good. The idea commonly held today that health is a matter of individual life style choices and treatments determined privately by patients and physicians would have seemed insufficient in the eighteenth century. Government always had attempted to protect public health, and it always would. Whether one endorsed a republican theory of communal virtue or a liberal theory of self-interest, pragmatism compelled the same conclusion. Public health was a prerequisite to public safety. It constituted a part of the common good. As a result, under social contract theory, government was not only entitled, but also obligated, to protect public health.

The different schools of thought would have framed the issue from different theoretical perspectives. Those influenced by classical republican thought accepted communal obligations and their primacy over individual rights. With such a view, in a time of repeated epidemics which could regularly kill a large percentage of the population, protection of public health fit easily within understanding of the public good. Moreover, the classical republican emphasis on self-government would also have pointed to a further relationship between the public health and the common good. As the framing generation knew only too well, self-government becomes

insecure under the threat of epidemics. Colonial history, in which governments repeatedly had to adjourn in the face of epidemics, would have suggested to the Framers the dangers disease posed to self-rule. . . . Public
health, therefore, would have been a necessary part of the common good
because it was a precondition to maintaining the republic wherein that
good could flourish. . . .

In a time of frequent epidemics, the preservation of self and property
almost inevitably would have been seen as requiring public efforts to
prevent the spread of disease. As individuals came into contact with
each other, as commerce and population grew, epidemics developed. Individuals faced death, commerce was destroyed, and property was
threatened. The preservation of individual interests thus necessarily required efforts to prevent disease. Whether contagionist or sanitarian,
pragmatism—not benevolence—ultimately required the care of those
who could not afford to care for themselves. Without provision for the
poor, including their treatment during times of illness, and steps such as
inoculation designed to prevent illness, other individual interests would
have remained insecure. Thus, individual preservation was inextricably
linked to public health policies. . . .

## SOCIAL CONTRACT THEORY AND PUBLIC HEALTH PROTECTION

Social contract theory, in both its individualistic and republican forms,
[assumed] . . . that the public good required the protection of health.
As a result, the state was not only empowered to protect the public's
health, but was obligated to do so, at least under natural, if not positive, law. A government that failed to protect health violated the terms
of its compact and had no right to expect obedience. A government's
authority was a function of its fulfillment of its duties.

Under social contract theory, individuals gave obedience or consent
to society on the understanding that they would receive protection from
it. Far from endorsing a *laissez faire* understanding of the relationship
between individual and state, as is often mistakenly assumed, social
contract theory in its eighteenth century form actually assumed a re-
ciprocal relationship between individual rights and governmental duties. . . .

In society, as opposed to the state of nature, individuals did not have
unlimited or absolute control over themselves or their property. Their
rights were necessarily limited by social obligation. This fully accorded
with the common law's understanding of property, especially the law of
nuisance which limited property rights in the public interest. It also ac-

corded with the experiences of a mercantilist society in which regulation, not free enterprise, was the norm. Most importantly, this view of rights would have been compatible with the era's public health practices, which limited and even impounded property in order to protect the public health. The framing generation would have had no reason to see a conflict between rights of property and public health protection. Even opponents of redistribution, such as Madison, would not have seen public health measures as redistributive.

To Locke and the Framers, the social compact was a way of theoretically delineating the necessary relationship between individual, society, and the state. Individual rights were curtailed not because they were not recognized or respected, but only because they were ultimately to be realized by achieving the common good which government was obligated by compact to fulfill. As a result, the sharp distinction that exists under modern doctrine between positive and negative rights could not have existed in the framing era with respect to public health care. . . .

Thus, the pattern of colonial and early federalist public health laws accords with the understanding of rights and liberties, obligations and duties, prevailing at the time of the Constitution's framing. Governments were not only empowered to protect the public health, but were expected to do so. When crises occurred, they were expected to act. Their authority to do so was unquestioned. Individual rights of property, travel, and even access to one's home gave way before the public health power. Those restraints were not seen as violations of individual liberties, as we might see them today. Rather, they were part and parcel of the relationship under the social or governmental contract: a construct which gave society a claim upon individuals only in return for the fulfillment of its obligation to provide care and protection. Thus, when ships arrived from plague-infested ports, they could be quarantined. Homes could be impounded; privies regulated. When individuals were sick, they were cared for. When they could not afford care, it was usually provided. As members of the society, individuals lacked absolute rights; instead, they received the benefits of the epidemics or plagues that were prevented by the authority of government acting to preserve the common good. . . .

My conclusion that the framing generation assumed a governmental obligation to protect the public is compatible with the practice and theory of the time. A mystery, however, remains. Why does the Constitution not simply say "the government is obligated to protect the health of citizens?" The answer to that question may lie in the self-evident nature of the public health obligation from the Framers' perspective. The duty was not controversial and was not a subject of debate. States and local governments acted to protect the public health. Their authority and obligation to do so was not on the table.

Recognition of the Framers' views about the public health obligation casts into question the conventional assumptions that underpin constitutional health law. Much of contemporary constitutional law is predicated on the constitutional tradition of *laissez faire*, providing only negative rights. Existing doctrine presupposes that the starting point or baseline of analysis is that government has no obligations at all. Constitutional rights are predominantly negative: limiting the scope of governmental authority and preserving individual freedom.

An examination of the public health activities and social contract theories . . . demonstrates that while *laissez faire* may or may not be an appropriate ideal, it was not our nation's historical starting point. Contrary to the perceived history, active government did not emerge for the first time during the Progressive and New Deal eras. In the area of public health, government was highly active long before the framing of the Constitution. The public health status quo of 1787 was a regulatory one, supported by the prevailing political theories and even by the early liberalism of the era. The age of *laissez faire* came later, if at all. . . .

[Public health jurisprudence] bring[s] into sharp focus the very reasons for having governments and law: to care for and protect each other, as best we can, without intruding too gravely upon the autonomy of each. By forgetting what the framing generation understood—that our own health is ultimately dependent on the care we give each other—we threaten the legitimacy of the state, and, in the final analysis, of our laws.

---

\*     \*     \*     \*     \*

The tragic case of Joshua DeShaney, a victim of child abuse, sets the backdrop for a landmark Supreme Court decision that limits the responsibility of government to protect the health of citizens. Georgetown law professors Louis M. Seidman and Mark V. Tushnet (1996, 52) describe the facts of the *DeShaney* case as follows:

> In Joshua DeShaney's first year of life, his parents divorced, and a court granted custody of the infant to his father, Randy DeShaney. For the next

four years, the child lived through a nightmare of pain and violence. Randy DeShaney beat his son repeatedly and with increasing savagery. Eventually, the toddler fell into a life-threatening coma, and emergency brain surgery revealed injuries, inflicted over an extended period, that left Joshua permanently and severely retarded.

As these tragic events unfolded, many of them came to the attention of county officials in the Wisconsin community where the DeShaneys lived. A battery of judges, lawyers, pediatricians, psychologists, police officers, and social workers became involved in Joshua's case. With Kafkaesque efficiency, these functionaries performed their particular assigned task within the social welfare bureaucracy. They held hearings, filed reports, completed forms. Yet despite all the purposeful bustling and the show of activity and concern, no one actually intervened to stop the violence until it was too late.

After the damage had already been done, Joshua and his mother filed an action against [Winnebago] county in United States District Court. They argued that county officials had deprived Joshua of his liberty without due process of law, thereby violating his rights under the Fourteenth Amendment.

If government officials had beaten Joshua themselves, his suit—even against their employers—might well have succeeded. Supreme Court decisions have made it clear that government agents who unjustifiably inflict physical injury violate the Due Process Clause. But because Joshua and his mother could not claim that the injury was directly inflicted by state officials, the suit foundered on the so-called "state action" requirement.

The Supreme Court's decision expresses a vision of a "negative" constitution where the judiciary is highly reluctant to impose on government an affirmative duty to safeguard the well-being of its citizens. The dissenting opinion of Justice Harry A. Blackmun conveys an alternative view of the constitutional obligation to protect vulnerable citizens. This dissent also expresses a sense of moral outrage at the notion that government cannot be held accountable for a failure to act in the interest of a citizen's health. As Blackmun said, simply, "Poor Joshua."

When reading *DeShaney*, consider whether the history and text genuinely support the view that the Constitution rarely imposes a responsibility on government to protect individuals and populations. Even if the Constitution imposes no affirmative obligations, is there a reason, based on principle, for the distinction between government's acts and omissions? Suppose a public health department, knowing there is a high risk of an infectious disease outbreak, does nothing to inform the public or intervene. Should the agency's failure to prevent the outbreak be actionable under the due process clause of the Fourteenth Amendment? Finally, if government does act to establish a protective agency (e.g., child welfare or public health), should citizens reasonably be able to rely on that agency to safeguard their health and safety?

---

### DeShaney v. Winnebago
### County Department of Social Services*
*Supreme Court of the United States*
*Decided February 22, 1989*

Chief Justice REHNQUIST delivered the opinion of the Court.

Petitioner [Joshua DeShaney] sued respondents [Winnebago County social workers and other officials] claiming that their failure to act deprived him of his liberty in violation of the Due Process Clause of the Fourteenth Amendment to the United States Constitution. We hold that it did not. . . .

The Due Process Clause of the Fourteenth Amendment provides that "[n]o State shall . . . deprive any person of life, liberty, or property, without due process of law." Petitioners contend that the State deprived Joshua of his liberty interest in "free[dom] from . . . unjustified intrusions on personal security," *Ingraham v. Wright,* 430 U.S. 651, 673 (1977), by failing to provide him with adequate protection against his father's violence. The claim is one invoking the substantive rather than the procedural component of the Due Process Clause; petitioners do not claim that the State denied Joshua protection without according him appropriate procedural safeguards, but that it was categorically obligated to protect him in these circumstances. . . .

[N]othing in the language of the Due Process Clause itself requires the State to protect the life, liberty, and property of its citizens against invasion by private actors. The Clause is phrased as a limitation on the State's power to act, not as a guarantee of certain minimal levels of safety and security. It forbids the State itself to deprive individuals of life, liberty, or property without "due process of law," but its language cannot fairly be extended to impose an affirmative obligation on the State to ensure that those interests do not come to harm through other means. Nor does history support such an expansive reading of the con-

---

*489 U.S. 189 (1989).

stitutional text. Like its counterpart in the Fifth Amendment, the Due Process Clause of the Fourteenth Amendment was intended to prevent government "from abusing [its] power, or employing it as an instrument of oppression," *Davidson v. Cannon,* 474 U.S. 344, 348 (1986). . . . Its purpose was to protect the people from the State, not to ensure that the State protected them from each other. The Framers were content to leave the extent of governmental obligation in the latter area to the democratic political processes.

Consistent with these principles, our cases have recognized that the Due Process Clause generally confers no affirmative right to governmental aid, even where such aid may be necessary to secure life, liberty, or property interests of which the government itself may not deprive the individual. . . . As we said in *Harris v. McRae:* "Although the liberty protected by the Due Process Clause affords protection against unwarranted government interference . . . , it does not confer an entitlement to such [governmental aid] as may be necessary to realize all the advantages of that freedom." 448 U.S. 297, 317–18 (1980). If the Due Process Clause does not require the State to provide its citizens with particular protective services, it follows that the State cannot be held liable under the Clause for injuries that could have been averted had it chosen to provide them. As a general matter, then, we conclude that a State's failure to protect an individual against private violence simply does not constitute a violation of the Due Process Clause.

Petitioners contend, however, that even if the Due Process Clause imposes no affirmative obligation on the State to provide the general public with adequate protective services, such a duty may arise out of certain "special relationships" created or assumed by the State with respect to particular individuals. Petitioners argue that such a "special relationship" existed here because the State knew that Joshua faced a special danger of abuse at his father's hands, and specifically proclaimed, by word and by deed, its intention to protect him against that danger. Having actually undertaken to protect Joshua from this danger—which petitioners concede the State played no part in creating—the State acquired an affirmative "duty," enforceable through the Due Process Clause, to do so in a reasonably competent fashion. Its failure to discharge that duty, so the argument goes, was an abuse of governmental power that so "shocks the conscience," *Rochin v. California,* 342 U.S. 165 (1952), as to constitute a substantive due process violation.

We reject this argument. It is true that in certain limited circumstances the Constitution imposes upon the State affirmative duties of care and protection with respect to particular individuals. In *Estelle v. Gamble*, 429 U.S. 97 (1976), we recognized that the Eighth Amendment's prohibition against cruel and unusual punishment, made applicable to the States through the Fourteenth Amendment's Due Process Clause, requires the State to provide adequate medical care to incarcerated prisoners. We reasoned that because the prisoner is unable "by reason of the deprivation of his liberty [to] care for himself," it is only "just" that the State be required to care for him. 429 U.S. at 103–04.

In *Youngberg v. Romeo*, 457 U.S. 307 (1982), we extended this analysis beyond the Eighth Amendment setting, holding that the substantive component of the Fourteenth Amendment's Due Process Clause requires the State to provide involuntarily committed mental patients with such services as are necessary to ensure their "reasonable safety" from themselves and others. . . .

Taken together, [these cases] stand only for the proposition that when the State takes a person into its custody and holds him there against his will, the Constitution imposes upon it a corresponding duty to assume some responsibility for his safety and general well-being. . . . [W]hen the State by the affirmative exercise of its power so restrains an individual's liberty that it renders him unable to care for himself, and at the same time fails to provide for his basic human needs—*e.g.*, food, clothing, shelter, medical care, and reasonable safety—it transgresses the substantive limits on state action set by the Eighth Amendment and the Due Process Clause. The affirmative duty to protect arises . . . from the limitation which it has imposed on his freedom to act on his own behalf. In the substantive due process analysis, it is the State's affirmative act of restraining the individual's freedom to act on his own behalf—through incarceration, institutionalization, or other similar restraint of personal liberty—which is the "deprivation of liberty" triggering the protections of the Due Process Clause, not its failure to act to protect his liberty interests against harms inflicted by other means. . . .

[This] analysis simply has no applicability in the present case. Petitioners concede that the harms Joshua suffered occurred . . . while he was in the custody of his natural father, who was in no sense a state actor. While the State may have been aware of the dangers that Joshua faced in the free world, it played no part in their creation, nor did it do anything to render him any more vulnerable to them. That the State once took temporary custody of Joshua does not alter the analysis, for when it returned him to his father's custody, it placed him in no worse position than that in which he would have been had it not acted at all; the State does not become the permanent guarantor of an individual's safety by having once offered him shelter. Under these circumstances, the State had no constitutional duty to protect Joshua . . . [and] its failure to do so—though calamitous in hindsight—simply does not constitute a violation of the Due Process Clause.

Judges and lawyers, like other humans, are moved by natural sympathy in a case like this to find a way for Joshua and his mother to receive adequate compensation for the grievous harm inflicted upon them. But before yielding to that impulse, it is well to remember once again that the harm was inflicted not by the State of Wisconsin, but by Joshua's father. The most that can be said of the state functionaries in this case is that they stood by and did nothing when suspicious circumstances dictated a more active role for them. In defense of them it must also be said that had they moved too soon to take custody of the son away from the father, they would likely have been met with charges of improperly intruding into the parent-child relationship, charges based on the same Due Process Clause that forms the basis for the present charge of failure to provide adequate protection.

The people of Wisconsin may well prefer a system of liability which would place upon the State and its officials the responsibility for failure to act in situations such as the present one. They may create such a system, if they do not have it already, by changing the tort law of the State in accordance with the regular lawmaking process. But they should not have it thrust upon them by this Court's expansion of the Due Process Clause of the Fourteenth Amendment.

Affirmed.

Justice BLACKMUN, dissenting.

Today, the Court purports to be the dispassionate oracle of the law, unmoved by "natural sympathy." But, in this pretense, the Court itself retreats into a sterile formalism which prevents it from recognizing either the facts of the case before it or the legal norms that should apply to those facts. As Justice Brennan demonstrates, the facts here involve not mere passivity, but active state intervention in the life of Joshua DeShaney— intervention that triggered a fundamental duty to aid the boy once the State learned of the severe danger to which he was exposed.

The Court fails to recognize this duty because it attempts to draw a sharp and rigid line between action and inaction. But such formalistic reasoning has no place in the interpretation of the broad and stirring Clauses of the Fourteenth Amendment. Indeed, I submit that these Clauses were designed, at least in part, to undo the formalistic legal reasoning that infected antebellum jurisprudence.

Like the antebellum judges who denied relief to fugitive slaves, the Court today claims that its decision, however harsh, is compelled by existing legal doctrine. On the contrary, the question presented by this case is an open one, and our Fourteenth Amendment precedents may be read more broadly or narrowly depending upon how one chooses to read them. Faced with the choice, I would adopt a "sympathetic" reading, one which comports with dictates of fundamental justice and recognizes that compassion need not be exiled from the province of judging.

Poor Joshua! Victim of repeated attacks by an irresponsible, bullying, cowardly, and intemperate father, and abandoned by respondents who placed him in a dangerous predicament and who knew or learned what was going on, and yet did essentially nothing except, as the Court revealingly observes, "dutifully recorded these incidents in [their] files." It is a sad commentary upon American life, and constitutional principles—so full of late of patriotic fervor and proud proclamations about "liberty and justice for all"—that this child, Joshua DeShaney, now is assigned to live out the remainder of his life profoundly retarded. Joshua and his mother, as petitioners here, deserve—but now are denied by this Court—the opportunity to have the facts of their case considered in the light of . . . constitutional protection.

---

## II. FEDERAL PUBLIC HEALTH POWERS

Although the Supreme Court has been loath to find affirmative constitutional obligations to protect individuals and the public, it certainly has upheld a wide range of public health powers. The readings in the remaining part of this chapter explore public health powers—at the federal and state levels.

The national government has only those powers expressly enumerated in the Constitution. The foremost powers for public health purposes are the power to tax and spend for the general welfare and to regulate interstate commerce. These powers provide Congress with independent authority to raise revenue for public health services and to regulate, both directly and indirectly, private activities that endanger the public's health. The Constitution also affords Congress additional powers. For example, Congress has the power to enforce the civil rights amendments passed during the Reconstruction era (the Thirteenth, Fourteenth, and Fifteenth Amendments); and it has the power to "promote the Progress of Science" by securing inventors the exclusive right to their discoveries through the granting of patents (U.S. CONST. art. I, § 8, cl. 8).

The "necessary and proper" clause in Article I, Section 8 of the Constitution permits Congress to employ all means reasonably appropriate to achieve the objectives of enumerated national powers. Chief Justice John Marshall's famous remark in *McCulloch v. Maryland,* 17 U.S. (4 Wheat.) 316, 421 (1819), illustrates the potentially expansive powers of Congress: "Let the end be legitimate, let it be within the scope of the constitution, and all means which are appropriate, which are plainly adapted to that end, which are not prohibited, but consistent with the letter and spirit of the constitution, are constitutional."

This "implied powers" doctrine has enabled the national government to expand into public health regulation, traditionally a state-level responsibility. Federal regulation now reaches broad aspects of public health such as air and water quality, food and drug safety, pesticide production and sales, consumer product safety, occupational health and safety, and medical care.

American federalism, then, provides the federal government with enumerated powers that the Supreme Court has, until recently, construed liberally. James G. Hodge, Jr. (1997), of the Center for Law and the Public's Health at Georgetown and Johns Hopkins Universities, explains the distribution of powers among the national government and the states (for a discussion of federalism in the context of environmental regulation, see Steinzor [2000]):

> In the context of public health, the federal Constitution "acts as both a fountain and a levee. It controls the flow of governmental power between state and federal governments to preserve the public health, and subsequently curbs that power to protect individual freedoms" (Areen, King, Goldberg, and Gostin 1996, 520). If the Constitution is a fountain from which powers flow to the states, federalism represents the partition in the pool from which the states' fountain draws [see Figure 3 in the companion text]. It divides the available pool of legislative power into two segments of

government, national and state. As a principle of law and governmental design, American federalism preserves a constitutional balance of power between state and national authorities.

In practice, federalism distinguishes between the powers exercised by federal and state governments. The federal government has those limited powers granted pursuant to the . . . Constitution, including the power to enact laws in its jurisdiction. The remaining sovereign powers of government are reserved to the states via the Tenth Amendment. . . . [T]hese powers, collectively known as police powers, allow states to broadly regulate matters affecting the health, safety, and general welfare of the public. They are the original and primary authority of government to regulate matters that affect the public health. . . .

Federalism requires us to ask which level of government has the responsibility for passing, enforcing, and adjudicating which public health laws. The answer is not an absolute. Federal and state governments can share jurisdiction in the field. Yet where federal and state powers intersect, struggles over the exercise of limited governmental powers occur. The resolution of such disputes is uniquely within the province of federalism. States' traditional [abilities] to control and maintain public health remain contingent on the scope of their police powers, and the extent of federal intrusion. This, in turn, depends on the emphasis placed on federalism: when enforced, federalism protects police powers of the states by curbing federal infringements on such powers. It simultaneously restricts the federal government's ability to regulate in the interests of public health, since such regulation traditionally has been the responsibility of state governments. In the balance of these observations rest the very goals of public health that rely on the interpretation of federalism.

Having discussed federalism generally, it will be helpful to explore three important aspects of national power: federal preemption, Congress's power to tax and spend, and Congress's power to regulate interstate commerce.

## A.  FEDERAL PREEMPTION:
### THE POWER TO SUPERSEDE STATE REGULATION

Conflicts between national and state regulation (assuming that national power is exercised validly) are resolved in favor of the federal government because federal law is supreme. The supremacy clause declares that the "Constitution, and the Laws of the United States . . . and all Treaties made . . . shall be the supreme law of the Land" (U.S. CONST. art. VI). Federal preemption occurs in many aspects of public health regulation.

The Supreme Court in 2000–2001 issued three decisions on preemption, demonstrating the powerful effects of federal supremacy over state public health regulation. In *Geier v. American Honda Motor Co., Inc.,* 529

U.S. 861 (2000), Alexis Geier sought damages under District of Columbia tort law for injuries he incurred in a crash while driving a 1987 Honda Accord that did not have an airbag. Pursuant to its authority under the National Traffic and Motor Vehicle Safety Act of 1966, the Department of Transportation required automobile manufacturers to equip some, but not all, of their 1987 vehicles with passive restraints. The Supreme Court held that the Act preempts a state common law tort action in which the plaintiff claims that the auto manufacturer, who was in compliance with the standard, should nonetheless have equipped the car with airbags. The Court reasoned that the "no airbag" lawsuit conflicts with the objectives of the federal law. The Court in *Geier* stressed that the key concern is whether imposing state tort liability will conflict with the federal scheme.

In *Lorillard Tobacco Co. v. Reilly,* 121 S. Ct. 2404 (2001) (posted on the *Reader* web site), manufacturers and sellers challenged Massachusetts regulations restricting the sale, promotion, and labeling of tobacco products. The Court held that the portion of the regulations governing outdoor and point-of-sale cigarette advertising were preempted by the Federal Cigarette Labeling and Advertising Act (FCLAA). The FCLAA prescribes mandatory health warnings for cigarette packaging and advertising. Its preemption provision prohibits (1) requiring cigarette packages to bear any "statement relating to smoking and health" (other than required health warnings) and (2) any "requirement or prohibition based on smoking and health . . . imposed under state law with respect to the advertising or promotion of [cigarettes]." The Court said that Massachusetts's argument that the regulations are not "based on smoking and health" since they do not involve health-related content, but instead target youth exposure to cigarette advertising, is unpersuasive. At bottom, the youth exposure concern is intertwined with the smoking and health concern. 121 S. Ct. at 2417–18. (For a discussion of the commercial speech aspects of *Lorillard,* see chapter 11.)

Finally, in *Buckman Co. v. Plaintiff's Legal Committee,* 531 U.S. 341 (2001), the Court held that state common law claims asserting that a medical device manufacturer committed fraud on the Food and Drug Administration (FDA) conflicts with the FDA's statutory responsibility to police fraud in its regulatory role. The tort action, therefore, was impliedly preempted by the Medical Device Amendments to the Food, Drug, and Cosmetic Act.

*Geier, Lorillard,* and *Buckman* demonstrate the potentially broad sweep of federal supremacy that enables Congress to override state regulation to promote the public's health.

## B. THE POWER TO TAX AND SPEND IS THE POWER TO INFLUENCE STATE AND PRIVATE BEHAVIOR

The power to tax and spend is found in the constitutional phrase: "Congress shall have Power To lay and collect Taxes, Duties, Imposts and Excises, to pay the Debts and provide for the common Defence and general Welfare of the United States" (art. I, § 8, cl. 1). On its face, the power to tax and spend has a single, overriding purpose: to raise revenue to provide for the good of the community, including services such as medical care to the poor, sanitation, and environmental protection. The taxing and spending power, while affording government the financial resources to provide services, has another, equally important purpose. The power to tax and spend is also the authority to regulate risk behavior and influence health-promoting activities. Through its taxing powers, government can create incentives to engage in beneficial activities (e.g., employer-sponsored health plans) or disincentives to engage in risk behaviors (e.g., smoking cigarettes). Alternatively, by setting "conditions" on the granting of funds, the United States can induce states to adopt federal regulatory standards.

The spending power has been challenged by states claiming that, when used inappropriately, the federal government coerces states and violates state sovereignty. This issue came before the Supreme Court in *South Dakota v. Dole*, which addressed the federal government's ability to encourage states to raise the minimum drinking age by setting conditions on the receipt of federal highway funds. *Dole* illustrates the Supreme Court's permissive view of the conditional spending power used to achieve a public health objective. However, the scope of Congress's spending power is being challenged in the lower courts (see discussion of the spending power and sovereign immunity later in this chapter).

---

### South Dakota v. Dole*

*Supreme Court of the United States*
*Decided June 23, 1987*

Chief Justice REHNQUIST delivered the opinion of the Court.

[In South Dakota, persons nineteen years of age or older are permitted to purchase beer containing up to 3.2 percent alcohol. Title 23

---

*483 U.S. 203 (1987).

U.S.C. § 158 directs the Secretary of Transportation to withhold federal highway funds from states that allow persons under the age of twenty-one years to purchase and possess alcohol. The State of South Dakota argues that § 158 violates the constitutional limitations on congressional spending power under Article I, Section 8, Clause 1 (tax-and-spend power) of the Constitution and violates the Tenth Amendment (among other constitutional arguments)].

Incident to [the tax-and-spend power], Congress may attach conditions on the receipt of federal funds, and has repeatedly employed the power "to further broad policy objectives by conditioning receipt of federal moneys upon compliance by the recipient with federal statutory and administrative directives." Fullilove v. Klutznick, 448 U.S. 448, 474 (1980). . . . [Even those] objectives not thought to be within Article I's "enumerated legislative fields" may nevertheless be attained through the use of the spending power and the conditional grant of federal funds.

The spending power is of course not unlimited, but is instead subject to several general restrictions articulated in our cases. The first of these limitations is derived from the language of the Constitution itself: the exercise of the spending power must be in pursuit of "the general welfare." In considering whether a particular expenditure is intended to serve general public purposes, courts should defer substantially to the judgment of Congress. Second, we have required that if Congress desires to condition the States' receipt of federal funds, it "must do so unambiguously . . . , enabl[ing] the States to exercise their choice knowingly, cognizant of the consequences of their participation." Pennhurst State Sch. and Hosp. v. Halderman, 451 U.S. 1, 17 (1981). Third, our cases have suggested (without significant elaboration) that conditions on federal grants might be illegitimate if they are unrelated "to the federal interest in particular national projects or programs." Massachusetts v. United States, 435 U.S. 444, 461 (1978) (plurality opinion). . . .

South Dakota does not seriously claim that § 158 is inconsistent with any of the first three restrictions mentioned above. We can readily conclude that the provision is designed to serve the general welfare, especially in light of the fact that "the concept of welfare or the opposite is shaped by Congress. . . ." Helvering v. Davis, 301 U.S. 619, 645 (1937). Congress found that the differing drinking ages in the States created particular incentives for young persons to combine their desire to drink with their ability to drive, and that this interstate problem required a national solution. The means it chose to address this dangerous situation were reasonably calculated to advance the general welfare. The conditions upon which States receive the funds, moreover, could not be more clearly stated by Congress. And the State itself, rather than challenging the germaneness of the condition to federal purposes, admits that it "has never contended that the congressional action was . . . unrelated to a national concern in the absence of the Twenty-first Amendment" (Brief for Petitioner, 6). Indeed, the condition imposed by Congress is directly related to one of the main purposes for which highway funds are expended—safe interstate travel. This goal of the interstate highway system had been frustrated by varying drinking ages among the States. A Presidential commission appointed to study alcohol-related accidents and fatalities on the Nation's highways concluded that the lack of uniformity in the States' drinking ages created "an incentive to drink and drive" because "young persons commut[e] to border States where the drinking age is lower." (Presidential Commission 1983, 11). By enacting § 158, Congress conditioned the receipt of federal funds in a way reasonably calculated to address this particular impediment to a purpose for which the funds are expended. . . .

We have also held that a perceived Tenth Amendment limitation on congressional regulation of state affairs did not concomitantly limit the range of conditions legitimately placed on federal grants. . . . [W]e think that . . . the [spending] power may not be used to induce the States to engage in activities that would themselves be unconstitutional. Thus, for example, a grant of federal funds conditioned on invidiously discriminatory state action or the infliction of cruel and unusual punishment would be an illegitimate exercise of the Congress's broad spending power. But no such claim can be or is made here. Were South Dakota to succumb to the blandishments offered by Congress and raise its drinking age to 21, the State's action in so doing would not violate the constitutional rights of anyone.

Our decisions have recognized that in some circumstances the financial inducement offered by Congress might be so coercive as to pass the point at which "pressure turns into compulsion." Steward Machine Co. v. Davis, 301 U.S. 548, 590 (1937). Here, however, Congress has directed only that a State desiring to establish a minimum drinking age lower than 21 lose a relatively small percentage of certain federal highway funds. Petitioner contends that the coercive nature of this program is evident from the degree of success it has achieved. We cannot conclude, however, that a conditional grant of federal money of this sort is unconstitutional simply by reason of its success in achieving the congressional objective.

When we consider, for a moment, that all South Dakota would lose if she adheres to her chosen course as to a suitable minimum drinking age is 5% of the funds otherwise obtainable under specified highway grant programs, the argument as to coercion is shown to be more rhetoric than fact. . . . Here Congress has offered relatively mild encouragement to the States to enact higher minimum drinking ages than they would otherwise choose. But the enactment of such laws remains the prerogative of the States not merely in theory but in fact. Even if Congress might lack the power to impose a national minimum drinking age directly, we conclude that encouragement to state action found in § 158 is a valid use of the spending power.

## C. CONTROLLING THE STREAM OF INTERSTATE COMMERCE IS THE POWER TO REGULATE

The commerce clause, more than any other enumerated power, affords Congress potent regulatory authority. Article I, Section 8, Clause 3 states that "[t]he Congress shall have the power . . . to regulate Commerce with foreign Nations, and among the several states, and with the Indian Tribes." Since Franklin Delano Roosevelt's New Deal era, the Supreme Court has interpreted the commerce clause broadly, giving Congress the ability to regulate in almost any area of activity as long as the activity has national effects. However, the Rehnquist Court has begun to rethink the breadth of commerce power, shifting regulatory authority back to the states for activities that are primarily intrastate. In *United States v. Lopez*, the Court was faced with a popular statute in which Congress had restricted gun possession in school zones. Chief Justice Rehnquist's opinion does not question the importance of firearm control as a legitimate public health function. Rather, he argues that controlling the mere possession of guns in schools is outside the sphere of federal commerce power.

In its 1999–2000 term, the Supreme Court struck down the private civil remedy provision of the Violence Against Women Act because it exceeded Congress's authority under the commerce clause. United States v. Morrison, 529 U.S. 598 (2000). The act created a civil rights remedy, permitting survivors to bring federal lawsuits against perpetrators of sexually motivated crimes of violence. Congress proclaimed that violence impairs women's abilities to work, harms businesses, and increases national health care costs. But the Court, reiterating its arguments in *Lopez,* found no national effects.

Similarly, in the Court's 2000–2001 term, Chief Justice Rehnquist declared that there were "significant constitutional questions" raised by a challenge to federal jurisdiction under the Clean Water Act. Solid Waste Agency of Northern Cook County v. United States Army Corps of Engineers, 531 U.S. 159 (2001) (posted on the *Reader* web site). The Army Corps of Engineers asserted jurisdiction over isolated wetlands, including seasonal ponds and small lakes that are not connected to navigable interstate waterways but serve as habitats for migratory birds. Although the Court ultimately avoided deciding on the commerce clause question, it reiterated its position that "the grant of authority to Congress under the commerce clause, though broad, is not unlimited." *Id.* at 173. (See further discussion of *Solid Waste* in chapter 8.)

---

### United States v. Lopez*
*Supreme Court of the United States*
*Decided April 26, 1995*

Chief Justice REHNQUIST delivered the opinion of the Court.

In the Gun-Free School Zones Act of 1990, Congress made it a federal offense "for any individual knowingly to possess a firearm at a place that the individual knows, or has reasonable cause to believe, is a school zone." 18 U.S.C. § 922(q)(1)(A) (1988 ed., Supp. V). The Act neither regulates a commercial activity nor contains a requirement that the possession be connected in any way to interstate commerce. We hold that the Act exceeds the authority of Congress "[t]o regulate Commerce . . . among the several States. . . ." U.S. CONST., art. I, § 8, cl. 3. . . .

[W]e have identified three broad categories of activity that Congress may regulate under its commerce power. First, Congress may regulate the use of the channels of interstate commerce. Second, Con-

---

*514 U.S. 549 (1995).

gress is empowered to regulate and protect the instrumentalities of interstate commerce, or persons or things in interstate commerce, even though the threat may come only from intrastate activities. Finally, Congress's commerce authority includes the power to regulate those activities having a substantial relation to interstate commerce, *i.e.*, those activities that substantially affect interstate commerce. . . .

Within this final category, admittedly, our case law has not been clear whether an activity must "affect" or "substantially affect" interstate commerce in order to be within Congress's power to regulate it under the Commerce Clause. We conclude, consistent with the great weight of our case law, that the proper test requires an analysis of whether the regulated activity "substantially affects" interstate commerce.

We now turn to consider the power of Congress, in the light of this framework, to enact § 922(q). The first two categories of authority may be quickly disposed of: § 922(q) is not a regulation of the use of the channels of interstate commerce, nor is it an attempt to prohibit the interstate transportation of a commodity through the channels of commerce; nor can § 922(q) be justified as a regulation by which Congress has sought to protect an instrumentality of interstate commerce or a thing in interstate commerce. Thus, if § 922(q) is to be sustained, it must be under the third category as a regulation of an activity that substantially affects interstate commerce. . . .

Section 922(q) is a criminal statute that by its terms has nothing to do with "commerce" or any sort of economic enterprise, however broadly one might define those terms. Section 922(q) is not an essential part of a larger regulation of economic activity, in which the regulatory scheme could be undercut unless the intrastate activity were regulated. It cannot, therefore, be sustained under our cases upholding regulations of activities that arise out of or are connected with a commercial transaction, which viewed in the aggregate, substantially affect interstate commerce.

Second, § 922(q) contains no jurisdictional element which would ensure, through case-by-case inquiry, that the firearm possession in question affects interstate commerce. . . .

The Government's essential contention . . . [is] that § 922(q) is valid because possession of a firearm in a local school zone does indeed substantially affect interstate commerce. The Government argues that possession of a firearm in a school zone may result in violent crime and that violent crime can be expected to affect the functioning of the national economy in two ways. First, the costs of violent crime are substantial, and, through the mechanism of insurance, those costs are spread throughout the population. Second, violent crime reduces the willingness of individuals to travel to areas within the country that are perceived to be unsafe. The Government also argues that the presence of guns in schools poses a substantial threat to the educational process by threatening the learning environment. A handicapped educational process, in turn, will result in a less productive citizenry. That, in turn, would have an adverse effect on the Nation's economic well-being. As a result, the Government argues that Congress could rationally have concluded that § 922(q) substantially affects interstate commerce.

. . . [U]nder the Government's "national productivity" reasoning, Congress could regulate any activity that it found was related to the economic productivity of individual citizens. . . [I]t is difficult to perceive any limitation on federal power, even in areas such as criminal law enforcement or education where States historically have been sovereign. Thus, if we were to accept the Government's arguments, we are hard pressed to posit any activity by an individual that Congress is without power to regulate. . . .

The possession of a gun in a local school zone is in no sense an economic activity that might, through repetition elsewhere, substantially affect any sort of interstate commerce. Respondent was a local student at a local school; there is no indication that he had recently moved in interstate commerce, and there is no requirement that his possession of the firearm [has] any concrete tie to interstate commerce.

To uphold the Government's contentions here, we would have to pile inference upon inference in a manner that would bid fair to convert congressional authority under the Commerce Clause to a general police power of the sort retained by the States. Admittedly, some of our prior cases have taken long steps down that road, giving great deference to congressional action. The broad language in these opinions has suggested the possibility of additional expansion, but we decline here to proceed any further. To do so would require us to conclude that the Constitution's enumeration of powers does not presuppose something not enumerated, and that there never will be a distinction between what is truly national and what is truly local. This we are unwilling to do.

## III. STATE POLICE POWERS:
## PROTECTING HEALTH, SAFETY, AND MORALS

As explained previously, the United States is a government of limited power, whose acts, to be valid, must be authorized by the Constitution. The states, by contrast, retain the power they possessed as sovereign governments before the Constitution was ratified. Consequently, the states do not need a grant of constitutional authority before they may act. The Tenth Amendment enunciates the plenary power retained by the states: "The powers not delegated to the United States by the Constitution, nor prohibited by it to the States, are reserved to the States respectively, or to the people."

The "reserved powers" doctrine holds that states may exercise all the powers inherent in government—that is, all the authority necessary to govern that is neither granted to the federal government nor prohibited to the states. The police power expresses the state's inherent sovereignty to safeguard the community's welfare (Hodge 1998). In the companion text (48), I define police power as "the inherent authority of the state (and, through delegation, local government) to enact laws and promulgate regulations to protect, preserve, and promote the health, safety, morals, and general welfare of the people. To achieve these communal benefits, the state retains the power to restrict, within federal and state constitutional limits, private interests—personal interests in autonomy, privacy, association, and liberty as well as economic interests in freedom to contract and uses of property."

Chief Justice John Marshall, in *Gibbons v. Ogden*, 22 U.S. 1, 87 (1824), was the first Supreme Court justice to refer to the police powers. Marshall conceived of state police powers as "that immense mass of legislation, which embraces every thing within the territory of a State, not surrendered to the general government: all which can be most advantageously exercised by the States themselves. Inspection laws, quarantine laws, health laws of every description, as well as laws for regulating the internal commerce of a State, and those which respect turnpike roads, ferries, are component parts of this mass."

In the following reading, University of Chicago historian William J. Novak talks about the rich linguistic and historical origins of the "police power." More important, he reminds us that, far from the laissez-faire philosophy often attributed to early America, the nation was truly a "well-regulated" society, and the locus of this regulation was principally at the state and local levels. For a further discussion of police powers, see *Jacobson v. Massachusetts*, excerpted in chapter 7.

## Governance, Police, and American Liberal Mythology*
*William J. Novak*

> She starts old, old, wrinkled and writhing
> In an old skin. And there is a gradual sloughing
> off of the old skin, towards a new youth.
> It is the myth of America.
>
> D. H. Lawrence

A distinctive and powerful governmental tradition devoted in theory and practice to the vision of a well-regulated society dominated United States social and economic policymaking from 1787 to 1877. With deep and diverse roots in colonial, English, and continental European customs, laws, and public practices, that tradition matured into a full-fledged science of government by midcentury. At the heart of the well-regulated society was a plethora of bylaws, ordinances, statutes, and common law restrictions regulating nearly every aspect of early American economy and society, from Sunday observance to the carting of offal. These laws—the work of mayors, common councils, state legislators, town and county officers, and powerful state and local judges—comprise a remarkable and previously neglected record of governmental aspiration and practice. Taken together they explode tenacious myths about nineteenth-century government (or its absence) and demonstrate the pervasiveness of regulation in early American versions of the good society: regulations for *public safety* and security (protecting the very existence of the population from catastrophic enemies like fire and invasion); the construction of a *public economy* (determining the rules by which the people would acquire and exchange food and goods); the policing of *public space*

---

*Reprinted from *The People's Welfare: Law and Regulation in Nineteenth-Century America* (Chapel Hill: University of North Carolina Press, 1996).

(defining common rights in roads, rivers, and public squares); all-important restraints on *public morals* (establishing the social and cultural conditions of public order); and the open-ended regulatory powers granted to public officials to guarantee *public health* (securing the population's well-being, longevity, and productivity). Public regulation—the power of the state to restrict individual liberty and property for the common welfare—colored all facets of early American development. It was the central component of a reigning theory and practice of governance committed to the pursuit of the people's welfare and happiness in a well-ordered society and polity.

These laws [are] what I collectively refer to as "the well-regulated society.". . . To the omnipresent and skeptical social-historical question, Were such laws enforced?, the thousand cases examined here testify simply and unequivocally, yes. A second question is more interesting, more complicated, and more controversial: Why is this governmental regulatory practice so invisible in our traditional accounts of nineteenth-century American history? Why is it at all surprising to discover the pivotal role played by public law, regulation, order, discipline, and governance in early American society? . . .

America's nineteenth-century regulatory past remains something of a trade secret. No comprehensive history of antebellum regulation exists, and the mention of an American regulatory heritage prompts a familiar incredulity if not outright denial. Why? The culprit is a set of four interrelated and surprisingly resilient myths about nineteenth-century America challenged by this [essay]: the myth of statelessness, the myth of liberal individualism, the myth of the great transformation, and the myth of American exceptionalism. . . .

[The author discusses these four myths].

Together these four organizing myths constitute a master narrative of American political development in which liberty *against* government serves as the fulcrum of a constant and distinctively American liberal-constitutional tradition. The reigning paradigms of American politics (self-interested liberalism), law (constitutionalism), and economics (neoclassical market theory) conspire with this mythic historiography to produce a gross overemphasis on individual rights, constitutional limitations, and the invisible hand; and a terminal neglect of the positive activities and public responsibilities of American government over time. . . .

The well-regulated society confronts the myths of statelessness, individualism, transformation, and exceptionalism with four distinguishing principles of positive governance: public spirit, local self-government, civil liberty, and law. While very much at odds with modern conceptions of the sovereign state and the rights-bearing individual, these principles were the heart of the nineteenth-century vision of a well-regulated society.

*Public spirit. Salus populi* (the people's welfare) is . . . an abridgment of the influential common law maxim *salus populi suprema lex est* (the welfare of the people is the supreme law) and one of the fundamental ordering principles of the early American polity. Nineteenth-century America was a *public* society in ways hard to imagine after the invention of twentieth-century privacy. Its governance was predicated on the elemental assumption that public interest was superior to private interest. Government and society were not created to protect pre-existing private rights, but to further the welfare of the whole people and community. . . . Historians of civic republicanism have alerted us to the prominence in early American thought of an autonomous conception of the public good between the extremes of abstract idealism and crude utilitarianism. But the *salus populi* tradition was not so much a product of formal political philosophizing . . . as a product of governance. It was embedded in the practices of local institutions and common laws. This political moment owed much more to magistracy than to Machiavelli.

*Local self-government.* Despite the jilting of the Articles of Confederation and the new supremacy clause in the federal Constitution, nineteenth-century American governance remained decidedly local. Towns, local courts, common councils, and state legislatures were the basic institutions of governance, and they continued to function in ways not unlike their colonial and European forebears. . . . But self-government implied more than a particular level for the exertion of public authority. It was part of a broader, more substantive understanding of the freedoms and obligations accorded citizens as contributing members of self-regulating communities. Though its anti-despotic thrust is often mistaken for liberal individualism, local self-government conceived of liberty and autonomy as collective attributes—badges of participation, things achieved in common through social and political interaction with others. The independent law-making authority of local communities . . . was to be defended from usurpation by despots, courtly mandarins, or other central powers. But within communities, individuals were expected to conform their behavior to local rules and expectations. No community was deemed free without the power and right of members to govern themselves, *that is,* to determine the rules under which the locality as a whole would be organized and regulated. Such open-ended local regulatory power was simply a necessary attribute of any truly popular sovereignty. . . .

*Civil liberty.* Integral to local self-government was a unique conception of civil or regulated liberty. In an 1853 treatise *The Science of Government,* Charles B. Goodrich (219) effectively captured its meaning: "Liberty is a relative term. Some persons regard it as a right in every individual to act in accordance with his own judgment. Such liberty is unknown to, and cannot be found in connection with or as a result of government, or of the law of society. Government and societies are established for the *regulation of* social intercourse, of social institutions." Civil liberty consisted only in those freedoms consistent with the laws of the land. Such liberty was never absolute, it always had to conform to the superior power of self-governing communities to legislate and regulate in the public interest. From time immemorial, as the common law saying went, this liberty was subject to local bylaws for the promotion and maintenance of community order, comfort, safety, health, and well-being. Freedom and regulation in this tradition were not viewed as antithetical but as complementary and mutually reinforcing. At the Constitutional Convention, James Wilson could argue without any sense of contradiction: "The state governments ought to be preserved—the *freedom of the people* and their *internal good police* depends on their existence in full vigor" (Farrand 1966, 157) (emphasis added).

*Law.* By definition, any history of early American government must also be a legal history. . . . As Thomas Paine (1945, 29) noted, "In America the law is king." John Adams famously added (invoking James Harrington) that this was "a government of laws" (Paine 1945, 29). . . . But the content of the common legal tradition undergirding the well-regulated society runs counter to some classic interpretations of American bench and bar that emphasize solely devotion to private (usually economic) interests and hostility to government. The legal doctrines and practices guaranteeing the rights of municipalities to regulate social and economic life were testaments to the importance of nonconstitutional public law to the American polity. The nineteenth century was not simply an age of private contract and public constitutional limitations. It was an epoch in which strong common law notions of public prerogatives and the duties and obligations of government persisted amid a torrent of private adjudication and constitution writing. The rule of law, a distinctly public and social ideal antedating both Lockean liberalism and Machiavellian civic humanism, dominated most thinking about governance in the nineteenth century. . . .

Public spirit, local self-government, civil liberty, and common law were part of a worldview decidedly different from our own and from the one we have imposed on an unsuspecting past. Their reference point was the relationship of a citizen to a republic rather than an individual subject to a sovereign nation-state. But *salus populi* and well-regulated governance entailed more than a particular legal-political worldview. It was a governmental practice embedded in some of the most important public policies and initiatives of the nineteenth century. In particular, the four principles outlined here found clearest expression in countless nineteenth-century exertions of what is known in legal parlance as *state police power.* . . .

The state police power is one of the most enigmatic phenomena in American legal and political history. To begin with, the phrase "state police power" is triply misleading. First, police power has little to do with our modern notion of a municipal police force. Second, the triumph of this particular legal terminology was part of a late nineteenth-century effort to rein in, constitutionalize, and centralize the disparate powers of states and localities. Using the term to describe earlier developments thus risks importing some anachronistic assumptions. Finally, despite being a "state" power, the police power was usually exercised by local officials.

Generations of judges and scholars have suggested that, in fact, state police power is undefinable. Ernst Freund (1904, iii), author of the most important treatises on regulatory and administrative law, made the bravest attempt, defining it in 1904 as "the power of promoting the public welfare by restraining and regulating the use of liberty and property." Lewis Hockheimer (1897, 158), Freund's contemporary, added that "The police power is the inherent plenary power of a State . . . to prescribe regulations to preserve and promote the public safety, health, and morals, and to prohibit all things hurtful to the comfort and welfare of society." Together these definitions cover three essential components of police power: law, regulation, and people's welfare. Police power was the ability of a state or locality to enact and enforce public laws regulating or even destroying private right, interest, liberty, or property for the common

good (i.e., for the public safety, comfort, welfare, morals, or health).
Such broad compass has led some to conclude that state police
power was the essence of governance, the hallmark of sovereignty
and statecraft.

The American constitutional basis of state police power was the
Tenth Amendment, reserving to the states all power not explicitly delegated or prohibited in the Constitution. But more significant than
this formal constitutional sanction were the substantive roots of state
regulatory power in early modern notions of police or *Polizei*. A product of the epochal transfer of civil power from church and lord to
polity that dominated Europe after the Reformation, police took on a
multiplicity of forms by the eighteenth century. . . . What all had in
common was a focus on the polity's newfound responsibility for the
happiness and welfare of its population. Police was a science and
mode of governance where the polity assumed control over, and became implicated in, the basic conduct of social life. . . . Police aspirations also included enriching population and state, increasing agricultural yields, minimizing threats to health and safety, promoting
communication and commerce, and improving the overall quality of
the people's existence.

Such sweeping objectives required the intense regulation and public monitoring of economy and society. Indeed the effect of police
was a vast proliferation of regulatory intrusions into the remotest
corners of public and private activity. As Michel Foucault (1979,
248) suggested, "The *police* includes everything." . . . Delamare's
initial treatise laid out eleven expansive categories of police regulation and administration: (1) religion, (2) manners (and morals),
(3) health, (4) provisions, (5) travel (roads and highways), (6) public
tranquillity and safety, (7) the sciences and liberal arts, (8) commerce
and trade, (9) manufactures and mechanical arts, (10) labor, and
(11) the poor. No aspect of human intercourse remained outside the
purview of police science. . . .

The vast, largely unwritten history of American governance and
police regulation suggests that it is time to refocus attention on [a] . .
. founding paradox—the myth of American liberty. For . . . the sto-
ried history of liberty in the United States, with its vaunted rhetoric of
unprecedented rights of property, contract, mobility, privacy, and
bodily integrity, was built directly upon a strong and consistent willingness to employ the full, coercive, and regulatory powers of law and

government. The public conditions of private freedom remain the
great problem of American governmental and legal history.

---

## IV. NEW FEDERALISM

As explained at the beginning of this chapter, public health functions
are carried out at multiple levels of government (federal, state, tribal,
and local). Some of the most significant, and politically contentious,
disputes occur when governments at each of these levels lay claim to
particular public health issues. In divisive areas such as gun control,
smoking, and the environment, the federal government may choose to
act. It is in this context that the Supreme Court may have to decide
whether national public health regulations are invading a sphere of
state sovereignty.

"New federalism" is a principle of political change, spurred by conservative activism, that seeks to limit federal authority and return power
to the states (Hodge 1997). New federalism has taken on significant political importance in public health with contentious debates over which
level of government should set standards, as well as perform and pay for
services. The Rehnquist Court has systematically contributed to altering
the balance between the supremacy of federal law and the separate sovereignty of the states. *United States v. Lopez*, excerpted earlier, is one
prominent example of new federalism jurisprudence. In *Lopez*, the
Supreme Court narrowed the scope of the commerce power in a case involving the regulation of firearms near schools.

This section discusses two important issues in American federalism:
Congress's power to require state government to implement federal
standards and Congress's power to waive a state's sovereign immunity.

### A. "COMMANDEERING" STATES
### TO IMPLEMENT FEDERAL REGULATION

The Rehnquist Court's federalism jurisprudence has extended well beyond
the commerce clause. Even if the Congress is acting validly within the
commerce power, the Court has held that it cannot directly coerce states
to comply with federal regulatory standards. In *New York v. United
States*, a federal program regulating radioactive waste removal was held
unconstitutional because it "commandeered" state governments to imple-

ment federal programs in violation of the Tenth Amendment. In this and other cases, the Court held that the federal government may not coerce state legislative or executive bodies to act according to federal standards. See *Printz v. United States*, 521 U.S. 898 (1997) (holding that a provision in the federal Brady Bill regulating background checks for firearm purchases was unconstitutional because it "commandeered" local executive officials to administer a federal program) (posted on the *Reader* web site).

---

**New York v. United States***
*Supreme Court of the United States*
*Decided June 19, 1992*

Justice O'CONNOR delivered the opinion of the Court.

[In 1985, Congress enacted the Low Level Radioactive Waste Policy Amendments Act of 1985 (the "Act") amid fears that the nation would be left without any disposal sites for low-level radioactive waste. The Act was intended to encourage states to establish and operate disposal facilities for low level radioactive waste over the next several years, acting either by themselves or with other states in regional compacts. The Act obligated states to provide for disposal of waste produced within each state's borders and provided three types of incentives to encourage compliance. The first were monetary incentives, the second were access incentives, and the final "incentives" were a take title provision. The take title provision mandates that if a state is not able to provide for the disposal of waste generated within its borders, it is obligated, upon request of the generator of the waste, to take possession of that waste. Should the state fail to take possession, it will be liable for all damages incurred by the waste generator as a result. Petitioner, the State of New York, claimed that the Act is inconsistent with the Tenth Amendment.]

These cases implicate one of our Nation's newest problems of public policy and perhaps our oldest question of constitutional law. The public policy issue involves the disposal of radioactive waste. . . . The constitutional question is as old as the Constitution: It consists of discerning the proper division of authority between the Federal Government and the

---

*505 U.S. 144 (1992).

States. We conclude that while Congress has substantial power under the Constitution to encourage the States to provide for the disposal of the radioactive waste generated within their borders, the Constitution does not confer upon Congress the ability simply to compel the States to do so. We therefore find that only two of the Act's three provisions at issue are consistent with the Constitution's allocation of power to the Federal Government. . . .

While no one disputes the proposition that "the Constitution created a Federal Government of limited powers," *Gregory v. Ashcroft*, 501 U.S. 452, 457 (1991); and while the Tenth Amendment makes explicit that "the powers not delegated to the United States by the Constitution, nor prohibited by it to the States, are reserved to the States respectively, or to the people"; the task of ascertaining the constitutional line between federal and state power has given rise to many of the Court's most difficult and celebrated cases. At least as far back as *Martin v. Hunter's Lessee*, 1 Wheat. 304, 324 (1816), the Court has resolved questions "of great importance and delicacy" in determining whether particular sovereign powers have been granted by the Constitution to the Federal Government or have been retained by the States. . . .

If a power is delegated to Congress in the Constitution, the Tenth Amendment expressly disclaims any reservation of that power to the States; if a power is an attribute of state sovereignty reserved by the Tenth Amendment, it is necessarily a power the Constitution has not conferred on Congress. . . .

[T]he Tenth Amendment confirms that the power of the Federal Government is subject to limits that may, in a given instance, reserve power to the States. The Tenth Amendment thus directs us to determine, as in this case, whether an incident of state sovereignty is protected by a limitation on an Article I power. . . .

The actual scope of the Federal Government's authority with respect to the States has changed over the years, therefore, but the constitutional structure underlying and limiting that authority has not. In the end, just as a cup may be half empty or half full, it makes no difference whether one views the question at issue in these cases as one of ascertaining the limits of the power delegated to the Federal Government under the affirmative provisions of the Constitution or one of discerning the core of sovereignty retained by the States under the Tenth Amendment. Either way, we must determine whether any of the three challenged provisions of the Act oversteps the boundary between federal and state authority.

Petitioners do not contend that Congress lacks the power to regulate the disposal of low level radioactive waste. . . . Petitioners contend only that the Tenth Amendment limits the power of Congress to regulate in the way it has chosen. Rather than addressing the problem of waste disposal by directly regulating the generators and disposers of waste, petitioners argue, Congress has impermissibly directed the States to regulate in this field. . . .

As an initial matter, Congress may not simply "commandeer the legislative processes of the States by directly compelling them to enact and enforce a federal regulatory program." Hodel v. Virginia Surface Mining & Reclamation Ass'n, Inc., 452 U.S. 264, 288 (1981). . . . While Congress has substantial powers to govern the Nation directly, including in areas of intimate concern to the States, the Constitution has never been understood to confer upon Congress the ability to require the States to govern according to Congress's instructions. . . .

In providing for a stronger central government, the Framers explicitly chose a Constitution that confers upon Congress the power to regulate individuals, not States. As we have seen, the Court has consistently respected this choice. We have always understood that even where Congress has the authority under the Constitution to pass laws requiring or prohibiting certain acts, it lacks the power directly to compel the States to require or prohibit those acts.

This is not to say that Congress lacks the ability to encourage a State to regulate in a particular way, or that Congress may not hold out incentives to the States as a method of influencing a State's policy choices. Our cases have identified a variety of methods, short of outright coercion, by which Congress may urge a State to adopt a legislative program consistent with federal interests. Two of these methods are of particular relevance here.

First, under Congress's spending power, "Congress may attach conditions on the receipt of federal funds." South Dakota v. Dole [excerpted earlier]. Such conditions must (among other requirements) bear some relationship to the purpose of the federal spending; otherwise, of course, the spending power could render academic the Constitution's other grants and limits of federal authority. Where the recipient of federal funds is a State, as is not unusual today, the conditions attached to the funds by Congress may influence a State's legislative choices. . . .

Second, where Congress has the authority to regulate private activity under the Commerce Clause, we have recognized Congress's power to offer States the choice of regulating that activity according to federal standards or having state law pre-empted by federal regulation. . . .

By either of these methods, as by any other permissible method of encouraging a State to conform to federal policy choices, the residents of the State retain the ultimate decision as to whether or not the State will comply. If a State's citizens view federal policy as sufficiently contrary to local interests, they may elect to decline a federal grant. If state residents would prefer their government to devote its attention and resources to problems other than those deemed important by Congress, they may choose to have the Federal Government rather than the State bear the expense of a federally mandated regulatory program, and they may continue to supplement that program to the extent state law is not pre-empted. Where Congress encourages state regulation rather than compelling it, state governments remain responsive to the local electorate's preferences; state officials remain accountable to the people.

By contrast, where the Federal Government compels States to regulate, the accountability of both state and federal officials is diminished. If the citizens of New York, for example, do not consider that making provision for the disposal of radioactive waste is in their best interest, they may elect state officials who share their view. That view can always be pre-empted under the Supremacy Clause if it is contrary to the national view, but in such a case it is the Federal Government that makes the decision in full view of the public, and it will be federal officials that suffer the consequences if the decision turns out to be detrimental or unpopular. But where the Federal Government directs the States to regulate, it may be state officials who will bear the brunt of public disapproval, while the federal officials who devised the regulatory program may remain insulated from the electoral ramifications of their decision. Accountability is thus diminished when, due to federal coercion, elected state officials cannot regulate in accordance with the views of the local electorate in matters not pre-empted by federal regulation. . . .

[The Court upholds the first two sets of incentives under the commerce and spending powers]. The take title provision is of a different character. This third so-called "incentive" offers States, as an alternative to regulating pursuant to Congress's direction, the option of taking title to and possession of the low level radioactive waste generated within their borders and becoming liable for all damages waste generators suffer as a result of the States' failure to do so promptly. In this provision, Congress has crossed the line distinguishing encouragement from coercion. . . . The take title provision offers state governments a "choice" of either accepting ownership of waste or regulating according to the instructions of Congress. . . .

Because an instruction to state governments to take title to waste, standing alone, would be beyond the authority of Congress, and because a direct order to regulate, standing alone, would also be beyond the authority of Congress, it follows that Congress lacks the power to offer the States a choice between the two. Unlike the first two sets of incentives, the take title incentive does not represent the conditional exercise of any congressional power enumerated in the Constitution. In this provision, Congress has not held out the threat of exercising its spending power or its commerce power; it has instead held out the threat, should the States not regulate according to one federal instruction, of simply forcing the States to submit to another federal instruction. A choice between two unconstitutionally coercive regulatory techniques is no choice at all. Either way, "the Act commandeers the legislative processes of the States by directly compelling them to enact and enforce a federal regulatory program," *Hodel,* 452 U.S. at 288, an outcome that has never been understood to lie within the authority conferred upon Congress by the Constitution. . . .

The take title provision appears to be unique. No other federal statute has been cited which offers a state government no option other than that of implementing legislation enacted by Congress. Whether one views the take title provision as lying outside Congress's enumerated powers, or as infringing upon the core of state sovereignty reserved by the Tenth Amendment, the provision is inconsistent with the federal structure of our Government established by the Constitution.

Respondents . . . observe that public officials representing the State of New York lent their support to the Act's enactment. . . . [and] then pose what appears at first to be a troubling question: How can a federal statute be found an unconstitutional infringement of state sovereignty when state officials consented to the statute's enactment?

The answer follows from an understanding of the fundamental purpose served by our Government's federal structure. The Constitution does not protect the sovereignty of States for the benefit of the States or state governments as abstract political entities, or even for the benefit of the public officials governing the States. To the contrary, the

Constitution divides authority between federal and state governments for the protection of individuals. . . .

State officials thus cannot consent to the enlargement of the powers of Congress beyond those enumerated in the Constitution. Indeed, the facts of these cases raise the possibility that powerful incentives might lead both federal and state officials to view departures from the federal structure to be in their personal interests. Most citizens recognize the need for radioactive waste disposal sites, but few want sites near their homes. As a result, while it would be well within the authority of either federal or state officials to choose where the disposal sites will be, it is likely to be in the political interest of each individual official to avoid being held accountable to the voters for the choice of location. If a federal official is faced with the alternatives of choosing a location or directing the States to do it, the official may well prefer the latter, as a means of shifting responsibility for the eventual decision. If a state official is faced with the same set of alternatives—choosing a location or having Congress direct the choice of a location—the state official may also prefer the latter, as it may permit the avoidance of personal responsibility. The interests of public officials thus may not coincide with the Constitution's intergovernmental allocation of authority. Where state officials purport to submit to the direction of Congress in this manner, federalism is hardly being advanced.

---

## B. SOVEREIGN IMMUNITY: CONGRESS'S POWER TO AUTHORIZE INDIVIDUAL SUITS AGAINST THE STATES

The Supreme Court's federalism jurisprudence has included a prolonged examination of the doctrine of sovereign immunity. The Eleventh Amendment immunizes states from federal court suits by private individuals without the state's consent. The Supreme Court has held that Congress can abrogate a state's sovereign immunity only if it unequivocally signals its intent to do so and acts pursuant to a valid grant of constitutional authority. Seminole Tribe of Florida v. Florida, 517 U.S. 44 (1996). The courts have examined whether Congress may validly abrogate states' sovereign immunity when acting under the commerce power, the power to enforce the Reconstruction amendments, and the spending power.

The Supreme Court has said that Congress lacks the power when acting under the commerce clause to abrogate states' sovereign immunity in federal court. This means that the federal government may not authorize private individuals to sue states. In 1999 the Court said for the first time that states also cannot be sued without their consent by private parties in the state's own courts for violations of federal law. Alden v. Maine, 527 U.S. 706 (1999). In 2000 the Court continued to limit federal power under the sovereign immunity doctrine by holding that the federal government may not authorize suits against the states under the Age Discrimination in Employment Act. Kimel v. Board of Regents, 528 U.S. 62 (2000).

Although Congress may not base abrogation of state immunity upon its commerce powers, it may subject nonconsenting states to suit in federal court when it does so pursuant to a valid exercise of its power under Section 5 of the Fourteenth Amendment, which authorizes Congress to enforce the equal protection clause through "appropriate legislation." The Court, however, has begun to take a narrow view of the breadth of legislation validly authorized under the Fourteenth Amendment. In 2001 the Court held that state employees cannot sue their employers for damages in federal court under Title I of the Americans with Disabilities Act (ADA). Board of Trustees of the University of Alabama v. Garrett, 121 S. Ct. 955 (2001) (posted on the *Reader* web site). In a 5-4 decision, the Court held that Congress exceeded its power under the Fourteenth Amendment when it applied the ADA to state workers (citing *City of Cleburne v. Cleburne Living Center*, reproduced in chapter 7 of the *Reader*). The Court reasoned that Congress failed to identify "a history and pattern of irrational employment discrimination by the states against the disabled."

The Court in *Garrett* dismissed the 300 examples of state discrimination cited by the dissenting justices. Justice Breyer, in dissent, said "the powerful evidence of discriminatory treatment throughout society in general, including discrimination by private persons and local governments, implicates state governments as well, for state agencies form part of that same larger society." The Supreme Court, with a razor-thin majority, is significantly diminishing Congress's power to combat discrimination by authorizing persons to sue states for violation of individual rights.

In theory, Congress may require a waiver of state sovereign immunity as a condition of receiving federal funds, even though it may not order the waiver directly. College Savings Bank v. Florida Prepaid Postsecondary Education Expense Board, 119 S. Ct. 2219, 2231 (1999).

However, a debate is brewing in the lower courts over the extent of Congress's power to require a waiver under the spending clause. In *Jim C. v. United States*, 235 F.3d 1079 (8th Cir. 2000), a panel of the circuit court reviewed a decision of Circuit Judge Bowman that § 504 of the Rehabilitation Act (which prohibits discrimination against persons with disabilities) was an invalid exercise of Congress's spending power because the conditions for funding were too broad and therefore coercive. The panel overturned the decision, holding that § 504 is a valid exercise of Congress's spending power and that Arkansas waived its immunity to § 504 suits by accepting federal funds.

The Eleventh Amendment creates a major hurdle for persons seeking to enforce federal public health or antidiscrimination laws against state governments. The issue of sovereign immunity, however, would not be as grave a matter if plaintiffs were permitted to sue state officials rather than the state itself. *Ex parte Young*, 209 U.S. 123 (1908), permits injunctive relief against state officials in certain circumstances, even when the state itself is immune from suit. However, in *Westside Mothers v. Haveman*, 133 F. Supp. 2d 549 (E.D. Mich. 2001), a federal district court held that the *Ex parte Young* doctrine does not apply to congressional enactments under the spending power. In a controversial ruling, the court reasoned that spending programs such as Medicaid are contracts consensually entered into by the states with the federal government and are not "supreme authority of the United States." The Court of Appeals decision in *Westside Mothers* will be posted on the *Reader* web site.

## C. FEDERALISM AND PUBLIC HEALTH POLICY

The readings in this chapter illustrate the complexity of constitutional law in creating government powers and duties to preserve the public's health and safety. Generally speaking, the Court sees few affirmative obligations, but does permit wide-ranging powers to act for the common good. The federal government possesses enumerated powers that enable it to regulate in virtually all areas of public health. The states retain the police powers that provide inherent authority to safeguard the health, safety, and morals of the community. Perhaps the most divisive issues in constitutional law involve matters of federalism. In recent years, the Court has shifted the balance of power, denying the national government the authority to invade a sphere of state sovereignty.

As a society, we have to seriously consider the competing claims of the national and state governments in matters of public health. If the states refuse to deal effectively with divisive public health issues such as gun control, violence against women, or tobacco, will the courts allow the federal government to intervene?

Another matter has preoccupied and divided the country every bit as much as American federalism: the claim of government to act for the welfare of the population and the countervailing claim of individuals to be free from government interference. The Constitution, of course, has a great deal to say about the competing interests of communal goods and individual rights. That is the topic of the next chapter.

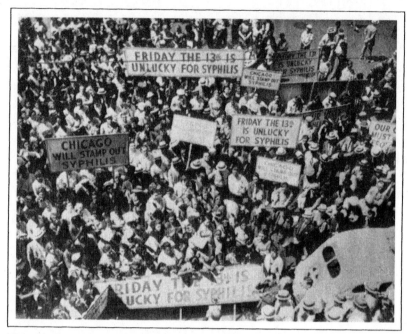

This march, sponsored by the National Youth Association in Chicago on Friday, August 13, 1937, encouraged city residents to get tested for syphilis.

# SEVEN

# Public Health and the Protection of Individual Rights

Government has a long tradition of regulating for the community's welfare. Regulations target individuals (e.g., infectious disease powers), professionals and institutions (e.g., licenses), and businesses (e.g., inspections and safety standards). The previous chapter emphasized the broad *powers and duties* of government to safeguard the public's health. This chapter and the next consider the *restraints* on government power to protect individual interests in autonomy, privacy, liberty, and property.

The cases and reflective readings in this chapter trace the evolution in judicial thought on the balance between public health power and protection of individual rights. It is important to emphasize that judicial review is neither static nor immune from political and social influences. Rather, judicial review of public health interventions has changed over time, depending on the current composition of the Supreme Court. These changes, moreover, often reflect prevailing social and political thought. For example, much of the Warren Court's defense of civil liberties can be traced to heightened awareness of individual rights and liberties relating to African Americans and women in the 1960s. Many federalism decisions by the Rehnquist Court, as excerpted in chapter 6, are influenced by the modern emphasis on states' rights and against large central government.

Several different meanings may be attributed to constitutional adjudication (see Figure 11). Some see the primary role of the Constitution

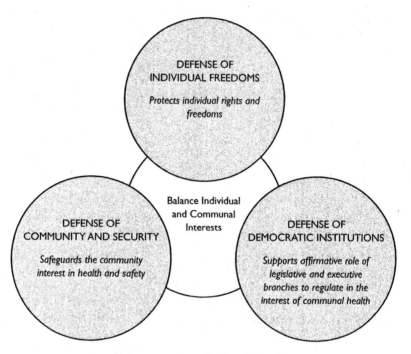

Figure 11.  Constitutional functions.

as a defense of freedom, others see it as a defense of community and security, and still others see it as a defense of democratic institutions. It is
possible to perceive the various phases of Supreme Court decision making as a vindication, or repudiation, of each of these values.

Many people perceive the Constitution's primary purpose as the protection of individual rights against excessive government interference.
Under this view, people are born free with inalienable interests in liberty and property that may not be impeded absent a highly persuasive
governmental justification. This perspective limits public health power
and flexibility. It assumes that one value—freedom—ought to prevail
over other values—health and security—except in unusual cases.
Courts that adhere to this view more closely scrutinize the exercise of
public health powers. Public health officials, knowing they are subject
to intense scrutiny, may shy away from aggressive use of power. The result may be firm protection of individual rights but diminished protection of the community's health and safety.

Others perceive the Constitution's primary purpose as the defense of common goods. Under this view, the principal purpose of government is to safeguard communal interests in health and security, even at the expense of individual interests. This perspective affords public health officials the most extensive and flexible authority. It assumes that public health powers are legitimately exercised unless they further an insubstantial purpose or unjustifiably trample individual interests. Courts that adhere to this view adopt a low level of constitutional scrutiny. Public health officials, knowing they are immune from careful scrutiny, may be inclined to exercise a broad range of powers.

Relatedly, some perceive the Constitution's primary purpose as the defense of democratic institutions. Under this view, the formulation and enforcement of policy are effectively left to the democratic branches of government. It assumes that public health powers involve highly complex policy choices that are best made by lawmakers and agency officials. Not only do these branches have greater policy expertise, they are also politically accountable. If the electorate is displeased with the decision of a legislator or public health official, it usually has a remedy at the ballot box. If the public is displeased with a court's decision based on a constitutional principle, the electoral remedy is not as clear. Courts that adhere to this view are highly deferential to legislatures and executive agencies, giving them wide latitude in formulating and executing public health policy.

Many judges reject these highly charged political explanations, claiming simply and objectively to read the text and history of the Constitution. To these jurists, the primary task is to discover the original intent of the Framers.

It is helpful to underscore that the power of public health officials is virtually unequaled. Few actors in the American system of government exercise such discretionary powers and experience this level of respect and deference. This public trust should vest a responsibility in public health officials to exercise their powers wisely and justly.

This chapter contains two sections—one relating to early constitutional limits on police powers, and the other on modern limits. Both are important not only because they give a sense of history and tradition, but also because they articulate judicial principles on the rightful exercise of public health authority. After excerpting two classic public health cases from the early twentieth century, *Jacobson v. Massachusetts* and *Jew Ho v. Williamson,* this chapter discusses modern constitutional doctrine. In the modern era, the courts have enunciated several overlapping standards of constitutional scrutiny that are clearly explained by Justice White in *City of Cleburne v. Cleburne Living Center*. The judiciary has also explored the idea of procedural justice, insisting that individuals receive a fair hearing prior to deprivation of important liberty and property interests. The United States Supreme Court in *Mathews v. Eldridge* explains the concept of procedural due process, and the West Virginia Supreme Court in *Greene v. Edwards* applies that concept in a case involving isolation of an individual with tuberculosis (TB).

## I.  EARLY-TWENTIETH-CENTURY
## LIMITS ON THE POLICE POWER

The story of public health law often begins with the refusal of Henning Jacobson to comply with an early-twentieth-century Cambridge, Massachusetts, ordinance compelling smallpox vaccination. The resulting case, *Jacobson v. Massachusetts,* is perhaps the most important Supreme Court opinion in the history of American public health law.

---

### Jacobson v. Massachusetts*
*Supreme Court of the United States*
*Decided February 20, 1905*

Justice HARLAN delivered the opinion of the Court.

[The board of health of the City of Cambridge, pursuant to a Massachusetts statute, adopted an ordinance providing for mandatory vaccination for smallpox of all city inhabitants over the age of twenty-one who had not been recently vaccinated. The board passed the ordinance due to an increasing prevalence of smallpox in the city. The vaccinations would be provided to the citizens free of charge. Those citizens who do not comply with the regulation would be subject to a fine of $5. Jacobson refused to be vaccinated, and as a result, he was criminally charged. He alleged, *inter alia,* that the ordinance was unconstitutional as a violation of the due process, equal protection, and privileges and immunities clauses of the Fourteenth Amendment.]

---

*197 U.S. 11 (1905).

This case involves the validity, under the Constitution of the United States, of certain provisions in the statutes of Massachusetts relating to vaccination. . . .

The authority of the state to enact this statute is to be referred to what is commonly called the police power, a power which the state did not surrender when becoming a member of the Union under the Constitution. Although this court has refrained from any attempt to define the limits of that power, yet it has distinctly recognized the authority of a state to enact quarantine laws and "health laws of every description" [Gibbons v. Ogden, 22 U.S. 1, 87 (1824)]; indeed, all laws that relate to matters completely within its territory and which do not by their necessary operation affect the people of other states. According to settled principles, the police power of a state must be held to embrace, at least, such reasonable regulations established directly by legislative enactment as will protect the public health and the public safety. It is equally true that the state may invest local bodies called into existence for purposes of local administration with authority in some appropriate way to safeguard the public health and the public safety. The mode or manner in which those results are to be accomplished is within the discretion of the state, subject, of course, so far as Federal power is concerned, only to the condition that no rule prescribed by a state, nor any regulation adopted by a local governmental agency acting under the sanction of state legislation, shall contravene the Constitution of the United States, nor infringe any right granted or secured by that instrument. A local enactment or regulation, even if based on the acknowledged police powers of a state, must always yield in case of conflict with the exercise by the general government of any power it possesses under the Constitution, or with any right which that instrument gives or secures.

We come, then, to inquire whether any right given or secured by the Constitution is invaded by the statute as interpreted by the state court. The defendant insists that his liberty is invaded when the state subjects him to fine or imprisonment for neglecting or refusing to submit to vaccination; that a compulsory vaccination law is unreasonable, arbitrary, and oppressive, and, therefore, hostile to the inherent right of every freeman to care for his own body and health in such way as to him seems best; and that the execution of such a law against one who objects to vaccination, no matter for what reason, is nothing short of an assault upon his person. But the liberty secured by the Constitution of the United States to every person within its jurisdiction does not import an absolute right in each person to be, at all times and in all circumstances, wholly freed from restraint. There are manifold restraints to which every person is necessarily subject for the common good. Real liberty for all could not exist under the operation of a principle which recognizes the right of each individual person to use his own, whether in respect of his person or his property, regardless of the injury that may be done to others. This court has more than once recognized it as a fundamental principle that "persons and property are subjected to all kinds of restraints and burdens in order to secure the general comfort, health, and prosperity of the state; of the perfect right of the legislature to do which no question ever was, or upon acknowledged general principles ever can be, made, so far as natural persons are concerned." Hannibal & St. J. R. Co. v. Husen, 95 U.S. 465, 471 (1877). In *Crowley v. Christensen*, 137 U.S. 86, 89 (1890), we said: "The possession and enjoyment of all rights are subject to such reasonable conditions as may be deemed by the governing authority of the country essential to the safety, health, peace, good order, and morals of the community. Even liberty itself, the greatest of all rights, is not unrestricted license to act according to one's own will. It is only freedom from restraint under conditions essential to the equal enjoyment of the same right by others. It is, then, liberty regulated by law." In the Constitution of Massachusetts adopted in 1780 it was laid down as a fundamental principle of the social compact that the whole people covenants with each citizen, and each citizen with the whole people, that all shall be governed by certain laws for "the common good," and that government is instituted "for the common good, for the protection, safety, prosperity, and happiness of the people, and not for the profit, honor, or private interests of any one man, family, or class of men." The good and welfare of the commonwealth, of which the legislature is primarily the judge, is the basis on which the police power rests in Massachusetts.

Applying these principles to the present case, it is to be observed that the legislature of Massachusetts required the inhabitants of a city or town to be vaccinated only when, in the opinion of the board of health, that was necessary for the public health or the public safety. The authority to determine for all what ought to be done in such an emergency must have been lodged somewhere or in some body; and surely it was appropriate for the legislature to refer that question, in the first instance, to a board of health composed of persons residing in the locality affected, and appointed, presumably, because of their fitness to determine such questions. To invest such a body with authority over such matters was not an unusual, nor an unreasonable or arbitrary, requirement. Upon the principle of self-defense, of paramount necessity, a community has the right to protect itself against an epidemic of disease which threatens the safety of its members. It is to be observed that when the regulation in question was adopted smallpox, according to the recitals in the regulation adopted by the board of health, was prevalent to some extent in the city of Cambridge, and the disease was increasing. If such was the situation—and nothing is asserted or appears in the record to the contrary—if we are to attach any value whatever to the knowledge which, it is safe to affirm, is common to all civilized peoples touching smallpox and the methods most usually employed to eradicate that disease, it cannot be adjudged that the present regulation of the board of health was not necessary in order to protect the public health and secure the public safety. Smallpox being prevalent and increasing at Cambridge, the court would usurp the functions of another branch of government if it adjudged, as matter of law, that the mode adopted under the sanction of the state, to protect the people at large was arbitrary, and not justified by the necessities of the case. We say necessities of the case, because it might be that an acknowledged power of a local community to protect itself against an epidemic threatening the safety of all might be exercised in particular circumstances and in reference to particular persons in such an arbitrary, unreasonable manner, or might go so far beyond what was reasonably required for the safety of the public, as to authorize or compel the courts to interfere for the protection of such persons. . . . If the mode adopted by the commonwealth of Massachusetts for the protection of its local communities against smallpox proved to be distressing, inconvenient, or objectionable to some—if nothing more could be reasonably affirmed of the statute in question—the answer is that it was the duty of the constituted authorities primarily to keep in view the welfare, comfort, and safety of the many, and not permit the interests of the many to be subordinated to the wishes or convenience of the few. There is, of course, a sphere within which the individual may assert the supremacy of his own will, and rightfully dispute the authority of any human government, especially of any free government existing under a written constitution, to interfere with the exercise of that will. But it is equally true that in every well-ordered society charged with the duty of conserving the safety of its members the rights of the individual in respect of his liberty may at times, under the pressure of great dangers, be subjected to such restraint, to be enforced by reasonable regulations, as the safety of the general public may demand. . . . The liberty secured by the 14th Amendment, this court has said, consists, in part, in the right of a person "to live and work where he will" [Allgeyer v. Louisiana, 165 U.S. 578 (1897)]; and yet he may be compelled, by force if need be, against his will and without regard to his personal wishes or his pecuniary interests, or even his religious or political convictions, to take his place in the ranks of the army of his country, and risk the chance of being shot down in its defense. It is not, therefore, true that the power of the public to guard itself against imminent danger depends in every case involving the control of one's body upon his willingness to submit to reasonable regulations established by the constituted authorities, under the sanction of the state, for the purpose of protecting the public collectively against such danger.

It is said, however, that the statute, as interpreted by the state court, although making an exception in favor of children certified by a registered physician to be unfit subjects for vaccination, makes no exception in case of adults in like condition. But this cannot be deemed a denial of the equal protection of the laws to adults; for the statute is applicable equally to all in like condition, and there are obviously reasons why regulations may be appropriate for adults which could not be safely applied to persons of tender years.

Looking at the propositions embodied in the defendant's rejected offers of proof, it is clear that they are more formidable by their number than by their inherent value. Those offers in the main seem to have had no purpose except to state the general theory of those of the medical profession who attach little or no value to vaccination as a means of preventing the spread of smallpox, or who think that vaccination causes other diseases of the body. What everybody knows the court must know, and therefore the state court judicially knew, as this court knows, that an opposite theory accords with the common belief, and is maintained by high medical authority. We must assume that, when the statute in question was passed, the legislature of Massachusetts was not unaware of these opposing theories, and was compelled, of necessity, to choose between them. It was not compelled to commit a matter involving the public health and safety to the final decision of a court or jury. It is no part of the function of a court or a jury to determine which one of two modes was likely to be the most effective for the protection of the public against disease. That was for the legislative department to determine in the light of all the information it had or could obtain. It could not properly abdicate its function to guard the public health and safety. The state legislature proceeded upon the theory which recognized vaccination as at least an effective, if not the best-known, way in which to meet and suppress the evils of a smallpox epidemic that imperiled an entire population. Upon what sound principles as to the relations existing between the different departments of government can the court review this action of the legislature? If there is any such power in the judiciary to review legislative action in respect of a matter affecting the general welfare, it can only be when that which the legislature has done comes within the rule that, if a statute purporting to have been enacted to protect the public health, the public morals, or the public safety, has no real or substantial relation to those objects, or is, beyond all question, a plain, palpable invasion of rights secured by the fundamental law, it is the duty of the courts to so adjudge, and thereby give effect to the Constitution.

Whatever may be thought of the expediency of this statute, it cannot be affirmed to be, beyond question, in palpable conflict with the Constitution. Nor, in view of the methods employed to stamp out the disease of smallpox, can anyone confidently assert that the means prescribed by the state to that end has no real or substantial relation to the protection of the public health and the public safety. Such an assertion would not be consistent with the experience of this and other countries whose authorities have dealt with the disease of smallpox. And the principle of vaccination as a means to prevent the spread of smallpox has been enforced in many states by statutes making the vaccination of children a condition of their right to enter or remain in public schools.

The latest case upon the subject of which we are aware is *Viemester v. White* [72 N.E. 97 (N.Y. Ct. App. 1904)], decided very recently by the court of appeals of New York. That case involved the validity of a statute excluding from the public schools all children who had not been vaccinated. One contention was that the statute and the regulation adopted in exercise of its provisions was inconsistent with the rights, privileges, and liberties of the citizen. The contention was overruled, the court saying, among other things:

> Smallpox is known of all to be a dangerous and contagious disease. If vaccination strongly tends to prevent the transmission or spread of this disease, it logically follows that children may be refused admission to the public schools until they have been vaccinated. The appellant claims that vaccination does not tend to prevent smallpox, but tends to bring about other diseases, and

that it does much harm, with no good. It must be conceded that some lay-men, both learned and unlearned, and some physicians of great skill and re-pute, do not believe that vaccination is a preventive of smallpox. The com-mon belief, however, is that it has a decided tendency to prevent the spread of this fearful disease, and to render it less dangerous to those who contract it. While not accepted by all, it is accepted by the mass of the people, as well as by most members of the medical profession. It has been general in our state, and in most civilized nations for generations. It is generally accepted in theory, and generally applied in practice, both by the voluntary action of the people, and in obedience to the command of law. Nearly every state in the Union has statutes to encourage, or directly or indirectly to require, vaccina-tion; and this is true of most nations of Europe. . . . A common belief, like common knowledge, does not require evidence to establish its existence, but may be acted upon without proof by the legislature and the courts. . . . The fact that the belief is not universal is not controlling, for there is scarcely any belief that is accepted by everyone. The possibility that the belief may be wrong, and that science may yet show it to be wrong, is not conclusive; for the legislature has the right to pass laws which, according to the common be-lief of the people, are adapted to prevent the spread of contagious diseases. In a free country, where the government is by the people, through their cho-sen representatives, practical legislation admits of no other standard of ac-tion, for what the people believe is for the common welfare must be accepted as tending to promote the common welfare, whether it does in fact or not. Any other basis would conflict with the spirit of the Constitution, and would sanction measures opposed to a Republican form of government. While we do not decide, and cannot decide, that vaccination is a preventive of small-pox, we take judicial notice of the fact that this is the common belief of the people of the state, and, with this fact as a foundation, we hold that the statute in question is a health law, enacted in a reasonable and proper exer-cise of the police power.

[*Id.* at 98–99]

Since, then, vaccination, as a means of protecting a community against smallpox, finds strong support in the experience of this and other countries, no court, much less a jury, is justified in disregarding the action of the legislature simply because in its or their opinion that particular method was—perhaps, or possibly—not the best either for children or adults.

Did the offers of proof made by the defendant present a case which entitled him, while remaining in Cambridge, to claim exemp-tion from the operation of the statute and of the regulation adopted by the board of health? We have already said that his rejected offers, in the main, only set forth the theory of those who had no faith in vaccination as a means of preventing the spread of smallpox, or who thought that vaccination, without benefitting the public, put in peril the health of the person vaccinated. But there were some offers which it is contended embodied distinct facts that might properly have been considered. Let us see how this is.

The defendant offered to prove that vaccination "quite often" caused serious and permanent injury to the health of the person vaccinated; that the operation "occasionally" resulted in death; that it was "impossible" to tell "in any particular case" what the results of vaccination would be, or whether it would injure the health or result in death; that "quite often" one's blood is in a certain condition of impurity when it is not prudent or safe to vaccinate him; that there is no practical test by which to determine "with any degree of certainty" whether one's blood is in such condition of impurity as to render vaccination necessarily unsafe or dangerous; that vaccine matter is "quite often" impure and dangerous to be used, but whether impure or not cannot be ascertained by any known practical test; that the defendant refused to submit to vaccination for the reason that he had, "when a child," been caused great and extreme suffering for a long period by a disease produced by vaccination; and that he had witnessed a similar result of vaccination, not only in the case of his son, but in the cases of others.

These offers, in effect, invited the court and jury to go over the whole ground gone over by the legislature when it enacted the statute in question. The legislature assumed that some children, by reason of their condition at the time, might not be fit subjects of vaccination; and it is suggested—and we will not say without reason—that such is the case with some adults. But the defendant did not offer to prove that, by reason of his then condition, he was in fact not a fit subject of vaccination at the time he was informed of the requirement of the regulation adopted by the board of health. It is entirely consistent with his offer of proof that, after reaching full age, he had become, so far as medical skill could discover, and when informed of the regulation of the board of health was, a fit subject of vaccination, and that the vaccine matter to be used in his case was such as any medical practitioner of good standing would regard as proper to be used. The matured opinions of medical men everywhere, and the experience of mankind, as all must know, negative the suggestion that it is not possible in any case to determine whether vaccination is safe. Was defendant exempted from the operation of the statute simply because of his dread of the same evil results experienced by him when a child, and which he had observed in

the cases of his son and other children? Could he reasonably claim such
an exemption because "quite often," or "occasionally," injury had resulted from vaccination, or because it was impossible, in the opinion of
some, by any practical test, to determine with absolute certainty
whether a particular person could be safely vaccinated?

It seems to the court that an affirmative answer to these questions
would practically strip the legislative department of its function to care
for the public health and the public safety when endangered by epidemics of disease. Such an answer would mean that compulsory vaccination could not, in any conceivable case, be legally enforced in a community, even at the command of the legislature, however widespread
the epidemic of smallpox, and however deep and universal was the belief of the community and of its medical advisers that a system of general vaccination was vital to the safety of all.

We are not prepared to hold that a minority, residing or remaining in
any city or town where smallpox is prevalent, and enjoying the general
protection afforded by an organized local government, may thus defy the
will of its constituted authorities, acting in good faith for all, under the
legislative sanction of the state. If such be the privilege of a minority, then
a like privilege would belong to each individual of the community, and
the spectacle would be presented of the welfare and safety of an entire
population being subordinated to the notions of a single individual who
chooses to remain a part of that population. We are unwilling to hold it
to be an element in the liberty secured by the Constitution of the United
States that one person, or a minority of persons, residing in any community and enjoying the benefits of its local government, should have the
power thus to dominate the majority when supported in their action by
the authority of the state. While this court should guard with firmness
every right appertaining to life, liberty, or property as secured to the individual by the supreme law of the land, it is of the last importance that
it should not invade the domain of local authority except when it is
plainly necessary to do so in order to enforce that law. The safety and the
health of the people of Massachusetts are, in the first instance, for that
commonwealth to guard and protect. They are matters that do not ordinarily concern the national government. So far as they can be reached by
any government, they depend, primarily, upon such action as the state, in
its wisdom, may take; and we do not perceive that this legislation has invaded any right secured by the Federal Constitution.

Before closing this opinion we deem it appropriate, in order to prevent
misapprehension as to our views, to observe—perhaps to repeat a thought

already sufficiently expressed, namely—that the police power of a state, whether exercised directly by the legislature, or by a local body acting under its authority, may be exerted in such circumstances, or by regulations so arbitrary and oppressive in particular cases, as to justify the interference of the courts to prevent wrong and oppression. Extreme cases can be readily suggested. Ordinarily such cases are not safe guides in the administration of the law. It is easy, for instance, to suppose the case of an adult who is embraced by the mere words of the act, but yet to subject whom to vaccination in a particular condition of his health or body would be cruel and inhuman in the last degree. We are not to be understood as holding that the statute was intended to be applied to such a case, or, if it was so intended, that the judiciary would not be competent to interfere and protect the health and life of the individual concerned. "All laws," this court has said, "should receive a sensible construction. General terms should be so limited in their application as not to lead to injustice, oppression, or an absurd consequence. It will always, therefore, be presumed that the legislature intended exceptions to its language which would avoid results of this character. The reason of the law in such cases should prevail over its letter." United States v. Kirby, 74 U.S. 482 (1868). Until otherwise informed by the highest court of Massachusetts, we are not inclined to hold that the statute establishes the absolute rule that an adult must be vaccinated if it be apparent or can be shown with reasonable certainty that he is not at the time a fit subject of vaccination, or that vaccination, by reason of his then condition, would seriously impair his health, or probably cause his death. No such case is here presented. It is the case of an adult who, for aught that appears, was himself in perfect health and a fit subject of vaccination, and yet, while remaining in the community, refused to obey the statute and the regulation adopted in execution of its provisions for the protection of the public health and the public safety, confessedly endangered by the presence of a dangerous disease.

We now decide only that the statute covers the present case, and that nothing clearly appears that would justify this court in holding it to be unconstitutional and inoperative in its application to the plaintiff in error.

*   *   *   *   *

The Supreme Court in *Jacobson* defends the communal values of health and security and exhibits deference to the legislature and public health authorities. Beyond its passive acceptance of state legislative discretion in matters of public health, however, is the Court's first systematic statement of the constitutional limitations imposed on public health authorities. The *Jacobson* Court establishes four constitutional standards.

The first standard, *public health necessity,* suggests that public health powers can be exercised only where necessary to prevent an avoidable harm. Justice Harlan insisted that police powers must be based on the "necessity of the case" and cannot be exercised in "an arbitrary, unreasonable manner" or go "beyond what was reasonably required for the safety of the public." *Jacobson,* 197 U.S. at 28.

The second standard, *reasonable means,* suggests that the methods used must be designed to prevent or ameliorate a health threat. Even though the objective of the legislature may be valid and beneficent, the methods adopted must have a "real or substantial relation" to protection of the public health, and cannot be "a plain, palpable invasion of rights." *Id.* at 31.

The third standard, *proportionality,* suggests that a public health regulation may be unconstitutional if the burden imposed is wholly disproportionate to the expected benefit. "[T]he police power of a state," said Justice Harlan, "may be exerted in such circumstances, or by regulations so arbitrary and oppressive in particular cases, as to justify the interference of the courts to prevent wrong, . . . injustice, oppression, or an absurd consequence." *Id.* at 38, 39.

The fourth standard, *harm avoidance,* suggests that the control measure should not pose an undue health risk to its subject. Justice Harlan emphasized that Henning Jacobson was a "fit person" for smallpox vaccination, but asserted that requiring a person to be immunized who would be harmed is "cruel and inhuman in the last degree." *Id.* at 38, 39. If there had been evidence that the vaccination would seriously impair Jacobson's health, he may have prevailed in this historic case. The courts have required safe and habitable environments for persons subject to isolation on the theory that public health powers are designed to promote well-being, and not to punish the individual. See, for example, *Kirk v. Wyman,* excerpted in chapter 13 (disallowing isolation in a pest house where "even temporary isolation . . . would be a serious affliction and peril to an elderly lady, enfeebled by disease").

During the same time period as *Jacobson,* the judiciary expressed its displeasure with governmental action motivated by animus against an ethnic group. In *Yick Wo v. Hopkins,* 118 U.S. 356 (1886), the Supreme Court found unlawful discrimination when a San Francisco ordinance prohibiting washing of clothes in public laundries after 10 P.M. was enforced only against Chinese owners.

By 1900 public health authorities were implementing a quarantine in San Francisco within a twelve-block district known as Chinatown housing a population of 12,000. Police, moreover, closed businesses owned only by nonwhite persons. The federal Court of Appeals held the quarantine unconstitutional on grounds that it was unfair—health authorities acted with an "evil eye and an unequal hand." *Jew Ho* (excerpted next) serves as a reminder that public health measures can be used as an instrument of prejudice and subjugation.

---

### Jew Ho v. Williamson*
*Circuit Court, Northern District of California*
*Decided June 15, 1900*

Circuit Judge MORROW delivered the opinion of the court (orally).

[The board of health of San Francisco adopted a resolution authorizing the board to quarantine twelve city blocks after nine people in the area died of bubonic plague. The complainant, who resided within the limits of the quarantined district, alleged, *inter alia*, that the resolution was enforced only against persons of Chinese race and nationality, and not against persons of other races. Additionally, the complainant alleged that there were not any cases of bubonic plague within the limits of the quarantined district within the thirty days preceding the filing of this complaint.]

[It is] contended that the acts of the defendants in establishing a quarantine district in San Francisco are authorized by the general police power of the state, intrusted to the city of San Francisco. . . . [T]he question therefore arises as to whether or not the quarantine established by the defendants in this case is reasonable, and whether it is necessary, under the circumstances of this case. As I had occasion to say in the former case (Wong Wai v. Williamson, 103 Fed. 1 (C.C.N.D. Cal. 1900)), this court will, of course, uphold any reasonable regulation that may be imposed for the purpose of protecting the people of the city from the invasion of epidemic disease. In the presence of a great calamity, the court will go to the greatest extent, and give the widest discretion, in construing the regulations that may be adopted by the board of health or the board of supervisors. But is the regulation in this case a reasonable one? Is it a proper regulation,

---

*103 F. 10 (C.C.N.D. Cal. 1900).

directed to accomplish the purpose that appears to have been in view? That is a question for this court to determine. . . .

The purpose of quarantine and health laws and regulations with respect to contagious and infectious diseases is directed primarily to preventing the spread of such diseases among the inhabitants of localities. In this respect these laws and regulations come under the police power of the state, and may be enforced by quarantine and health officers, in the exercise of a large discretion, as circumstances may require. . . .

This is a system of quarantine that is well recognized in all communities, and is provided by the laws of the various states and municipalities: That, when a contagious or infectious disease breaks out in a place, they quarantine the house or houses first; the purpose being to restrict spread to other people in the same locality. It must necessarily follow that, if a large section or a large territory is quarantined, intercommunication of the people within that territory will rather tend to spread the disease than to restrict it. . . .

The quarantined district comprises 12 blocks. It is not claimed that in all the 12 blocks of the quarantined district the disease has been discovered. There are, I believe, 7 or 8 blocks in which it is claimed that deaths have occurred on account of what is said to be this disease. In 2 or 3 blocks it has not appeared at all. Yet this quarantine has been thrown around the entire district. The people therein obtain their food and other supplies, and communicate freely with each other in all their affairs. They are permitted to go from a place where it is said that the disease has appeared, freely among the other 10,000 people in that district. It would necessarily follow that, if the disease is there, every facility has been offered by this species of quarantine to enlarge its sphere and increase its danger and its destructive force. . . . The court cannot ignore this evidence and the condition it describes. The court cannot but see the practical question that is presented to it as to the ineffectiveness of this method of quarantine against such a disease as this. So, upon that ground, the court must hold that this quarantine is not a reasonable regulation to accomplish the purposes sought. It is not in harmony with the declared purpose of the board of health or of the board of supervisors.

But there is still another feature of this case that has been called to the attention of the court, and that is its discriminating character; that is to say, it is said that this quarantine discriminates against the Chinese population of this city, and in favor of the people of other races. . . . The evidence here is clear that this is made to operate against the Chinese population only, and the reason given for it is that the Chinese may communicate the disease from one to the other. That explanation, in the judgment of the court, is not sufficient. It is, in effect, a discrimination, and it is the discrimination that has been frequently called to the attention of the federal courts where matters of this character have arisen with respect to Chinese. . . .

In the case at bar, assuming that the board of supervisors had just grounds for quarantining the district which has been described, it seems that the board of health, in executing the ordinance, left out certain persons, members of races other than Chinese. This is precisely the point noticed by the Supreme Court of the United States, namely, the administration of a law "with an evil eye and an unequal hand." Yick Wo v. Hopkins, 118 U.S. 356 (1886). Wherever the courts of the United States have found such an administration of the law . . . [with] the purpose to enforce it "with an evil eye and an unequal hand," then it is the duty of the court to interpose, and to declare the ordinance discriminating in its character, and void under the constitution of the United States. . . .

It follows from the remarks that I have made that this quarantine cannot be continued, by reason of the fact that it is unreasonable, unjust, and oppressive, and therefore contrary to the laws limiting the police powers of the state and municipality in such matters; and, second, that it is discriminating in its character, and is contrary to the provisions of the fourteenth amendment of the constitution of the United States. The counsel for complainant will prepare an injunction, which shall, however, permit the board to maintain a quarantine around such places as it may have reason to believe are infected by contagious or infectious diseases, but that the general quarantine of the whole district must not be continued, and that the people residing in that district, so far as they have been restricted or limited in their persons and their business, have that limitation and restraint removed.

## II. PUBLIC HEALTH POWERS IN THE MODERN CONSTITUTIONAL ERA

The Supreme Court changed markedly during the two decades beginning in the late 1950s. This was a time when the ideology of rights and freedoms became salient. The Warren Court revitalized and strengthened the Court's position on issues of equality and civil liberties. It set a liberal agenda that prized personal freedom and nondiscrimination (Stoddard and Rieman 1990).

Broadly speaking, it is possible to identify two different kinds of restraint on police powers. The first restraint is substantive in nature,
requiring government to provide a plausible explanation for the intrusion
on individual interests. As the restriction on rights or liberties intensifies,
the government must offer an increasingly strong justification. To accomplish this objective, the Supreme Court has developed a "tiered" approach to constitutional law, where it adopts various levels of scrutiny
depending on the importance of the individual interest at stake—strict
scrutiny, intermediate scrutiny, or minimum rationality. *City of Cleburne
v. Cleburne Living Center* represents one of the Warren Court's clearest
expressions of this layered approach to constitutional adjudication.

The second restraint on police powers is procedural in nature. Here
the Supreme Court requires government to provide a fair hearing before
depriving individuals of important liberty or property interests. An expansive literature exists on the nature of the liberty or property interest
that triggers a procedural due process requirement. Police powers that
affect important interests may be exercised only with procedural due
process—for example, a liberty interest denied by isolation or a property
interest denied by confiscation of dangerous possessions. Once the court
determines that the government must provide procedural due process,
the issue becomes "what process is due?"—that is, how elaborate must
the procedures be to satisfy the due process requirement? The Supreme
Court in *Mathews v. Eldridge* discussed this issue and set modern standards for procedural due process. The West Virginia Supreme Court applied these standards in the public health context in *Greene v. Edwards*.

## A.  SUBSTANTIVE DUE PROCESS AND EQUAL
##     PROTECTION OF THE LAWS: LEVELS OF SCRUTINY

---

### City of Cleburne v. Cleburne Living Center*
*Supreme Court of the United States*
*Decided July 1, 1985*

Justice WHITE delivered the opinion of the Court.

A Texas city denied a special use permit for the operation of a group
home for the mentally retarded, acting pursuant to a municipal zoning or-

---

*473 U.S. 432 (1985).

dinance requiring permits for such homes. The Court of Appeals for the Fifth Circuit held that mental retardation is a "quasi-suspect" classification and that the ordinance violated the Equal Protection Clause because it did not substantially further an important governmental purpose. We hold that a lesser standard of scrutiny is appropriate, but conclude that under that standard the ordinance is invalid as applied in this case. . . .

The Equal Protection Clause of the Fourteenth Amendment commands that no State shall "deny to any person within its jurisdiction the equal protection of the laws," which is essentially a direction that all persons similarly situated should be treated alike. Plyler v. Doe, 457 U.S. 202, 216 (1982). Section 5 of the Amendment empowers Congress to enforce this mandate, but absent controlling congressional direction, the courts have themselves devised standards for determining the validity of state legislation or other official action that is challenged as denying equal protection. The general rule is that legislation is presumed to be valid and will be sustained if the classification drawn by the statute is rationally related to a legitimate state interest. When social or economic legislation is at issue, the Equal Protection Clause allows the States wide latitude, and the Constitution presumes that even improvident decisions will eventually be rectified by the democratic processes.

The general rule gives way, however, when a statute classifies by race, alienage, or national origin. These factors are so seldom relevant to the achievement of any legitimate state interest that laws grounded in such considerations are deemed to reflect prejudice and antipathy—a view that those in the burdened class are not as worthy or deserving as others. For these reasons and because such discrimination is unlikely to be soon rectified by legislative means, these laws are subjected to strict scrutiny and will be sustained only if they are suitably tailored to serve a compelling state interest. Similar oversight by the courts is due when state laws impinge on personal rights protected by the Constitution.

Legislative classifications based on gender also call for a heightened standard of review. That factor generally provides no sensible ground for differential treatment. "[W]hat differentiates sex from such nonsuspect statuses as intelligence or physical disability . . . is that the sex characteristic frequently bears no relation to ability to perform or contribute to society." Frontiero v. Richardson, 411 U.S. 677, 686 (1973) (plurality opinion). Rather than resting on meaningful considerations, statutes distributing benefits and burdens between the sexes in different ways very likely reflect outmoded notions of the relative capabilities of men and women. A gender classification fails unless it is substantially related to a sufficiently important governmental interest. . . .

We have declined, however, to extend heightened review to differential treatment based on age:

> While the treatment of the aged in this Nation has not been wholly free of discrimination, such persons, unlike, say, those who have been discriminated against on the basis of race or national origin, have not experienced a "history of purposeful unequal treatment" or been subjected to unique disabilities on the basis of stereotyped characteristics not truly indicative of their abilities.

(Massachusetts Bd. of Retirement v. Murgia,
427 U.S. 307, 313 [1976])

The lesson of *Murgia* is that where individuals in the group affected by a law have distinguishing characteristics relevant to interests the State has the authority to implement, the courts have been very reluctant, as they should be in our federal system and with our respect for the separation of powers, to closely scrutinize legislative choices as to whether, how, and to what extent those interests should be pursued. In such cases, the Equal Protection Clause requires only a rational means to serve a legitimate end.

Against this background, we conclude for several reasons that the Court of Appeals erred in holding mental retardation a quasi-suspect classification calling for a more exacting standard of judicial review than is normally accorded economic and social legislation. [The Court gives reasons for concluding that mental retardation is not a quasi-suspect classification: persons with mental retardation are a diverse population, are materially different with less ability to cope, and have a certain level of public and political support.] . . .

Doubtless, there have been and there will continue to be instances of discrimination against the retarded that are in fact invidious, and that are properly subject to judicial correction under constitutional norms. But the appropriate method of reaching such instances is not to create a new quasi-suspect classification and subject all governmental action based on that classification to more searching evaluation. Rather, we should look to the likelihood that governmental action premised on a particular classification is valid as a general matter, not merely to the specifics of the case before us. Because mental retardation is a characteristic that the government may legitimately take into account in a wide range of decisions, and because both State and Federal Governments have recently committed themselves to assisting the retarded, we will not presume that any given legislative action, even one that disadvantages retarded individuals, is rooted in considerations that the Constitution will not tolerate.

Our refusal to recognize the retarded as a quasi-suspect class does not leave them entirely unprotected from invidious discrimination. To withstand equal protection review, legislation that distinguishes between the mentally retarded and others must be rationally related to a legitimate governmental purpose. This standard, we believe, affords government the latitude neces- sary both to pursue policies designed to assist the retarded in realizing their full potential, and to freely and efficiently engage in activities that burden the retarded in what is essentially an incidental manner. The State may not rely on a classification whose relationship to an asserted goal is so attenuated as to render the distinction arbitrary or irrational. Furthermore, some objec- tives—such as "a bare . . . desire to harm a politically unpopular group," *United States Dep't of Agric. v. Moreno,* 413 U.S. 528, 534 (1973), are not legitimate state interests. Beyond that, the mentally retarded, like others, have and retain their substantive constitutional rights in addition to the right to be treated equally by the law. [The Court goes on to hold that, although mental retardation is not a classification deserving "strict scrutiny," in this case denial of a zoning permit was unreasonable and unconstitutional.]

---

## B. PROCEDURAL DUE PROCESS

When government exercises its police powers, it must not only have a good reason. It must also provide fair procedures. In *Mathews v. Eldridge,* 424 U.S. 319, 321 (1976) (posted on the *Reader* web site), the Court set the modern standard for fair procedures under the due process clause:

> "(D)ue process is flexible and calls for such procedural protections as the particular situation demands." Morrissey v. Brewer, 408 U.S. 471, 481 (1972). Accordingly, resolution of the issue whether the administrative pro- cedures provided . . . are constitutionally sufficient requires analysis of the governmental and private interests that are affected. . . . More precisely, our prior decisions indicate that identification of the specific dictates of due process generally requires consideration of three distinct factors: First, the private interest that will be affected by the official action; second, the risk of an erroneous deprivation of such interest through the procedures used, and the probable value, if any, of additional or substitute procedural safeguards; and finally, the Government's interest, including the function involved and the fiscal and administrative burdens that the additional or substitute pro- cedural requirement would entail.

In *Greene v. Edwards,* the West Virginia Supreme Court applies that standard in the public health context of isolation for TB.

---

### Greene v. Edwards*
*Supreme Court of Appeals of West Virginia*
*Decided March 11, 1980*

PER CURIAM:

William Arthur Greene . . . is involuntarily confined in Pinecrest Hospital under an order of the Circuit Court of McDowell County entered pursuant to the terms of the West Virginia Tuberculosis Control Act, W. VA. CODE § 26-5A-1, et seq. He alleges, among other points, that the Tuberculosis Control Act does not afford procedural due process because: (1) it fails to guarantee the alleged tubercular person the right to counsel; (2) it fails to insure that he may cross-examine, confront and present witnesses; and (3) it fails to require that he be committed only upon clear, cogent and convincing proof. We agree. . . .

W. VA. CODE § 26-5A-5, the statute under which the commitment proceedings in this case were conducted, provides in part:

> If such practicing physician, public health officer, or chief medical officer having under observation or care any person who is suffering from TB in a communicable stage is of the opinion that the environmental conditions of such person are not suitable for proper isolation or control by any type of local quarantine as prescribed by the state health department, and that such person is unable or unwilling to conduct himself and to live in such a manner as not to expose members of his family or household or other persons with whom he may be associated to danger of infection, he shall report the facts to the department of health which shall forthwith investigate or have investigated the circumstances alleged. If it shall find that any such person's physical condition is a health menace to others, the department of health shall petition the circuit court of the county in which such person resides, or the judge thereof in vacation, alleging that such person is afflicted with communicable TB and that such person's physical condition is a health menace to others, and requesting an order of the court committing such person to one of the state institutions. Upon receiving the petition, the court shall fix a date for hearing thereof and notice of such petition and the time and place for hearing thereof shall be served personally, at least seven days before the hearing, upon the person who is afflicted with TB and alleged to be danger-

---

*263 S.E.2d 661 (W. Va. 1980).

ous to the health of others. If, upon such hearing, it shall appear that the complaint of the department of health is well founded, that such person is afflicted with communicable TB, and that such person is a source of danger to others, the court shall commit the individual to an institution maintained for the care and treatment of persons afflicted with TB. . . .

It is evident from an examination of this statute that its purpose is to prevent a person suffering from active communicable TB from becoming a danger to others. A like rationale underlies our statute governing the involuntary commitment of a mentally ill person, W. VA. CODE § 27-5-4.

In *State ex rel. Hawks v. Lazaro,* 202 S.E.2d 109 (W. Va. 1974), we examined the procedural safeguards which must be extended to persons charged under our statute governing the involuntary hospitalization of the mentally ill. We noted that Article 3, Section 10 of the West Virginia Constitution and the Fifth Amendment to the United States Constitution provide that no person shall be deprived of life, liberty, or property without due process of law. . . .

We concluded that due process required that persons charged under W. VA. CODE § 27-5-4, must be afforded: (1) an adequate written notice detailing the grounds and underlying facts on which commitment is sought; (2) the right to counsel; (3) the right to be present, cross-examine, confront and present witnesses; (4) the standard of proof to warrant commitment to be by clear, cogent and convincing evidence; and (5) the right to a verbatim transcript of the proceeding for purposes of appeal.

Because the Tuberculosis Control Act and the Act for the Involuntary Hospitalization of the Mentally Ill have like rationales, and because involuntary commitment for having communicable TB impinges upon the right to "liberty, full and complete liberty" no less than involuntary commitment for being mentally ill, we conclude that the procedural safeguards set forth in *State ex rel. Hawks v. Lazaro,* must, and do, extend to persons charged under W. VA. CODE § 26-5A-5. . . .

We noted in *State ex rel. Hawks v. Lazaro,* that where counsel is to be appointed in proceedings for the involuntary hospitalization of the mentally ill, the law contemplates representation of the individual by the appointed guardian in the most zealous, adversary fashion consistent with the Code of Professional Responsibility. Since this decision, we have concluded that appointment of counsel immediately prior to a trial in a criminal case is impermissible since it denies the defendant effective assistance of counsel. It is obvious that timely appointment and reasonable opportunity for adequate preparation are prerequisites for fulfillment of appointed counsel's constitutionally assigned role in representing persons charged under W. Va. Code § 26-5A-5, with having communicable TB.

In the case before us, counsel was not appointed for Mr. Greene until after the commencement of the commitment hearing. Under the circumstances, counsel could not have been properly prepared to defend Mr. Greene. For this reason, he must be accorded a new hearing. . . .

[Mr. Greene's discharge is hereby delayed for a period of thirty days during which time the State may entertain further proceedings to be conducted in accordance with the principles expressed herein. . . .]

---

\*    \*    \*    \*    \*

The government has considerable power to safeguard the health and well-being of its citizens. However, this power has limits in a constitutional democracy. The state may regulate in the name of public health, but it may not overreach. It may act on the basis of scientific evidence, but not arbitrarily or with animus. Seen in this way, society seeks a reasonable balance between the common goods of public health regulation and individual rights or freedoms. To ensure that we reach a fair balance of interests, the Constitution requires government to have a good reason for public health interventions. And when government does intervene, the Constitution requires that individuals subject to coercion receive procedural due process.

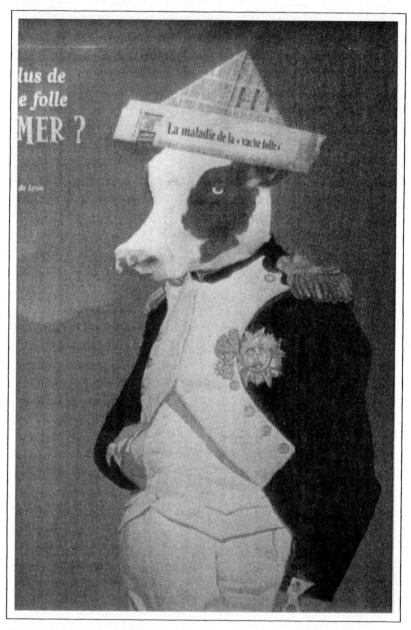

This modern painting depicts French emperor Napoleon with the head of a cow and a newspaper hat reading "mad cow disease." It was part of a November 2000 exhibition at a natural history museum in Lyon, France, presenting differing points of view of the population's response to the disease. (Patric Gardin, AP/Wide World Photos, 11/24/00.)

# EIGHT

# Public Health Regulation of Property and the Professions

Chapter 7 focused on the limits on government power to protect personal freedoms: autonomy, privacy, bodily integrity, and liberty. Individuals, however, do not want only personal freedom, but also economic liberty. They claim the liberty to own and use private property, run businesses, enter into contracts, and pursue trades, livelihoods, or professions.

Market capitalism and the profit incentive are salient values in modern America. Citizens sometimes see government as an obstacle to achieving their financial dreams. They assert a right to freedom from government bureaucracy, taxation, and burdensome regulation. Market economists believe that regulation, if desirable at all, should redress market failures rather than restrain free enterprise.

Market economists often claim that historical precedent supports the notion of minimal governmental intervention in the economy, asserting that the free enterprise system was the prevailing value in early America. William J. Novak (1993, 1, 2), a history professor at the University of Chicago, disputes this claim:

> The relationship of law, state, and economy in America has been the center of legal-historical research for almost 50 years now. But basic assumptions about state regulation and economics have remained surprisingly static. First, regulation and the economy are seen as diametrical opposites. Regulation is a contrived and public interference in a field of invisible economic

relations otherwise natural and private. Second, American regulation is un-derstood as a relatively recent invention. . . .

Through a historical reconstruction of 19th century notions of "public economy" and the "well-ordered market," I hope to establish the predomi-nance in theory and practice of an approach to economic life in early Amer-ica antithetical to the classical separation of market and state. [Numerous] cases, statutes, and ordinances suggest that early Americans understood the economy as simply another part of their "well-regulated society," inter-twined with public safety, health, morals, and welfare and subject to the same kinds of legal controls. Far from viewing the state and the economy as adversarial, the notion of "public economy" was part of a worldview slow to separate public and private, government and society. It understood com-merce, trade, and economics, like health and morals, as fundamentally pub-lic in nature, created, shaped, and *regulated* by the polity via public law.

Through an analysis of nineteenth-century inspection laws, licens-ing cases and regulations, and controls on the urban marketplace, Novak argues that economic regulation was deeply rooted in Amer-ican life and law throughout the pre–Civil War era. The pervasive-ness of these regulations and accompanying rationales steeped in a vision of a "well-regulated society" call into question historical de-scriptions of this period as the golden age of market capitalism and individualism. (See further Novak's essay on the police power in chapter 6.)

Public health advocates strongly oppose unfettered private enterprise and are suspicious of free-market solutions to social problems. They see numerous areas of economic life that require careful regulation, such as occupational health and safety risks, defective consumer products, im-pure food and water, ineffective or dangerous pharmaceuticals and medical devices, and degradation of the environment. From a public health perspective, the community can benefit from living in a well-regulated society that promotes health and prevents injury and disease. Although individuals have to forgo a certain amount of economic freedom, they are able to obtain the benefits of safer and healthier com-munities.

To achieve many of the advantages of communal health and safety, governments have formed specialized agencies, usually in the executive branch. This chapter examines commercial regulation by these agencies. Section I, "Public Health Agencies and the Rise of the Administrative State," examines the role of public health agencies in modern society. An understanding of public health agencies requires an examination of ad-ministrative law principles. Despite its position in the executive branch of government, the modern public health agency possesses wide authority to make rules, enforce health and safety standards, and adjudicate disputes (see Figure 12). Administrative law helps to determine when public health agencies are acting openly, fairly, and within the scope of their legislative mandates.

Section II, "Regulatory Tools of Public Health Agencies," examines the various techniques of commercial regulation. This section discusses several public health powers that are integral parts of civil society and staples of public health practice. Public health agencies license professionals, businesses, and institutions to ensure adequate qualifications and standards. They inspect premises and commercial establishments to identify unsanitary conditions, unsafe environments, or impure products. Agencies also possess the power to order individuals and companies to abate nuisances that pose unreasonable hazards to people in the community.

Although commercial regulation achieves important societal benefits, it also interferes with a variety of economic freedoms. Section III, "Constitutional Rights and Normative Values of Economic Liberty," examines individual claims to economic freedom. This section reviews constitutional theories of economic due process, freedom of contract, and government "takings." Those who advocate free enterprise often turn to the Constitution to justify their libertarian claims. Throughout this chapter, the key normative issue concerns the appropriate weight to be afforded to economic freedom. When government acts for the common good, how concerned should we be about impeding commercial and professional opportunities? Do economic freedoms have the same moral importance as political and civil liberties?

## I. PUBLIC HEALTH AGENCIES AND THE RISE OF THE ADMINISTRATIVE STATE

Public health problems pose complex, highly technical challenges that require expertise, flexibility, and deliberative study over the long term. Solutions cannot be found within traditional governmental structures such as representative assemblies or governors' offices. As a result, governments at the federal, state, and local (e.g., city and county) levels have formed specialized agencies to pursue the goals of population health and safety. These administrative agencies form the bulwark for public health activities in America. For an account of the policies, practices, and funding of public health agencies, see Wall (1998) and Atchison, Barry, Kanarek, and Gebbie (2000).

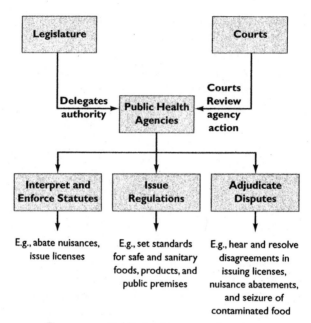

Figure 12.   Public health agency functions.

The legal status of the modern public health agency is highly complex, informed by a vast body of administrative law. Although it is not possible to discuss the breadth of administrative law doctrines here, it is helpful to study briefly the functions of public health agencies and the important legal concepts that apply. (For a more detailed discussion, see chapter 9 of the companion text.)

The modern public health agency resides within the executive branch of government but exercises powers to issue regulations, interpret statutes, and adjudicate disputes. In short, agencies possess not only executive power, but also quasi-legislative and quasi-judicial power. The lines between lawmaking, enforcement, and adjudication (inherent in the doctrine of separation of powers) have become blurred with the rise of the administrative state.

The following court cases review two major administrative law doctrines relevant to public health agencies: (1) Agencies must act within the scope of their legislative authorizations, and (2) representative assemblies may not delegate purely legislative functions to administrative agencies.

## A. AGENCY ACTION MUST BE WITHIN THE SCOPE OF LEGISLATIVE AUTHORITY

Legislatures are the policy-making arm of government and form public health agencies to carry out legislative policy. Consequently, administrative agencies have only those powers that are delegated by the legislature. The judiciary reviews statutory grants of power to ensure that agencies act within the scope of their authority. The central question for the courts is whether the legislature intended to grant the power exercised by the public health agency.

The judiciary often affords public health agencies deference in decision making. For example, if the agency asserts that it has the delegated authority to act in a certain area, or the agency interprets the authorizing statute in a certain way, the courts tend to defer. Chevron U.S.A., Inc. v. Natural Resources Defense Council, Inc., 467 U.S. 837 (1984).

The measure of deference to an agency administering its own statute varies with the circumstances. The courts have looked to the degree of agency care, its consistency, formality, and relative expertise, and the persuasiveness of the agency's position. United States v. Mead Corp., 121 S. Ct. 2164, 2171 (2001).

There are at least two circumstances in which courts will not grant agencies what is known as *Chevron* deference. The first, discussed in *Food and Drug Administration v. Brown & Williamson Tobacco Corp.* (excerpted next), is where congressional intent is clear. If the statute unambiguously does not permit the agency to act, courts will not grant it deference.

The second circumstance in which the courts will not grant deference is if the agency action raises significant constitutional questions. In *Solid Waste Agency of Northern Cook County v. United States Army Corps of Engineers*, 531 U.S. 159 (2001), the Supreme Court held that the Army Corps of Engineers exceeded its authority under the Clean Water Act when it regulated waste disposal in intrastate waters. (See further chapter 6.) The Court said that where an administrative interpretation of a statute invokes the outer limits of Congress's constitutional power, it is not entitled to *Chevron* deference. Concern that agency action exceeds the limits of power granted by Congress is heightened where the administrative interpretation alters the federal-state framework by permitting federal encroachment on a traditional state power.

## Food and Drug Administration v.
## Brown & Williamson Tobacco Corp.*

*Supreme Court of the United States*
*Decided March 21, 2000*

Justice O'CONNOR delivered the opinion of the Court.

[The Food and Drug Administration (FDA) has the power to regulate drugs and medical devices to ensure they are "safe and effective." Pursuant to this power, the FDA claimed jurisdiction to regulate tobacco products as a "nicotine delivery device." The question for the Supreme Court was whether Congress intended to give the agency the power to regulate.]

In 1996, the FDA, after having expressly disavowed any such authority since its inception, asserted jurisdiction to regulate tobacco products. The FDA concluded that nicotine is a "drug" within the meaning of the Food, Drug, and Cosmetic Act (FDCA or Act), 21 U.S.C. § 301 et seq., and that cigarettes and smokeless tobacco are "combination products" that deliver nicotine to the body. Pursuant to this authority, it promulgated regulations intended to reduce tobacco consumption among children and adolescents. The agency believed that, because most tobacco consumers begin their use before reaching the age of 18, curbing tobacco use by minors could substantially reduce the prevalence of addiction in future generations and thus the incidence of tobacco-related death and disease.

Regardless of how serious the problem an administrative agency seeks to address, however, it may not exercise its authority "in a manner that is inconsistent with the administrative structure that Congress enacted into law." ETSI Pipeline Project v. Missouri, 484 U.S. 495, 517 (1998). And although agencies are generally entitled to deference in the interpretation of statutes that they administer, a reviewing "court, as well as the agency, must give effect to the unambiguously expressed intent of Congress." Chevron U.S.A. Inc. v. Natural Resources Defense Council, Inc., 467 U.S. 837, 842–43 (1984). In this case, we believe that Congress has clearly precluded the FDA from asserting jurisdiction to regulate tobacco products. Such authority is inconsistent with the intent that Congress has expressed in the FDCA's overall regulatory

---

*529 U.S. 120 (2000).

scheme and in the tobacco-specific legislation that it has enacted subsequent to the FDCA. . . .

The FDCA grants the FDA . . . the authority to regulate, among other items, "drugs" and "devices." See 21 U.S.C. § 321(g)–(h), 393 (1994 ed. & Supp. III). The Act defines "drug" to include "articles (other than food) intended to affect the structure or any function of the body." *Id.* at § 321(g)(1)(c). It defines "device," in part, as "an instrument, apparatus, implement, machine, contrivance, . . . or other similar or related article, including any component, part, or accessory, which is . . . intended to affect the structure or any function of the body." *Id.* at § 321(h). The Act also grants the FDA the authority to regulate so-called "combination products," which "constitute a combination of a drug, device, or biologic product." *Id.* at § 353(g)(1). The FDA has construed this provision as giving it the discretion to regulate combination products as drugs, as devices, or as both. . . .

The FDA determined that nicotine is a "drug" and that cigarettes and smokeless tobacco are "drug delivery devices," and therefore it had jurisdiction under the FDCA to regulate tobacco products as customarily marketed—that is, without manufacturer claims of therapeutic benefit. First, the FDA found that tobacco products "affect the structure or any function of the body" because nicotine "has significant pharmacological effects." Fed. Reg. 44,418, 44,631 (1996). Specifically, nicotine "exerts psychoactive, or mood-altering, effects on the brain" that cause and sustain addiction, have both tranquilizing and stimulating effects, and control weight. *Id.* at 44,631–44,632. Second, the FDA determined that these effects were "intended" under the FDCA because they "are so widely known and foreseeable that [they] may be deemed to have been intended by the manufacturers," *id.* at 44,687; consumers use tobacco products "predominantly or nearly exclusively" to obtain these effects, *id.* at 44,807; and the statements, research, and actions of manufacturers revealed that they "have 'designed' cigarettes to provide pharmacologically active doses of nicotine to consumers," *id.* at 44,849. Finally, the agency concluded that cigarettes and smokeless tobacco are "combination products" because, in addition to containing nicotine, they include device components that deliver a controlled amount of nicotine to the body, *id.* at 45,208–45,216.

Having resolved the jurisdictional question, the FDA next explained the policy justifications for its regulations, detailing the deleterious health effects associated with tobacco use. It found that tobacco consumption was "the single leading cause of preventable death in the United States." *Id.* at 44,398. . . . The agency also determined that the only way to reduce the amount of tobacco-related illness and mortality was to reduce the level of addiction, a goal that could be accomplished only by preventing children and adolescents from starting to use tobacco. . . .

Based on these findings, the FDA promulgated regulations concerning tobacco products' promotion, labeling, and accessibility to children and adolescents. . . .

[The Court analyzes the FDA's assertion of authority to regulate tobacco products, specifically the agency's construction of the statute, which is governed by *Chevron,* 467 U.S. 837 (1984). Under *Chevron,* the Court determines whether Congress has directly spoken (the expressed intent of Congress). If Congress has not spoken, the Court must respect the agency's construction of the statute so long as it is permissible. Such deference is justified because the "responsibilities for assessing the wisdom of such policy choices and resolving the struggle between competing views of the public interest are not judicial ones," *id.* at 866, and because of the agency's greater familiarity with the ever-changing facts and circumstances surrounding the subjects regulated.]

We find that Congress has directly spoken to the issue here and precluded the FDA's jurisdiction to regulate tobacco products.

Viewing the FDCA as a whole, it is evident that one of the Act's core objectives is to ensure that any product regulated by the FDA is "safe" and "effective" for its intended use. . . . [T]he Act generally requires the FDA to prevent the marketing of any drug or device where the "potential for inflicting death or physical injury is not offset by the possibility of therapeutic benefit." United States v. Rutherford, 442 U.S. 544, 556 (1979).

In its rule making proceeding, the FDA quite exhaustively documented that "tobacco products are unsafe," "dangerous," and "cause great pain and suffering from illness." 61 Fed. Reg. 44,412 (1996). . . . These findings logically imply that, if tobacco products were "devices" under the FDCA, the FDA would be required to remove them from the market. . . .

Congress, however, has foreclosed the removal of tobacco products from the market. A provision of the United States Code currently in force states that "[t]he marketing of tobacco constitutes one of the greatest basic industries of the United States with ramifying activities which directly affect interstate and foreign commerce at every point, and stable conditions therein are necessary to the general welfare."

7 U.S.C. § 1311(a). More importantly, Congress has directly addressed the problem of tobacco and health through legislation on six occasions since 1965. . . . Congress has stopped well short of ordering a ban. Instead, it has generally regulated the labeling and advertisement of tobacco products, expressly providing that it is the policy of Congress that "commerce and the national economy may be . . . protected to the maximum extent consistent with [consumers] be[ing] adequately informed about any adverse health effects." 15 U.S.C. § 1331. . . . [T]he collective premise of these statutes is that cigarettes and smokeless tobacco will continue to be sold in the United States. A ban of tobacco products by the FDA would therefore plainly contradict congressional policy. . . .

Nonetheless, . . . the FDA found that, because of the high level of addiction among tobacco users, a ban would likely be "dangerous." 61 Fed. Reg. 44,413 (1996). In particular, current tobacco users could suffer from extreme withdrawal, the health care system and available pharmaceuticals might not be able to meet the treatment demands of those suffering from withdrawal, and a black market offering cigarettes even more dangerous than those currently sold illegally would likely develop. . . .

But the FDA's judgment that leaving tobacco products on the market "is more effective in achieving public health goals than a ban," *id.* at 44,398, is no substitute for the specific safety determinations required by the FDCA's various operative provisions. . . . In contrast, the FDA's conception of safety would allow the agency, with respect to each provision of the FDCA that requires the agency to determine a product's "safety" or "dangerousness," to compare the aggregate health effects of alternative administrative actions. This is a qualitatively different inquiry. Thus, although the FDA has concluded that a ban would be "dangerous," it has not concluded that tobacco products are "safe" as that term is used throughout the Act.

. . . To accommodate the FDA's conception of safety, however, one must read "any probable benefit to health" to include the benefit to public health stemming from adult consumers' continued use of tobacco products, even though the reduction of tobacco use is the *raison d'etre* of the regulations. In other words, the FDA is forced to contend that the very evil it seeks to combat is a "benefit to health." This is implausible. . . .

What the FDA may not do is conclude that a drug or device cannot be used safely for any therapeutic purpose and yet, at the same time, allow that product to remain on the market. Such regulation is incompatible with the FDCA's core objective of ensuring that every drug or device is safe and effective.

Considering the FDCA as a whole, it is clear that Congress intended to exclude tobacco products from the FDA's jurisdiction. A fundamental precept of the FDCA is that any product regulated by the FDA—but not banned—must be safe for its intended use. . . . Consequently, if tobacco products were within the FDA's jurisdiction, the Act would require the FDA to remove them from the market entirely. But a ban would contradict Congress's clear intent as expressed in its more recent, tobacco-specific legislation. The inescapable conclusion is that there is no room for tobacco products within the FDCA's regulatory scheme. If they cannot be used safely for any therapeutic purpose, and yet they cannot be banned, they simply do not fit.

In determining whether Congress has spoken directly to the FDA's authority to regulate tobacco, we must also consider in greater detail the tobacco-specific legislation that Congress has enacted over the past 35 years. . . .

Congress has enacted six separate pieces of legislation since 1965 addressing the problem of tobacco use and human health. Those statutes, among other things, require that health warnings appear on all packages and in all print and outdoor advertisements. . . .

In adopting each statute, Congress has acted against the backdrop of the FDA's consistent and repeated statements that it lacked authority under the FDCA to regulate tobacco absent claims of therapeutic benefit by the manufacturer. In fact, on several occasions over this period, and after the health consequences of tobacco use and nicotine's pharmacological effect had become well known, Congress considered and rejected bills that would have granted the FDA such jurisdiction. Under these circumstances, it is evident that Congress's tobacco-specific statutes have effectively ratified the FDA's long-held position that it lacks jurisdiction under the FDCA to regulate tobacco products. Congress has created a distinct regulatory scheme to address the problem of tobacco and health, and that scheme, as presently constructed, precludes any role for the FDA. . . .

Finally, our inquiry into whether Congress has directly spoken to the precise question at issue is shaped, at least in some measure, by the nature of the question presented. Deference under *Chevron* to an agency's construction of a statute . . . is premised on the theory that a statute's ambiguity constitutes an implicit delegation from Congress to the agency to fill in the statutory gaps. . . . Given this history and the breadth of the authority that the FDA has asserted, we are obliged to defer not to the agency's expansive construction of the statute, but to Congress's consistent judgment to deny the FDA this power. . . .

By no means do we question the seriousness of the problem that the FDA has sought to address. . . . Nonetheless, no matter . . . how likely the public is to hold the Executive Branch politically accountable, an administrative agency's power to regulate in the public interest must always be grounded in a valid grant of authority from Congress. . . . Reading the FDCA as a whole, as well as in conjunction with Congress's subsequent tobacco-specific legislation, it is plain that Congress has not given the FDA the authority that it seeks to exercise here.

* * * * *

To support its claim of jurisdiction, the FDA published voluminous evidence indicating that the industry manipulated the nicotine content of tobacco, designed cigarettes to deliver the drug to consumers, and knew that nicotine was a highly addictive substance. The agency also relied on the fact that cigarettes may not be lawfully marketed to children and adolescents. The FDA demonstrated that the industry had engaged in a persistent campaign of advertising to young persons. Should the Supreme Court have relied on these data to support the FDA's asserted jurisdiction? And, from a policy perspective, has Congress shirked its responsibility to safeguard the public's health? The Court made a pointed reference to the fact that "Congress has persistently acted to preclude a meaningful role for any administrative agency in making policy on the subject of tobacco and health." *Brown & Williamson*, 529 U.S. at 156.

## B. THE NONDELEGATION DOCTRINE

The Supreme Court, in *Brown & Williamson*, was concerned only with interpreting the statute granting the FDA regulatory power. The sole issue for the Court was whether Congress intended to grant the FDA jurisdiction to regulate tobacco products. Sometimes, however, even if the legislature does intend to delegate broad authority to administrative agencies, the courts may prohibit the delegation on constitutional grounds.

Conventionally, representative assemblies may not delegate legislative functions to the executive branch. Known as "nondelegation," this doctrine holds that policy-making functions should be undertaken by the legislative branch on the theory that only representative assemblies are politically accountable. Thus, even if the legislature intends to empower an agency to issue rules, it must do so with sufficient clarity. If the legislative grant of authority is so vague that the agency has no policy guidance, it may be unconstitutional.

The nondelegation doctrine has rarely been used by the federal courts to limit agency powers. In 1935 the Supreme Court invoked the doctrine to invalidate New Deal programs. *See* A.L.A. Schechter Poultry Corp. v. United States, 295 U.S. 495 (1935) (invalidating agency rules regarding maximum hours and minimum wages because the legislature did not provide clear standards). However, since that time the Court has not struck down a federal regulatory program on these grounds.

In 2001 the Supreme Court decided a much anticipated case about the allocation of authority in the modern administrative state. In *Whitman v. American Trucking Associations, Inc.*, 121 S. Ct. 903 (2001) (posted on the *Reader* web site), the Court refused to strike down the Environmental Protection Agency's (EPA) rules on air quality standards for ozone and particulate matter (developed pursuant to the Clean Air Act) based on a nondelegation doctrine challenge. Writing for the Court, Justice Scalia explained the nondelegation doctrine as follows:

> In a delegation challenge at the federal level, the constitutional question is whether the statute has delegated legislative power to the agency. Article I § 1 of the Constitution vests "all legislative Powers herein granted . . . in a Congress of the United States." This permits no delegation of those powers, . . . and so we have repeatedly said that when Congress confers decision-making authority upon agencies *Congress* must "lay down by legislative act an intelligible principle to which the person or body authorized to [act] is directed to conform" (*id.* at 912) (quoting J. W. Hampton, Jr. & Co. v. United States, 276 U.S. 394, 409 (1928)).

Justice Scalia ruled that the Clean Air Act's delegation of authority to the EPA to set national ambient air quality standards at a level "requisite to protect public health" was not an unconstitutional delegation of power. It contained an "intelligible principle" for setting air quality standards, and there was no necessity that the Act set precise upper limits for pollutants.

Even if the courts do not rigidly apply the nondelegation doctrine, they may use it as an aid to statutory construction, interpreting agency authority narrowly if the grant of rule-making power is vague. Recall the "Benzene case" discussed in chapter 5, in which the Supreme Court invalidated a federal agency rule that limited benzene in the workplace to no more than one part per million parts of air. The Court reasoned that the broad congressional delegation of power did not permit the Occupational Safety and Health Administration to impose health standards for exceptionally low risks with inordinately high economic costs.

The nondelegation doctrine has received varying interpretations at the state level; some jurisdictions liberally permit delegations, whereas others are more restrictive. In *Boreali v. Axelrod*, New York's highest court found unconstitutional a health department prohibition on smoking in public places because the legislature, not the health department, should make these "policy" choices.

---

**Boreali v. Axelrod***
*New York Court of Appeals*
*Decided November 25, 1987*

Judge TITONE delivered the opinion of the court.

We hold that the Public Health Council (PHC) overstepped the boundaries of its lawfully delegated authority when it promulgated a comprehensive code to govern tobacco smoking in areas that are open to the public. While the Legislature has given the Council broad authority to promulgate regulations on matters concerning the public health, the scope of the Council's authority under its enabling statute must be deemed limited by its role as an administrative, rather than a legislative, body. In this instance, the Council usurped the latter role and thereby exceeded its legislative mandate, when, following the Legislature's inability to reach an acceptable balance, the Council weighed the concerns of nonsmokers, smokers, affected businesses and the general public and, without any legislative guidance, reached its own conclusions about the proper accommodation among those competing interests. . . .

The growing concern about the deleterious effects of tobacco smoking led our State Legislature to enact a bill in 1975 restricting smoking in certain designated areas, specifically, libraries, museums, theaters and public transportation facilities. Efforts during the same year to

---

*517 N.E.2d 1350 (N.Y. Ct. App. 1987).

adopt more expansive restrictions on smoking in public areas were, however, unsuccessful. . . .

In late 1986, the PHC took action of its own. Purportedly acting pursuant to the broad grant of authority contained in its enabling statute (Public Health Law § 225[5][a]), the PHC published proposed rules, held public hearings and, in February of 1987, promulgated the final set of regulations prohibiting smoking in a wide variety of indoor areas that are open to the public, including schools, hospitals, auditoriums, food markets, stores, banks, taxicabs and limousines. . . .

The only dispute is whether the challenged restrictions were properly adopted by an administrative agency acting under a general grant of authority and in the face of the Legislature's apparent inability to establish its own broad policy on the controversial problem of passive smoking. . . .

Section 225(5)(a) of the Public Health Law authorizes the PHC to "deal with any matters affecting the . . . public health." At the heart of the present case is the question of whether this broad grant of authority contravened the oft-recited principle that the legislative branch of the government cannot cede its fundamental policy-making responsibility to an administrative agency. As a related matter, we must also inquire whether, assuming the propriety of the Legislative's grant of authority, the agency exceeded the permissible scope of its mandate by using it as a basis for engaging in inherently legislative activities. While the separation of powers doctrine gives the Legislature considerable leeway in delegating its regulatory powers, enactments conferring authority on administrative agencies in broad or general terms must be interpreted in light of the limitations that the Constitution imposes.

However facially broad, a legislative grant of authority must be construed, whenever possible, so that it is no broader than that which the separation of powers doctrine permits. Even under the broadest and most open-ended of statutory mandates, an administrative agency may not use its authority as a license to correct whatever societal evils it perceives. Here, we cannot say that the broad enabling statute in issue is itself an unconstitutional delegation of legislative authority. However, we do conclude that the agency stretched that statute beyond its constitutionally valid reach when it used the statute as a basis for drafting a code embodying its own assessment of what public policy ought to be. . . .

A number of coalescing circumstances that are present in this case persuade us that the difficult-to-define line between administrative rule-making and legislative policy-making has been transgressed. While none of these circumstances, standing alone, is sufficient to warrant the conclusion that the PHC has usurped the Legislature's prerogative, all of these circumstances, when viewed in combination, paint a portrait of an agency that has improperly assumed for itself . . . [a range of actions] which characterizes the elected Legislature's role in our system of government.

First, while generally acting to further the laudable goal of protecting nonsmokers from the harmful effects of "passive smoking," the PHC has, in reality, constructed a regulatory scheme laden with exceptions based solely upon economic and social concerns. . . . [T]hey demonstrate the agency's own effort to weigh the goal of promoting health against its social cost and to reach a suitable compromise. . . .

Striking the proper balance among health concerns, cost and privacy interests, however, is a uniquely legislative function. While it is true that many regulatory decisions involve weighing economic and social concerns against the specific values that the regulatory agency is mandated to promote, the agency in this case has not been authorized to structure its decision making in a "cost-benefit" model and, in fact, has not been given any legislative guidelines at all for determining how the competing concerns of public health and economic cost are to be weighed. Thus, [the agency] . . . was "acting solely on [its] own ideas of sound public policy" and was therefore operating outside of its proper sphere of authority. Matter of Picone v. Commissioner of Licenses, 149 N.E. 336 (N.Y. 1925). This conclusion is particularly compelling here, where the focus is on administratively created exemptions rather than on rules that promote the legislatively expressed goals, since exemptions ordinarily run counter to such goals and, consequently, cannot be justified as simple implementations of legislative values.

The second, and related, consideration is that in adopting the antismoking regulations challenged here the PHC did not merely fill in the details of broad legislation describing the over-all policies to be implemented. Instead, the PHC wrote on a clean slate, creating its own comprehensive set of rules without benefit of legislative guidance. . . .

A third indicator that the PCH exceeded the scope of the authority properly delegated to it by the Legislature is the fact that the agency acted in an area in which the Legislature had repeatedly tried—and failed—to reach agreement in the face of substantial public debate and vigorous lobbying by a variety of interested factions. . . .

In summary, we conclude that while Public Health Law §225(5)(a) is a valid delegation of regulatory authority, it cannot be construed to encompass the policy-making activity at issue here without running afoul of the constitutional separation of powers doctrine.

## II. REGULATORY TOOLS OF PUBLIC HEALTH AGENCIES

Public health agencies possess ample tools to regulate commercial activities to ensure the health and safety of the population. This section examines three of the most common regulatory powers: (1) licensing trades, professions, and institutions; (2) inspecting for violations of health and safety standards; and (3) abating public nuisances.

### A. LICENSES AND PERMITS

Public health agencies have the power to require persons, businesses, and institutions to obtain a license for the pursuit of an activity. A license provides formal permission from the government to perform certain activities, such as practicing a profession (e.g., medicine or nursing), conducting a business (e.g., food service or tattoo parlor), and operating an institution (e.g., hospital or nursing home). Licenses are part of a regulatory system that set standards for entering a field and monitor compliance.

In the following brief excerpt from a late-nineteenth-century case, the Supreme Court upheld the licensing of physicians on public health grounds in a ruling that is one of the most important licensing precedents.

---

**Dent v. West Virginia\***
*Supreme Court of the United States*
*Decided January 14, 1889*

Justice FIELD delivered the opinion of the Court.

[The petitioner was indicted for violating a West Virginia statute that requires a practitioner of medicine to obtain a certificate from the state board of health stating that he is a graduate of a reputable medical college, that he has practiced medicine for a specific period of time, or that he has otherwise been examined and found by the board to be qualified to practice medicine. The petitioner claimed that this statute was unconstitutional because it violates his rights to due process under the Fourteenth Amendment.]

---

*129 U.S. 114 (1889).

The power of the state to provide for the general welfare of its people authorizes it to prescribe all such regulations as in its judgment will secure or tend to secure them against the consequences of ignorance and incapacity, as well as deception and fraud. . . . The nature and extent of the qualifications required must depend primarily upon the judgment of the state as to their necessity. . . . It is only when they have no relation to such calling or profession, or are unattainable by such reasonable study and application, that they can operate to deprive one of his right to pursue a lawful vocation.

Few professions require more careful preparation by one who seeks to enter it than that of medicine. It has to deal with all those subtle and mysterious influences upon which health and life depend. . . . The physician must be able to detect readily the presence of disease and prescribe appropriate remedies for its removal. Everyone may have occasion to consult him, but comparatively few can judge of the qualifications of learning and skill which he possesses. Reliance must be placed upon the assurance given by his license, issued by an authority competent to judge in that respect, that he possesses the requisite qualifications. Due consideration, therefore, for the protection of society may well induce the state to exclude from practice those who have not such a license, or who are found upon examination not to be fully qualified. The same reasons which control in imposing conditions, upon compliance with which the physician is allowed to practice in the first instance, may call for further conditions as new modes of treating disease are discovered. . . . It would not be deemed a matter for serious discussion that a knowledge of the new acquisitions of the profession, as it from time to time advances in its attainments for the relief of the sick and suffering, should be required for continuance in its practice, but for the earnestness with which the plaintiff in error insists that by being compelled to obtain the certificate required, and prevented from continuing in his practice without it, he is deprived of his right and estate in his profession without due process of law. We perceive nothing in the statute which indicates an intention of the legislature to deprive one of any of his rights. No one has a right to practice medicine without having the necessary qualifications of learning and skill; and the statute only requires that whoever assumes, by offering to the community his service as a physician, that he possesses such learning and skill, shall present evidence of it by a certificate or license from a body designated by the state as competent to judge of his qualifications. . . .

It is sufficient, for the purposes of this case, to say that legislation is not open to the charge of depriving one of his rights without due process of law, if it be general in its operation upon the subjects to which it relates, and is enforceable in the usual modes established in the administration of government with respect to kindred matters; that is, by process or proceedings adapted to the nature of the case. The great purpose of the requirement is to exclude everything that is arbitrary and capricious in legislation affecting the rights of the citizen. . . .

There is nothing of an arbitrary character in the provisions of the statute in question. It applies to all physicians, except those who may be called for a special case from another state. It imposes no conditions which cannot be readily met; and it is made enforceable in the mode usual in kindred matters, that is, by regular proceedings adapted to the case. . . . If, in the proceedings under the statute, there should be any unfair or unjust action on the part of the board in refusing him a certificate, we doubt not that a remedy would be found in the courts of the state. But no such imputation can be made, for the plaintiff in error did not submit himself to the examination of the board after it had decided that the diploma he presented was insufficient.

. . . The law of West Virginia was intended to secure such skill and learning in the profession of medicine that the community might trust with confidence those receiving a license under authority of the state.

---

*     *     *     *     *

Licensing, as *Dent* suggests, can have important public health benefits by helping to ensure that only qualified individuals engage in a profession. Licensing, however, can be unfair because it parcels out a privilege based on the discretion of officials. This discretionary authority can be exercised in a discriminatory fashion against disfavored groups such as racial or religious minorities and women. Apart from blatant social and cultural discrimination, the legal conditions for issuing a license can operate to exclude the poor and minorities because they cannot meet educational and qualification standards that may be set artificially high. For example, when the American Medical Association co-opted medical licensing in the early twentieth century, it forced the closure of many existing black medical schools, resulting in marked declines in the number of

African-American physicians (Kessel 1970). Medical historian Todd L. Savitt (1984, 181–84) tells the story of Leonard Medical School of Shaw University in Raleigh, North Carolina:

> Failure rates on state licensure exams became the measure of a school's worth, once the American Medical Association began publishing this information in 1904. Leonard did not fare so well, either in comparison with other black schools or with other medical students around the country. . . . In the periodic inspections that the American Medical Association's Council on Medical Education made after 1904, Leonard always received C ratings. . . . [T]he school's administration tried desperately to keep up. . . . But still, at the core, lack of money wore Leonard down. . . . Leonard did not have the growth potential, the financial strength, or the strong faculty to meet the higher educational standards of a new era. . . . In 1918 Leonard Medical School closed its doors forever.

## B. ADMINISTRATIVE SEARCHES AND INSPECTIONS

States and localities have the power to inspect a product, business, or building to ascertain its authenticity (e.g., possession of a valid license), quality (e.g., purity and fitness for use), or condition (e.g., safety and sanitation). Inspection laws authorize and direct public health authorities to conduct administrative searches to ensure private conformance with health and safety standards.

The power of public health authorities to conduct administrative searches or inspections is among the oldest state powers, being mentioned expressly in Article I, Section 10, Clause 2 of the Constitution: States may lay imposts or duties on imports or exports, without the consent of Congress, where "absolutely necessary for executing its Inspections Laws." Inspections, however, also invade a sphere of privacy protected by the Fourth Amendment to the Constitution, which guarantees the "right of people to be secure in their persons, houses, papers, and effects, against unreasonable searches and seizures."

For most of the nation's history, public health inspections were rarely challenged and presumed to be constitutional. However, in 1967 the Supreme Court held that public health inspections are governed by the Fourth Amendment and are presumptively unreasonable if conducted without a warrant. In 1987 the Court made an exception to the warrant requirement for inspections of pervasively regulated industries. Searches without a warrant, the Court said, are reasonable only if necessary to achieve a substantial public interest.

### Camara v. Municipal Court*
Supreme Court of the United States
Decided June 5, 1967

Justice WHITE delivered the opinion of the Court.

Appellant brought this action in a California Superior Court alleging that he was awaiting trial on a criminal charge of violating the San Francisco Housing Code [§ 503] by refusing to permit a warrantless inspection of his residence, and that a writ of prohibition should issue to the criminal court because the ordinance authorizing such inspections is unconstitutional on its face. . . .

Appellant has argued throughout this litigation that § 503 is contrary to the Fourth and Fourteenth Amendments in that it authorizes municipal officials to enter a private dwelling without a search warrant and without probable cause to believe that a violation of the Housing Code exists therein. . . .

In *Frank v. State of Maryland*, 359 U.S. 360 (1955), this Court upheld the conviction of one who refused to permit a warrantless inspection of private premises for the purposes of locating and abating a suspected public nuisance. . . . To the *Frank* majority, municipal fire, health, and housing inspection programs "touch at most upon the periphery of the important interests safeguarded by the Fourteenth Amendment's protection against official intrusion," 359 U.S. at 367, because the inspections are merely to determine whether physical conditions exist which do not comply with minimum standards prescribed in local regulatory ordinances. . . .

We may agree that a routine inspection of the physical condition of private property is a less hostile intrusion than the typical policeman's search for the fruits and instrumentalities of crime. . . . But we cannot agree that the Fourth Amendment interests at stake in these inspection cases are merely "peripheral." . . . Like most regulatory laws, fire, health, and housing codes are enforced by criminal processes. In some cities, discovery of a violation by the inspector leads to a criminal complaint. Even in cities where discovery of a violation produces only an administrative compliance order, refusal to comply is a criminal offense, and the fact of compliance is verified by a second inspection,

---

*387 U.S. 523 (1967).

again without a warrant. Finally, as this case demonstrates, refusal to permit an inspection is itself a crime, punishable by fine or even by jail sentence.

The *Frank* majority suggested, and appellee reasserts, two other justifications for permitting administrative health and safety inspections without a warrant. First, it is argued that these inspections are "designed to make the least possible demand on the individual occupant." 359 U.S. at 367. The ordinances authorizing inspections are hedged with safeguards, and at any rate the inspector's particular decision to enter must comply with the constitutional standard of reasonableness even if he may enter without a warrant. In addition, . . . the warrant process could not function effectively in this field. The decision to inspect an entire municipal area is based upon legislative or administrative assessment of broad factors such as the area's age and condition. Unless the magistrate is to review such policy matters, he must issue a "rubber stamp" warrant which provides no protection at all to the property owner. . . .

Under the present system, when the inspector demands entry, the occupant has no way of knowing whether enforcement of the municipal code involved requires inspection of his premises, no way of knowing the lawful limits of the inspector's power to search, and no way of knowing whether the inspector himself is acting under proper authorization. . . . Yet, only by refusing entry and risking a criminal conviction can the occupant at present challenge the inspector's decision to search. . . . The practical effect of this system is to leave the occupant subject to the discretion of the official in the field. . . . We simply cannot say that the protections provided by the warrant procedure are not needed in this context; broad statutory safeguards are no substitute for individualized review, particularly when those safeguards may only be invoked at the risk of a criminal penalty.

The final justification suggested for warrantless administrative searches is that the public interest demands such a rule: it is vigorously argued that the health and safety of entire urban populations is dependent upon enforcement of minimum fire, housing, and sanitation standards, and that the only effective means of enforcing such codes is by routine systemized inspection of all physical structures. . . . In assessing whether the public interest demands creation of a general exception to the Fourth Amendment's warrant requirement, the question is not whether the public interest justifies the type of search in question, but whether the authority to search should be evidenced by a warrant, which in turn depends in part upon whether the burden of obtaining a warrant is likely to frustrate the governmental purpose behind the search. It has nowhere been urged that fire, health, and housing code inspection programs could not achieve their goals within the confines of a reasonable search warrant requirement. Thus, we do not find the public need argument dispositive. . . .

There is unanimous agreement among those most familiar with this field that the only effective way to seek universal compliance with the minimum standards required by municipal codes is through routine periodic inspections of all structures. It is here that the probable cause debate is focused, for the agency's decision to conduct an area inspection is unavoidable based on its appraisal of conditions in the area as a whole, not on its knowledge of conditions in each particular building. . . .

[S]uch programs have a long history of judicial and public acceptance. Second, the public interest demands that all dangerous conditions be prevented or abated, yet it is doubtful that any other canvassing technique would achieve acceptable results. . . . The warrant procedure is designed to guarantee that a decision to search private property is justified by a reasonable governmental interest. But reasonableness is still the ultimate standard. If a valid public interest justifies the intrusion contemplated, then there is probable cause to issue a suitably restricted search warrant.

---

\*     \*     \*     \*     \*

In a companion case to *Camara*, the Supreme Court held that a fire inspector who searched a business without consent or a warrant violated the Fourth Amendment: "The businessman, like the occupant of a residence, has a constitutional right to go about his business free from unreasonable official entries upon his private commercial property." *See v. City of Seattle*, 387 U.S. 541, 543 (1967).

Two decades after *Camara* and *See*, the Supreme Court recognized an exception to the warrant requirement for administrative inspections of closely regulated businesses. In *New York v. Burger*, 482 U.S. 691, 702–03 (1987), the Court held that because

> the owner or operator of commercial premises in a "closely regulated" industry has a reduced expectation of privacy, the warrant and probable cause requirements, which fulfill the traditional Fourth Amendment standard of reasonableness for a government search, have lessened application. . . . The warrantless inspection, however, . . . will be deemed to be reasonable only so long as three criteria are met.

First, there must be a "substantial" government interest that informs the regulatory scheme pursuant to which the inspection is made. Second, the warrantless inspections must be "necessary to further [the] regulatory scheme.". . . Finally, "the statute's inspection program, in terms of the certainty and regularity of its application, [must] provid[e] a constitutionally adequate substitute for a warrant."

Since *Burger*, the courts have permitted public health searches without warrants for a range of heavily regulated (and often hazardous) businesses, such as mining, firearms, and alcoholic beverages. They also permit inspections without warrants for licensed businesses with substantial public health significance, such as nursing homes and health care facilities. The judiciary permits administrative searches of pervasively regulated businesses without a warrant because of the importance of routine inspections in enforcing health and safety standards (warrants may afford owners time to conceal hazards) and the reduced expectation of privacy in highly regulated commercial activities.

## C. NUISANCE ABATEMENT

Public health authorities have the power to abate public nuisances. At common law, a public nuisance was an act or omission that obstructs or causes inconvenience or damage to the public in the exercise of rights common to all. Nuisance abatement has been one of the most important forms of public health regulation since the earliest days in American history (Tandy 1923a; Culhane and Egger 2001).

Today public nuisances are usually defined by the legislature. The legislative or administrative definition is often broad and virtually coterminous with the police power (e.g., "anything which is injurious to health, or indecent or offensive"). Public nuisances include all activities that harm the community or common pool resources (such as silence, clean air and water, or species diversity).

The judiciary has sustained a wide spectrum of traditional nuisance abatements, including diseased crops, hazardous waste, unsanitary or dangerous buildings, and even public meeting places that increase risks of sexually transmitted diseases (STDs). For example, in several cities public health agencies have used nuisance laws to close down bathhouses in response to the HIV epidemic, believing that they create opportunities for anonymous sex. The courts have usually sustained these closure orders. However, the Florida Supreme Court held that an apartment complex where two cocaine arrests had occurred within six months could not be considered a nuisance because there was no "record of persistent drug activity." Keshbro, Inc. v. City of Miami, 26 FLA. L. WKLY. 5469 (2001). The court then concluded that the owner had to be given just compensation in accordance with the takings clause because his property did not come under the nuisance exception in *Lucas v. South Carolina Coastal Council*, 505 U.S. 1003 (1992). (See discussion later in this chapter on the takings clause.)

In reading *New St. Mark's Baths* (excerpted next), think about the gay community's argument that closure infringes the freedom of association, whereas positive measures, such as education and condom distribution, would help prevent high-risk sexual behavior. Which policy option poses the greater health risk: closure of bathhouses, possibly leading to unsafe sex in alternative public gathering places, or regulation of bathhouses by making sex education and condoms available?

---

### New York v. New St. Mark's Baths*
*Supreme Court of New York*
*Decided June 6, 1986*

Judge WALLACH delivered the opinion of the court.

[New York City sought to close a bathhouse as a public nuisance pursuant to state regulation aimed at preventing the spread of AIDS. The court documents the prevalence of AIDS, particularly among gay men, and notes its transmissibility through sexual contact.]

The City has submitted ample supporting proof that high risk sexual activity has been taking place at St. Marks on a continuous and regular basis. Following numerous on site visits by City inspectors, over 14 separate days, these investigators have submitted affidavits describing 49 acts of high risk sexual activity. . . .This evidence of high risk sexual activity, all occurring either in public areas of St. Marks or in enclosed cubicles left visible to the observer without intrusion therein, demonstrates the inadequacy of self-regulatory procedures by the St. Marks attendant staff, and the futility of any less intrusive solution to the problem other than the closure.

With a demonstrated death rate from AIDS . . . plaintiffs and intervening State officers have demonstrated a compelling state interest in act-

---

*497 N.Y.S.2d 979 (1986).

ing to preserve the health of the population. Where such a compelling state interest is demonstrated even the constitutional rights of privacy and free association must give way provided, as here, it is also shown that the remedy adopted is the least intrusive reasonably available.

Furthermore, it is by no means clear that defendant's rights will, in actuality, be adversely affected in a constitutionally recognized sense by closure of St. Marks. The privacy protection of sexual activity conducted in a private home does not extend to commercial establishments simply because they provide an opportunity for intimate behavior or sexual release. . . . However the closure of this bath house does not extinguish their opportunities for unrestricted association in establishments which avoid creating a serious risk to the public health. . . .

To be sure, defendants and the intervening patrons challenge the soundness of the scientific judgments upon which the Health Council regulation is based, citing inter alia, the observation of the City's former Commissioner of Health in a memorandum dated October 22, 1985 that "closure of bathhouses will contribute little if anything to the control of AIDS." Defendants particularly assail the regulation's inclusion of fellatio as a high risk sexual activity, and argue that enforced use of prophylactic sheaths would be a more appropriate regulatory response. They go further and argue that facilities such as St. Marks, which attempts to educate its patrons with written materials, signed pledges, and posted notices as to the advisability of safe sexual practices, provide a positive force in combating AIDS, and a valuable communication link between public health authorities and the homosexual community. While these arguments and proposals may have varying degrees of merit, they overlook a fundamental principle of applicable law: "It is not for the courts to determine which scientific view is correct in ruling upon whether the police power has been properly exercised. . . ." Chiropractic Ass'n of NY v. Hilleboe, 12 N.Y.2d 109, 114 (1962). . . .

Accordingly, defendants' motion to dismiss the complaint is in all respects denied.

---

## III. CONSTITUTIONAL RIGHTS AND NORMATIVE VALUES OF ECONOMIC LIBERTY

The regulatory techniques used by public health authorities (e.g., licensing, inspection, and nuisance abatement), while protecting the public's health and safety, undoubtedly interfere with economic liberties.

The Framers clearly intended to protect economic liberties, as evidenced by several constitutional provisions. Notably, the Constitution forbids the state from depriving persons of property (or life or liberty) without due process of law (Fifth and Fourteenth Amendments), impairing the obligations of contracts (art. I, § 10), and taking private property for public use without just compensation (Fifth Amendment).

## A.  ECONOMIC DUE PROCESS AND FREEDOM OF CONTRACT

Recall the discussion in chapter 7 of the landmark case of *Jacobson v. Massachusetts,* in which the Supreme Court held that government had ample authority to safeguard the public's health, even if it meant a diminution in autonomy and bodily integrity. *Jacobson* was decided in the same term as *Lochner v. New York,* the beginning of the so-called Lochner era in constitutional law—from 1905 to 1937. During the Lochner era, the Supreme Court afforded individuals greater protection in the realm of economic affairs than in personal affairs.

---

### Lochner v. New York*
*Supreme Court of the United States*
*Decided April 17, 1905*

Justice PECKHAM delivered the opinion of the Court.

[A New York law prohibited the employment of bakery employees for more than 10 hours a day or 60 hours a week. Lochner was convicted and fined for permitting an employee to work in his Utica, N.Y., bakery for more than 60 hours in one week, or more than 10 hours in one day.]

[When] the [state], in the assumed exercise of its police powers, has passed an act which seriously limits the right to labor or the right of contract in regard to their means of livelihood between persons who are sui juris (both employer and employee), it becomes of great importance to determine which shall prevail—the right of the individual to labor for such time as he may choose, or the right of the State to prevent the individual from laboring [beyond] a certain time pre-

---

*198 U.S. 45 (1905).

scribed by the State. This court [has] upheld the exercise of the police powers of the States in many cases which might fairly be considered as border ones, and it [has] been guided by rules of a very liberal nature, the application of which has resulted, in numerous instances, in upholding the validity of state statutes thus assailed.

It must, of course, be conceded that there is a limit to the valid exercise of the police power by the state. There is no dispute concerning this general proposition. Otherwise the 14th Amendment would have no efficacy and the legislatures of the states would have unbounded power, and it would be enough to say that any piece of legislation was enacted to conserve the morals, the health, or the safety of the people; such legislation would be valid, no matter how absolutely without foundation the claim might be. The claim of the police power would be a mere pretext—become another and delusive name for the supreme sovereignty of the state to be exercised free from constitutional restraint. In every case that comes before this court, therefore, where legislation of this character is concerned, and where the protection of the Federal Constitution is sought, the question necessarily arises: Is this a fair, reasonable, and appropriate exercise of the police power of the state, or is it an unreasonable, unnecessary, and arbitrary interference with the right of the individual to his personal liberty, or to enter into those contracts in relation to labor which may seem to him appropriate or necessary for the support of himself and his family? . . .

There is no reasonable ground for interfering with the liberty of person or the right of free contract, by determining the hours of labor, in the occupation of a baker. There is no contention that bakers as a class are not equal in intelligence and capacity to men in other trades or manual occupations, or that they are not able to assert their rights and care for themselves without the protecting arm of the state, interfering with their independence of judgment and of action. They are in no sense wards of the state. Viewed in the light of a purely labor law, with no reference whatever to the question of health, we think that a law like the one before us involves neither the safety, the morals, nor the welfare, of the public, and that the interest of the public is not in the slightest degree affected by such an act. The law must be upheld, if at all, as a law pertaining to the health of the individual engaged in the occupation of a baker. It does not affect any other portion of the public than those who are engaged in that occupation. Clean and wholesome bread does not depend upon whether the baker works but ten hours per day or only sixty hours a week. The limitation of the hours of labor does not come within the police power on that ground. . . .

The mere assertion that the subject relates, though but in a remote degree, to the public health, does not necessarily render the enactment valid. The act must have a more direct relation, as a means to an end, and the end itself must be appropriate and legitimate, before an act can be held to be valid which interferes with the general right of an individual to be free in his person and in his power to contract in relation to his own labor. . . .

We think that there can be no fair doubt that the trade of a baker, in and of itself, is not an unhealthy one to that degree which would authorize the legislature to interfere with the right to labor, and with the right of free contract on the part of the individual, either as employer or employee. . . . It might be safely affirmed that almost all occupations more or less affect the health. There must be more than the mere fact of the possible existence of some small amount of unhealthiness to warrant legislative interference with liberty. . . . No trade, no occupation, no mode of earning one's living, could escape this all-pervading power, and the acts of the legislature in limiting the hours of labor in all employments would be valid, although such limitation might seriously cripple the ability of the laborer to support himself and his family. . . .

[W]e think that such a law as this, although passed in the assumed exercise of the police power, and as relating to the public health, or the health of the employees named, is not within that power, and is invalid. The act is not, within any fair meaning of the term, a health law, but is an illegal interference with the rights of individuals, both employers and employees, to make contracts regarding labor upon such terms as they may think best. . . .

Mr. Justice HARLAN dissenting:

It is plain that this statute was enacted in order to protect the physical well-being of those who work in bakery and confectionery establishments. . . . The constant inhaling of flour dust causes inflammation of the lungs and of the bronchial tubes. The eyes also suffer through this dust, which is responsible for the many cases of running eyes among the bakers. . . . The average age of a baker is below that of other workmen; they seldom live over their fiftieth year, most of them dying between the ages of forty and fifty. During periods of epidemic diseases the bakers are generally the first to succumb to the disease, and the number swept away during such periods far exceeds the number of other crafts in comparison to the men employed in the respective industries. . . .

There are many reasons of a weighty, substantial character, based upon the experience of mankind, in support of the theory that, all things considered, more than ten hours' steady work each day, from week to week, in a bakery or confectionery establishment, may endanger the health and shorten the lives of the workmen, thereby diminishing their physical and mental capacity to serve the state and to provide for those dependent upon them. . . .

Let the state alone in the management of its purely domestic affairs, so long as it does not appear beyond all question that it has violated the Federal Constitution. This view necessarily results from the principle that the health and safety of the people of a state are primarily for the state to guard and protect.

---

\*       \*       \*       \*       \*

The Lochner era posed deep concerns for those who realized that much of what public health does interferes with economic freedoms involving contracts, business relationships, the use of property, and the practice of trades and professions. *Lochner,* in the words of Justice Harlan, in dissent, "would seriously cripple the inherent power of the states to care for the lives, health, and well-being of their citizens." 198 U.S. at 73. So it was. In the next three decades, the Supreme Court struck down important health and social legislation setting minimum wages for women, protecting consumers from hazardous products, and licensing or regulating businesses.

By the time of the New Deal, the laissez faire philosophy that undergirded Lochnerism was challenged by those who believed that economic transactions were naturally constrained by unequal wealth and power relationships. This was also a time when people looked toward government to pursue actively the values of welfare, health, and greater social and economic equity. It was within this political and social context that the Supreme Court repudiated the principles of *Lochner:* "What is this freedom? The Constitution does not speak of freedom of contract. It speaks of liberty and prohibits the deprivation of liberty without due process of law." West Coast Hotel Co. v. Parrish, 300 U.S. 379, 391 (1937). The post–New Deal period led to a resurgence of a permissive judicial approach to public health regulation, irrespective of its effects on commercial and business affairs.

## B. REGULATORY "TAKINGS"

The federal government and the states have the power of eminent domain, which is the authority to confiscate private property for a governmental activity. However, the Fifth Amendment imposes a significant constraint on this power by requiring "just compensation" for private property taken for a public use. The theory behind the takings clause is that individuals should not have to bear public burdens that should be borne by the community as a whole.

Despite its just purposes, an expansive interpretation of the takings clause would shackle public health agencies by requiring them to provide compensation whenever regulation significantly reduced the value of private property. Since public health regulation restricts commercial property uses, it has become a focal point for a sustained conservative critique. For example, Charles Fried (1991, 181) said that Attorney General Meese in the Reagan administration had a "specific, aggressive, and it seemed to me, quite radical project in mind: to use the takings clause of the Fifth Amendment as a severe brake on federal and state regulation of business and property."

Government confiscation or physical occupation of property is a "possessory" taking that certainly requires compensation. During the early twentieth century, however, the Supreme Court held that government regulation that "reaches a certain magnitude" also is a taking requiring compensation. Pennsylvania Coal Co. v. Mahon, 260 U.S. 393 (1922). Initially, this idea of "regulatory" takings was not highly problematic for public health agencies because the Court suggested that government need not compensate property owners when regulating within the police power. However, regulatory takings took on public health significance in 1992.

---

**Lucas v. South Carolina Coastal Council***
*Supreme Court of the United States*
*Decided June 29, 1992*

Justice SCALIA delivered the opinion of the Court.

In 1986, petitioner David H. Lucas paid $975,000 for two residential lots on the Isle of Palms in Charleston County, South Carolina, on

---

*505 U.S. 1003 (1992).

which he intended to build single-family homes. In 1988, however, the South Carolina Legislature enacted the Beachfront Management Act, S.C. CODE ANN. § 48-39-250 et seq. (Supp. 1990), which had the direct effect of barring petitioner from erecting any permanent habitable structures on his two parcels. A state trial court found that this prohibition rendered Lucas's parcels "valueless." This case requires us to decide whether the Act's dramatic effect on the economic value of Lucas's lots accomplished a taking of private property under the Fifth and Fourteenth Amendments requiring the payment of "just compensation.". . .

Prior to Justice Holmes's exposition in *Pennsylvania Coal Co. v. Mahon,* 260 U.S. 393 (1922), it was generally thought that the Takings Clause reached only a "direct appropriation" of property, or the functional equivalent. Justice Holmes recognized in *Mahon,* however, that if the protection against physical appropriations of private property was to be meaningfully enforced, the government's power to redefine the range of interests included in the ownership of property was necessarily constrained by constitutional limits. If, instead, the uses of private property were subject to unbridled, uncompensated qualification under the police power, "the natural tendency of human nature [would be] to extend the qualification more and more until at last private property disappear[ed]." *Id.* at 415. These considerations gave birth in that case to the oft-cited maxim that "while property may be regulated to a certain extent, if regulation goes too far it will be recognized as a taking." *Id.*

Nevertheless, our decision in *Mahon* offered little insight into when, and under what circumstances, a given regulation would be seen as going "too far" for purposes of the Fifth Amendment. In 70-odd years of succeeding "regulatory takings" jurisprudence, we have generally eschewed any "set formula" for determining how far is too far, preferring to "engag[e] in . . . essentially ad hoc, factual inquiries." Goldblatt v. Hempstead, 369 U.S. 590, 594 (1962). We have, however, described at least two discrete categories of regulatory action as compensable without case-specific inquiry into the public interest advanced in support of the restraint. The first encompasses regulations that compel the property owner to suffer a physical "invasion" of his property. In general (at least with regard to permanent invasions), no matter how minute the intrusion, and no matter how weighty the public purpose behind it, we have required compensation. . . .

The second situation in which we have found categorical treatment appropriate is where regulation denies all economically beneficial or productive use of land. As we have said on numerous occasions, the Fifth Amendment is violated when land-use regulation "does not substantially advance legitimate state interests or denies an owner economically viable use of his land." Agins v. City of Tiburon, 447 U.S. 255, 260 (1980).

We have never set forth the justification for this rule. Perhaps it is simply, as Justice Brennan suggested, that total deprivation of beneficial use is, from the landowner's point of view, the equivalent of a physical appropriation. See San Diego Gas & Electric Co. v. San Diego, 450 U.S. 621, 652 (1981) (dissenting opinion). . . . [A]ffirmatively supporting a compensation requirement, is the fact that regulations that leave the owner of land without economically beneficial or productive options for its use—typically, as here, by requiring land to be left substantially in its natural state—carry with them a heightened risk that private property is being pressed into some form of public service under the guise of mitigating serious public harm. . . .

We think, in short, that there are good reasons for our frequently expressed belief that when the owner of real property has been called upon to sacrifice all economically beneficial uses in the name of the common good, that is, to leave his property economically idle, he has suffered a taking. . . .

In [the view of the South Carolina Supreme Court], the Beachfront Management Act was no ordinary enactment, but involved an exercise of South Carolina's "police powers" to mitigate the harm to the public interest that petitioner's use of his land might occasion. . . . In the court's view, [the] petitioner's challenge [came] within a long line of this Court's cases sustaining against Due Process and Takings Clause challenges the State's use of its "police powers" to enjoin a property owner from activities akin to public nuisances. . . .

Where the State seeks to sustain regulation that deprives land of all economically beneficial use, we think it may resist compensation only if the logically antecedent inquiry into the nature of the owner's estate shows that the proscribed use interests were not part of his title to begin with. This accords, we think, with our "takings" jurisprudence, which has traditionally been guided by the understandings of our citizens regarding the content of, and the State's power over, the "bundle of rights" that they acquire when they obtain title to property. It seems to us that the property owner necessarily expects the uses of his property to be restricted, from time to time, by various measures newly enacted by the State in legitimate exercise of its police powers; "[a]s long recognized, some values are enjoyed under an implied limitation and must yield to the police power." *Mahon*, 260 U.S. at 413. And in the case of personal property, by reason of the State's traditionally high degree of control over commercial dealings, he ought to be aware of the possibility that new regulation might even render his property economically worthless (at least if the property's only economically productive use is sale or manufacture for sale). In the case of land, however, we think the notion pressed by the Council that title is somehow held subject to the "implied limitation" that the State may subsequently eliminate all economically valuable use is inconsistent with the historical compact recorded in the Takings Clause that has become part of our constitutional culture.

Where "permanent physical occupation" of land is concerned, we have refused to allow the government to decree it anew (without compensation), no matter how weighty the asserted public interests involved — though we assuredly would permit the government to assert a permanent easement that was a pre-existing limitation upon the landowner's title. We believe similar treatment must be accorded confiscatory regulations, i.e., regulations that prohibit all economically beneficial use of land: Any limitation so severe cannot be newly legislated or decreed (without compensation), but must inhere in the title itself, in the restrictions that background principles of the State's law of property and nuisance already place upon land ownership. A law or decree with such an effect must, in other words, do no more than duplicate the result that could have been achieved in the courts — by adjacent landowners (or other uniquely affected persons) under the State's law of private nuisance, or by the State under its complementary power to abate nuisances that affect the public generally, or otherwise. . . .

In light of our traditional resort to existing rules or understandings that stem from an independent source such as state law to define the range of interests that qualify for protection as "property" under the Fifth and Fourteenth Amendments, this recognition that the Takings Clause does not require compensation when an owner is barred from putting land to a use that is proscribed by those "existing rules or understandings" is surely unexceptional. When, however, a regulation that declares "off-limits" all economically productive or beneficial uses of land goes beyond what the relevant background principles would dictate, compensation must be paid to sustain it.

The "total taking" inquiry we require today will ordinarily entail (as the application of state nuisance law ordinarily entails) analysis of, among other things, the degree of harm to public lands and resources, or adjacent private property, posed by the claimant's proposed activities, the social value of the claimant's activities and their suitability to the locality in question, and the relative ease with which the alleged harm can be avoided through measures taken by the claimant and the government (or adjacent private landowners) alike. The fact that a particular use has long been engaged in by similarly situated owners ordinarily imports a lack of any common-law prohibition (though changed circumstances or new knowledge may make what was previously permissible no longer so). So also does the fact that other landowners, similarly situated, are permitted to continue the use denied to the claimant.

It seems unlikely that common law principles would have prevented the erection of any habitable or productive improvements on petitioner's land; they rarely support prohibition of the essential use of land. The question, however, is one of state law to be dealt with on remand. . . . South Carolina must identify background principles of nuisance and property law that prohibit the uses he now intends in the circumstances in which the property is presently found. Only on this showing can the State fairly claim that, in proscribing all such beneficial uses, the Beachfront Management Act is taking nothing.

---

\*     \*     \*     \*     \*

Since *Lucas,* state and lower federal courts have been divided on the question of compensation resulting from environmental regulation. Some courts have used the "property rights" tenor of Justice Scalia's opinion to strike down important public health and environmental regulation. For example, in *Philip Morris, Inc. v. Reilly,* 113 F. Supp. 2d 129 (D. Mass. 2000), a federal district court held that a Massachusetts state law requiring manufacturers to disclose brand-specific ingredient lists to state regulators for eventual public dissemination effects an unconstitutional taking of trade secrets. The U.S. Court of Appeals for the First Circuit, however, overturned the decision. The Court of Appeals reasoned that tobacco manufacturers receive the economic benefit of permission to market their products in return for disclosing their ingredients. A dissent called the court's approach "alarming." Philip Morris Inc. v. Reilly, 70 U.S.L.W. 1254 (Oct. 30, 2001).

If the takings clause is to be used as a severe constraint on public health regulation, the outcome remains uncertain. Much depends on the direction of a divided Supreme Court which, at present, has four members apparently committed to expansion of the regulatory takings doctrine (Chief Justice Rehnquist and Justices Scalia, Thomas, and O'Connor) (Lazarus 1993). In 2001 these four justices were joined by Justice Kennedy in *Palazzolo v. Rhode Island*, 121 S. Ct. 2448 (2001), in a potentially important property rights case. The Court held that a landowner's knowledge of land use restrictions at the time he acquires property does not automatically preclude him from asserting a Fifth Amendment takings claim for compensation. The holding enabled the owner of waterfront property to proceed with a takings claim occasioned by coastal wetlands regulations affecting a portion of his property. A total taking of the property had not occurred because the nonwetlands portion could be developed, but the Court remanded the case for consideration of whether some compensation may be due.

## CONCLUSION

The court cases discussed in this chapter raise an important normative issue about the significance of economic liberty in our society. How important is unbridled freedom in property uses, financial relationships, and the pursuit of occupations? A market economy is important in its own right because it increases productivity and raises standards of living. Free enterprise also has public health significance because of the positive association between socioeconomic status and well-being. After all, it is possible to theorize that the free market will create wealth not only for entrepreneurs, but for the wider population.

Despite the value of the undeterred entrepreneur, should we strive for a well-regulated society that deters harmful commercial activities? Surely, no one would impose burdensome regulation gratuitously, but government does have an obligation to safeguard the health of people and their environment. Suppose it is more profitable for a manufacturer to make a product without a safety feature (e.g., automobiles without airbags) or to fail to control an emission (e.g., dumping toxic waste into a lake). Isn't it within the government's prerogative to regulate the activity? If the legislature makes a social choice that favors communal health and safety over economic freedom, arguably the courts should respect that judgment.

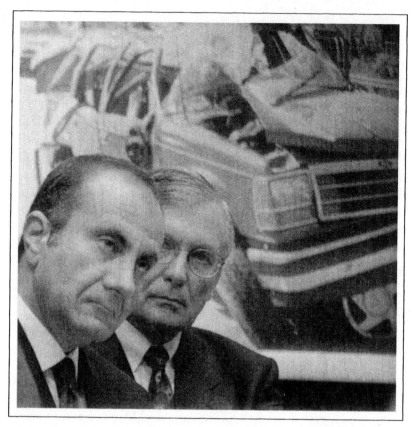

With a photograph of a wrecked Ford Explorer in the background, Ford Motor Co. executives listen to testimony on Capitol Hill on September 6, 2000, as part of a House Committee investigation of a national recall of Firestone tires. The tires, which Ford installed on many of its Explorers, had manufacturing defects. Over 140 individuals were killed in auto accidents allegedly caused by the defective tires. (Dennis Cook, AP/Wide World Photos, 9/6/00.)

# NINE

# Tort Litigation
# for the Public's Health

The levers of public health regulation are often viewed as being in the hands of legislatures and executive agencies. However, attorneys general and private citizens possess a powerful means of indirect regulation through the tort system. Tort litigation can be an effective method for reducing the burden of injury and disease. The courts help redress harms caused by pollution, toxic substances, unsafe pharmaceuticals or vaccines, and defective or hazardous consumer products. Figure 13 provides an image of tort law serving as a tool for reducing a variety of harms to the population's health.

The goals of tort law, although imperfectly achieved, are frequently consistent with public health objectives. The tort system aims to hold individuals and businesses accountable for their dangerous activities, compensate persons who are harmed, deter unreasonably hazardous conduct, and encourage innovation in product design, labeling, and advertising to reduce the risk of injury or disease. Civil litigation, therefore, can provide potent incentives for people and manufacturers to engage in safer, more socially conscious behavior. (For an insightful discussion of the functions of tort litigation, see Jacobson and Warner [1999].)

Tort law can be an effective method of advancing the public's health, but, like any form of regulation, it is not an unmitigated good. The tort system imposes economic costs and personal burdens on individuals and businesses, including transaction expenses (e.g., the court system

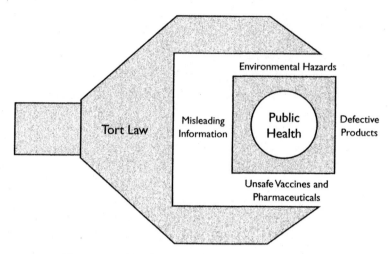

Figure 13.   Tort law as a tool in public health.

and attorneys' fees) and liability. Society may not be any the poorer if tort costs make it difficult for dangerous, socially unproductive enterprises (e.g., tobacco and firearms) to operate within the market. Tort costs, however, appear to be just as high for socially advantageous goods and services such as vaccines, pharmaceuticals, and medical devices.

Tort litigation, moreover, can be seen as antidemocratic and unfair. Critics argue that the political branches of government, not the judicial branch, should set health policy. Even though redress through the courts is an important right in a constitutional democracy, some observers do not believe that judges and juries should award substantial punitive damages against manufacturers. Critics also claim that the chief beneficiaries of the tort system are often a few plaintiffs and their attorneys, rather than the entire population that has been harmed. For example, some tobacco litigation has imposed substantial penalties on manufacturers but has disproportionately rewarded a relatively small number of smokers and trial lawyers.

Litigation as a form of regulation, then, holds enormous potential for improving the public's health, but also entails economic costs and unjust distribution of benefits and burdens. Like any form of regulation, we trade off the public goods resulting from civil litigation against the burdens and inequities.

This chapter takes a look at tort litigation as a tool of public health. (For those who are unfamiliar with the major theories of tort law, it will be helpful to read chapter 10 in the companion text.) First, this chapter generally discusses tort law as a prevention strategy. Many scholars and practitioners claim that civil litigation can be an important public health strategy in fields ranging from injury prevention to tobacco and firearm control (Parmet 1999; Christoffel and Gallagher 1999). Stephen P. Teret, a professor at Johns Hopkins University and a leading injury prevention scholar, perceives product liability litigation as a form of "vector control" comparable to control of rodents and mosquitoes: "Today, the vehicles for injury and disease are often manmade products, frequently transmitting energy as the etiologic agent of injury." (See the following excerpt.)

Second, this chapter examines the complex problems involving science and epidemiology in the courtroom. The courts have long struggled with the issue of scientific evidence and "proof" in public health litigation. What kind of evidence should be admissible in the courts? This is a crucial issue because it determines the degree of scientific rigor that the courts require of experts. If the judiciary adopts a permissive approach, this may result in what some people call "junk science" in the courtroom. If the judiciary adopts a restrictive approach, this may result in potentially relevant evidence being excluded.

A related question is the degree of proof needed to establish causality. If epidemiologists find an association, say, between exposure to a toxic substance and an increased rate of cancer, how do we know if that substance actually caused the harm about which the plaintiffs complain?

## I. TORT LAW AS A PREVENTION STRATEGY

The two brief selections in this section provide a general overview of tort litigation for the public's health. Their purpose is to show the unique role of the courts in public health regulation. The fundamental questions are how public health policy should be constructed and by which institutions: the market, the political system (i.e., the legislative and executive branches of government), or the courts? The articles discuss the advantages, and disadvantages, of policy making by the courts. In their unedited versions, they provide illustrations of particular public health problems. Teret emphasizes airbag, cigarette, and firearm litigation; Wendy E. Parmet and Richard A. Daynard, professors of law at Northeastern University, explain a matrix of the forms of legal action utilized in tobacco, firearm, and lead paint cases. These illustrations are deemphasized in the edited versions, but readers can find excellent discussions of tobacco (Jacobson and Warner 1999; Rabin 1992) and firearm (Vernick and Teret 1999) litigation elsewhere.

---

## Litigating for the Public Health*
*Stephen P. Teret*

Vector control has long been one of the basic tools of public health. When it was learned that rodents, mosquitoes, and other living organisms transmitted to man the etiologic agents for disease, the public health response was to control those vectors of disease. Today, the vehicles for injury and disease are often manmade products, frequently transmitting energy as the etiologic agent of injury. The public health response should similarly be the control of these vehicles by use of the law. But unlike rodents and mosquitoes, the modern day vehicles of injury and disease have vested interests, lobbyists and political action committees that sometimes thwart effective legislative and regulatory attempts to enhance the public's health. When this happens, public health advocates have turned to the third branch of government, the judiciary, to seek relief from juries.

Product liability litigation is now being used as an effective tool for public health advocacy. Its use is based on the premise that substantial settlements and verdicts against the manufacturer of an unnecessarily dangerous product will ultimately cause that manufacturer to invest in prevention rather than pay the penalty for neglect. Manufacturers, responding to the negative effect which large damage awards have on corporate profits and insurance premiums, have recalled and redesigned formerly unsafe products, and have developed testing methods and design strategies aimed at reducing the likelihood that a new product will injure its user.

But product liability litigation, or the specter thereof, may also retard the introduction of innovative products that can be beneficial to the public's health. Some manufacturers suggest that product liability exposure is great enough to warrant the withdrawal of products from the market, even if on balance the benefit of the product to the public clearly outweighs the risk of the product to an individual. . . . Thus, product liability litigation can be seen as a double-edged sword, to be used as a tool of public health

---

*Reprinted from *American Journal of Public Health* 76 (1986): 1027–29.

under carefully chosen circumstances, when more conventional forms of advocacy have not proven fruitful. . . .

Cars, cigarettes and guns have presented sizable problems to the public's health. Together, their annual death toll in the United States approaches half a million people. The fact that each of these products may be susceptible to product liability litigation is a reflection that jurors can find the hazards these products pose as unacceptable. Cigarettes and guns can be seen as low-benefit, high-risk products. Cars, although of great social benefit, are inadequately crashworthy with regard to foreseeable risk.

The solution to liability exposure should be the marketing of safe products. For some products, this may mean modification by the use of already existing devices such as air bags. For other products such as cigarettes, it may mean the end of manufacturing and marketing of the product altogether.

But instead of product changes, the perceived crisis of litigation has led many, under the banner of tort reform, to propose limiting monetary recoveries for people damaged from products. Some aspects of these proposals may have merit, particularly with regard to products which are now regulated. But for those products which have been able to avoid meaningful regulation, largely due to the political strength of lobbying groups, litigation represents the only de facto form of safety regulation. Limitation of the ability of injured and ill persons to seek compensation from the manufacturers of guns and cigarettes, for example, would permit the continuing damage these products cause to the public's health. The crisis involved with these products is not litigation, but the terrible burden of death and disability caused by these vehicles of injury and disease.

## The New Public Health Litigation*

Wendy E. Parmet and Richard A. Daynard

INTRODUCTION

One of the most remarkable developments of the last three decades has been the increasing use of litigation as a public health tool. Although courts have long been called on to review matters concerning public health, historically the courtroom was seldom the forum of choice for public health enthusiasts. Instead, it was the place where those who wished to resist

*Reprinted from Annual Review of Public Health 21 (2000): 437–54.

public health regulation, be they milk producers, bread makers, or parents who did not want their children to be vaccinated, went in the hope of limiting the authority of public health agencies. Although such litigants were usually not successful, public health had little to gain by the litigation. At best the regulation might be upheld; at worst, the right of the individual or business to refuse compliance might be proclaimed. The courtroom, in short, was a barrier that public health authorities sometimes needed to pass through on their way to protecting the public's health.

In recent years, however, the tables have turned. Increasingly, individuals and organizations concerned about public health have sought to use litigation to further their goals. In other words, courts are now being used affirmatively in an effort to make public health policy. Most notably, the tobacco control movement has pursued a litigation strategy, not simply to obtain compensation for tobacco's victims, but also to achieve a reduction in tobacco use. Likewise, groups concerned about gun violence have chosen to sue the gun industry. In similar fashion, the American Public Health Association has urged the use of litigation to hold paint manufacturers accountable for the injuries caused by lead paint. Litigation has also played a prominent role in the struggle to ensure access to health care for individuals infected with HIV. . . .

## TYPOLOGY OF PUBLIC HEALTH LITIGATION

Courts have always played a role in public health enforcement. If a public health agency ordered a warehouse with rotting food to close, the owner could go to court and seek review of the order. Similarly, if a manufacturer wanted to resist a government regulation, it could challenge that regulation in court. In the process of deciding these cases, courts inevitably help delineate the nature and extent of public health authority. . . .

What is different today is the increasing, and sometimes dominant, role played by public health concerns. In [earlier] cases, individuals sought either to limit public health authorities or to achieve monetary relief. The affirmative protection of the public's health was not often one of the plaintiff's major goals. But in the wake of the civil rights and other law reform movements, public health advocates have increasingly turned to the courts to achieve social change. . . .

## THE LITERATURE

Much of the literature analyzing the success of reform litigation has focused on litigation that [concerns] cases brought against governmental entities. One leading scholar on the impact of law reform litigation,

Rosenberg (1991), has concluded that much of the constitutional reform litigation of the 1950s, 1960s, and 1970s, including the litigation surrounding *Brown v. Board of Education*, resulted in far less change than is generally believed. . . . Other scholars have suggested that reform litigation may have an even more robust effect. The work of McCann (1992) is particularly relevant to a consideration of the impact of public health litigation. McCann believes that Rosenberg has focused too heavily on the impact of judicial decisions themselves rather than on the multidimensional process of litigation. From McCann's perspective, the focus must be not simply on court decisions and their direct impact but also on the litigation process, which may have a constitutive impact and "reshape perceptions of when and how particular values are realistically actionable."

Other scholars have considered the impact of product liability litigation, which often touches on questions of public health. For the most part, these scholars have used an economic perspective, asking whether such litigation is economically efficient, rather than whether it is capable of improving public health or influencing the public health agenda. Nevertheless, although these scholars have disagreed about the degree of deterrence achieved by product liability litigation, as well as its efficiency as a deterrent or compensation system, they have generally found that it creates some deterrent effect. . . .

[The authors discuss the effectiveness of tobacco litigation.]

## PUBLIC HEALTH LITIGATION AND DEMOCRATIC THEORY

A commonly made and potent criticism of litigation-centered reform movements is that they are fundamentally antidemocratic. If change is to occur in our laws, so the criticism goes, it should occur via legislation enacted by democratically accountable representatives. Situating policy development reform in the courts bypasses that political accountability in favor of less accountable judges and juries.

In public health litigation, a further related criticism may be made. In our market economy, individuals are presumed to have significant freedom as to what risks they wish to incur. To the extent that public health policies seek to reduce risks beyond the rate individuals would choose in the market, those policies may be described as inherently paternalistic and contrary to the prevailing individualistic/market ethos. When public health advocates seek to reduce those risks and achieve their aims not through legislation but via judicial decrees, they become particularly vulnerable to a charge of paternalism, for they may be seen

as trying to force the public to accept what neither it nor its representatives desire. . . .

Several responses may be made to the charge that public health litigation is both antidemocratic and paternalistic. The first and narrow-
est is that litigation often serves to further a democratically determined
policy. Even if we concede that interference with the market should be
the exception rather than the norm and that such exceptions should
be derived from politically accountable processes, a significant role remains for litigation. Democratically enacted laws still require interpretation and enforcement, and that often requires litigation. . . .

Another response to the antidemocratic critique recognizes that the
judicial law making that defines "the common law" has long been an
accepted part of our democratic polity. Indeed many public health policies in place today result from an interactive dialog between courts and
legislatures. For example, the doctrine of informed consent for medical
services originally emerged from litigation in which plaintiffs asked
courts to build on common-law doctrines of battery. . . .

A different response goes further to explain the use of litigation not
only in enforcing legislation but also in creating new public health policies. This response questions the assumption that the legislative process
itself is as democratic as the antidemocratic critique assumes. As the
Supreme Court recognized in the reapportionment cases of the 1960s,
there are situations in which, absent judicial intervention, structural
flaws in our political system prevent the popular will from being enacted as legislation.

This situation has arisen with some public health issues, owing to
campaign contributions by special interests. Because these contributions flow overwhelmingly to incumbents, making credible challenges
to their seats both difficult and rare, incumbents often refuse to enact
serious campaign reform. What the special interests exact in return for
their money is a de facto veto over legislation adverse to their interests.
Contributions by the tobacco, gun, and health care industries are cases
in point. . . .

There is another way in which litigation may be able to force regulation onto the legislative agenda, even if the affected special interest
demurs. Litigation makes compelling drama; lawsuits grab headlines,
are regularly featured on talk shows, and become part of ordinary
conversation. Lawsuits can therefore thwart the desire of the special
interest to restrict discussion of issues involving it to the halls of Congress, administrative agencies, and other venues where challenges to

established ways of dealing with the issues are unlikely. Once the public and the media are actively engaged in the issue, the political calculus, in Congress and elsewhere, may change. In other words, litigation may be used not only to achieve judicially imposed changes but also to change the political climate in which issues of public health are debated.

At times, the information obtained via civil litigation's discovery process may play a critical role in disclosing information and educating the public about the nature and causes of health risks, thus making the political process itself more informed. In her study of tobacco litigation, Mather (1998) chronicles the vital role that litigation-induced discovery of tobacco industry documents played in shifting the attitudes of both the public and policymakers about tobacco regulation. . . .

## THE EFFICIENCY AND EFFICACY OF PUBLIC HEALTH LITIGATION

One of the fundamental goals of civil litigation is the prevention of socially undesirable activities. In public health litigation . . . a key goal is deterring the injury-causing behavior of a private party. In terms of deterrence, product liability law seeks to reduce the cost of product-related injuries, whereas the partially overlapping area of toxic torts is intended to reduce the number and severity of illnesses caused by toxic substances. Product liability and toxic tort laws reduce injuries and illnesses by encouraging manufacturers and polluters either to make their products and by-products safer or to make fewer of them. The encouragement comes from their fear of having to pay large monetary damages if a jury decides they behaved irresponsibly (negligently, recklessly, fraudulently, etc.) in endangering the public. . . .

Some analysts of contemporary product liability law argue that, by awarding judgments to injured consumers, tort law may actually increase injuries by making the general public and potential plaintiffs less careful. It seems, however, extremely unlikely that many would-be reckless or even negligent drivers (or other users of consumer products) are deterred by the prospect that they or their estates may not be able to recover damages for their physical injuries or deaths. More plausible is the possibility that publicity surrounding product liability litigation may help educate the public about the dangers of hazardous products. But even if consumers do not change their behavior, product manufacturers are typically in a better position to anticipate and internalize the costs of accidents than is the consumer who may be harmed.

Other economic concerns arise from the significant transaction costs associated with litigation. In pure dollar terms, there is little doubt that litigation can be expensive. A 1984 RAND Corporation study determined that 61 cents of every dollar spent on the asbestos litigation went to lawyers' fees and expenses. The tobacco litigation has also been a costly affair. Estimates suggest that industry alone has spent at least $600 million a year on lawyers' fees. The multistate settlement reached by the attorneys general will also result in the industry's paying $500 million per year in attorneys' fees to plaintiffs' counsel for many years to come.

Several scholars have contended that the large transaction costs associated with medical malpractice litigation undermine its efficiency as a method for compensating injured patients. The question of litigation's efficiency as a compensation system, however, should not be confused with the question of whether the system can achieve adequate deterrence or public health improvements. Indeed, to some extent, the high costs of litigation can be assumed to abet public health goals because they increase the cost of accidents and add incentives to reduce injurious activities. Of course, this holds true only when the plaintiff or public health advocate can garner sufficient resources to commence and continue the litigation. . . .

There is the paradoxical concern that the very power of litigation to achieve public health goals may lead lawyers and others to forget that lawyers are not, per se, public health experts. The remedies lawyers seek and the settlements they agree to may not always constitute the optimal solution from a public health perspective. . . . [Nevertheless,] public health litigation itself benefits immensely from the expertise and support provided by public health authorities. To the extent that such litigation is successful in the courtroom, it is often only because it has worked in harmony with the policies of public health officials. The tobacco litigation would have been far less effective than it has been were there no Surgeon General's Reports.

## PUBLIC HEALTH LITIGATION AND THE NATURE OF RIGHTS

In recent years legal theorists across the political spectrum have questioned our culture's tendency to reduce issues of policy and politics to questions of legal rights. While some of these concerns focus on the capacity of legal decisions to actually effect change, an issue that has been considered previously, others focus on the nature of legal reasoning and the contours of legal doctrine and ask whether they are supportive or destructive of sound public policy and constructive political changes. Several of these concerns appear particularly pertinent to public health litigation. One set of issues relates to the strong preference in legal doctrine for viewing rights, those interests that the law protects, as negative. To a large degree, legal rights require that someone refrain from taking an action, rather than that someone or something undertake an action. Tort law, for example, will generally not hold an individual responsible for failing to come to the aid of another. . . .

## CONCLUSION

Advocates for public health are increasingly going to court to advance their concerns. Such affirmative public health litigation faces formidable obstacles and cannot always achieve its aims. Nevertheless, it may play a significant role in the advancement of public health. Public health litigation may form a critical part of a political struggle to achieve a public health agenda. It may also have a powerful deterrent effect on those individuals and organizations that create risks to the public health. Finally, litigation's articulation and recognition of individual rights can serve as a necessary foundation for more fully protecting the public health.

## II. SCIENCE IN THE COURTROOM: PROOF AND CAUSATION

Litigators using the court system as an instrument of public health advocacy inevitably confront the vexing questions of proof and causation. As Tom Christoffel and Stephen P. Teret explain, problems of proof and causation in mass tort litigation are materially different from those in traditional tort actions, such as motor vehicle accidents. If X hits Y, who then sustains an immediate injury, causality is readily established by a witness who observes the event and a medical expert who testifies that the harm resulted from the impact. What if a product (P) or activity (A) is associated with an increased rate of harm (H) in the population? How difficult is it to marshal scientific proof that A or P caused H?

### Epidemiology and the Law:
### Courts and Confidence Intervals*
*Tom Christoffel and Stephen P. Teret*

The law, wrote Oliver Wendell Holmes, Jr. (1881, 36), "is forever adopting new principles from life at one end, and it always retains old ones from history at the other." The common law (or case law), which was Holmes's subject, is continually recreated as existing legal principles are applied or modified to fit new fact patterns. And because the law deals with real-world facts, the legal system must keep appropriately abreast with new ways of seeing and understanding the world. This means that, as science develops increasingly more sophisticated and precise means of measurement and analysis, the nation's courts must struggle to decide how much legal weight to afford the never-ending stream of new scientific insights and techniques.

Earlier in this century, courts had to decide whether polygraph readings and paternity test results should be admitted as evidence in legal proceedings. Today's legal controversies include the admissibility of such new types of scientific evidence as DNA fingerprinting. In each case, the judicial concern is one of determining if a particular area of science offers results that are valid and reliable enough to meet accepted legal standards of proof.

Epidemiology provides another example of this interaction of law and science. With the swine flu litigation of the early 1980s, epidemiological evidence began to play an increasingly prominent role in helping courts determine whether a plaintiff's disease or other harm was caused by some activity of the defendant. The increasing judicial reliance on epidemiology is dramatic. . . .

## THE BASICS OF TORT LAW

The main force driving the increased use of epidemiology in the courtroom has been tort litigation. The law of torts determines when one person (or groups of persons, or corporation or government) must pay compensation for civil, noncontractual wrongs caused to others. The injuries addressed by tort law include specific types of intentionally inflicted wrongs (such as assault and battery, defamation, and invasion of privacy), as well as injuries inflicted unintentionally through failure to

*Reprinted from *American Journal of Public Health* 81 (December 1991): 1661–66.

exercise the care that could be expected of an ordinarily prudent person [negligence]. . . .

For a claimant to succeed in a lawsuit alleging unintentional, negligent harm, four requirements must be met. The plaintiff must prove that (1) the defendant owed the plaintiff a duty to act in a particular way, (2) the defendant failed to fulfill that duty, (3) the plaintiff suffered harm, and (4) the defendant's breach of duty was the *cause* of the plaintiff's harm. The plaintiff bears the burden of demonstrating the existence of all four elements. This need not be proven beyond a reasonable doubt, as in criminal prosecutions, but simply by a preponderance of evidence. If the plaintiff fails to prove any one of the four required elements by this criterion, the fact that the other elements have been satisfied will not matter; the plaintiff will lose.

## TOXIC TORTS

During most of this century, tort law was concerned predominantly with injuries for which the cause-effect association was clear-cut: a car ran into a pedestrian, a shopper fell on a store's slippery floor, or a baby choked on a toy with small parts. The injury and the facts surrounding it were evident. More recently, however, tort law has been used to seek compensation for injuries in which causation is not provable by mere eyewitness testimony regarding a specific causal event.

At the heart of such litigation has been a new and rapidly growing area of tort law, usually labeled "toxic torts" but perhaps more appropriately referred to as "mass-exposure" or "environmental-injury litigation." Exposure to asbestos, toxic waste, radiation, and pharmaceuticals have led to large numbers of lawsuits in the past 15 years. In a sense, toxic torts could be viewed as one response to the harmful health effects resulting from the careless or irresponsible use of modern technology.

The common element linking these various lawsuits is that some activity or product of the defendant is alleged to be associated with increased rates of a particular type of harm, and the causal relationship between the exposure and the harm is not amenable to eyewitness testimony. Some harmful agents that have been involved in such lawsuits are dioxin, Agent Orange, low-level radiation, contaminated groundwater, lead paint chips, tampons leading to toxic shock syndrome, asbestos, diethylstilbestrol (DES), and various pharmaceuticals (including polio and flu vaccines as well as Bendectin).

These noxious agents have several things in common: (1) all have been alleged to cause harm to humans, (2) this harm has resulted in lawsuits, (3) the causal connection between the agent and the specific harm has been the subject of some specific controversy, and (4) this combination of factors has resulted in epidemiology and epidemiologists being brought into the courtroom. Whether the defendant is selling a pharmaceutical product, is accused of contaminating groundwater, or is responsible for the release of radioactive debris into the atmosphere, epidemiological evidence may be critical to showing that the defendant's actions are causally associated with the plaintiff's damage.

Toxic tort lawsuits do not differ fundamentally from the more familiar motor vehicle injury and product liability lawsuits. There is a victim/plaintiff and an allegedly culpable defendant. The harmful outcome was not sought by the plaintiff. Further, in most cases, the injury was the result of exposure to some form of energy: kinetic, chemical, thermal, electrical, or ionizing radiation. . . .

With toxic tort injuries . . . there is usually a latency period between exposure and the development of noticeable harm. When harm becomes apparent decades after a toxic exposure, the documentation of a cause-effect relationship must rely on forms of proof that are new to the law. Greatly compounding this difficulty of proof is that few harms are limited to unique single-cause, single-effect connections. Most toxic tort harms can result from several causes, only one of which may involve the defendant. And the plaintiff may have been exposed to more than one noxious agent (e.g., tobacco and asbestos). Thus, it is not enough for toxic tort plaintiffs to show that factor X is capable of causing harm Y. Plaintiffs must also demonstrate that it is more likely than not that factor X caused *their* harm Y. The difficulty here is that, even when it is possible to demonstrate that factor X is responsible for a significant percentage of all cases of harm Y, it can rarely be proven that the harm Y suffered by a particular individual, the plaintiff, was one of the cases caused by factor X. This means that, even where it can be demonstrated that the defendant is responsible for a significant number of the cases of a particular harm, no plaintiff can prove that he or she is one of these particular cases.

A few harmful substances are closely associated with certain signature diseases, such as DES and adenocarcinoma; in such cases, the disease is known to occur rarely, if ever, absent the substance. But these cases are the exception. . . .

## "REASONABLY EXCLUSIVE FACTUAL CONNECTION"

The legal system has attempted to fit toxic torts into a standard tort framework, but that has proven difficult to do. Even if it can be shown that a defendant is responsible for a doubling or tripling of the number of cases of a particular disease or other harm, it is hard for individual plaintiffs suffering from that harm to demonstrate that theirs is one of the excess cases, rather than one of the cases that would have occurred absent the defendant. . . .

Proving that the defendant had contributed a factor that is directly associated with the type of harm suffered by the plaintiff does not complete the plaintiff's case unless it can also be shown that the factor is both a necessary and sufficient cause of such harm. If the direct association is one in which the defendant's factor is (1) a sufficient but not necessary cause, (2) a necessary but not sufficient cause, or even (3) neither a necessary nor sufficient—but still a possible—cause, the problem for the court is how to deal fairly with both plaintiff and defendant. . . .

## WHAT DOES THIS MEAN?

The expanding role of epidemiology in tort litigation serves to highlight an important and interesting contrast between the nature of scientific proof and of legal proof. Science is a matter of probabilities in a universe of randomness and uncertainty. From the scientist's point of view, . . . [t]o demand certainty would be to misunderstand the nature of scientific knowledge. The legal system, on the other hand, seeks finality in the resolution of disputes. Without such finality, the legal process would be one of continual litigation and relitigation. For this reason, concepts of legal causation have favored single-cause explanations. Tort law posits a direct chain of causation, and a tort defendant's conduct is held to be a cause of a particular event if the event would not have occurred "but for" that conduct or if the conduct was a "substantial factor" in bringing the event about. . . .

The job of the court is to come to the peaceful resolution of disputes. The court does not have the luxury of awaiting further scientific studies to approach the truth; it must come to a timely decision for the benefit of the litigants and the judicial system. Certainly the court would like its decision to be based on what it understands to be the truth, but what the true facts are is often exactly what is being contested. In the end, the court must act on uncertainties to resolve the dispute.

The idea of acting on uncertainty may cause discomfort to scientists, whose discipline allows them to admit that they have not yet achieved a complete understanding of the truth and that further investigation is necessary. When the work of scientists is being used as proof in court— for example, the use of epidemiological evidence in toxic tort cases— scientists may complain that undue weight is being attributed to inconclusive findings. The misperception, however, is in thinking that the conclusion sought by the court is the same conclusion sought by the scientist. The scientist's conclusion is achieved when truth is illuminated, and the level of certainty or proof required for this is very high. The court's conclusion is achieved when the best decision, given the weight of the evidence, is made for that case and the litigants' dispute has been resolved in a socially acceptable fashion. For this, the level of certainty need not be that of the scientist. . . .

## CONCLUSION

Epidemiologists need to recognize the growing involvement of their profession in complex tort litigation. . . . As a simple first step, epidemiology and the law should become a standard part of health law courses. On a more complex level, if one or two schools of public health established enough of a reputation in some of the areas being confronted by the courts in toxic tort litigation, these institutions could serve as valuable resource centers to the courts. Judges are free to pick court-appointed experts, but in the toxic tort area they most often do not know where to turn. The result is one of "hired guns" providing expertise for one or both sides of the litigation. . . . Whatever course is ultimately charted, it is clear that epidemiology and the law will be working closely together for some time to come.

---

\*     \*     \*     \*     \*

The problems of causation discussed by Christoffel and Teret can be overcome only if the judge admits scientific evidence into the court proceedings. It therefore becomes important to understand the criteria used by the judiciary to admit expert evidence. In *Frye v. United States*, 293 F. 1013 (D.C. Cir. 1923), a federal appeals court set a standard for the admissibility of scientific evidence that lasted for more than seventy years. *Frye*'s "general acceptance" test permitted into evidence only "a well recognized scientific principle or

discovery . . . sufficiently established to have gained general acceptance in the particular field." *Id.* at 1014. Thus, establishing a consensus within the scientific community was crucial to the admission
of expert testimony. In 1975 Congress enacted the Federal Rules of
Evidence, which reflected a more liberal attitude toward the admission of evidence: "If scientific, technical or other specialized knowledge will assist the trier of fact to understand the evidence . . . a witness qualified as an expert . . . may testify" (§ 702). The Federal
Rules favor the admission of relevant testimony, relying on the adversarial process to sort out strong from weak evidence.

    After 1975 courts began to divide on whether the restrictive *Frye*
test, or the permissive Federal Rules test, governed admissibility. This
disagreement led to one of the most important Supreme Court cases on
the admissibility of scientific evidence, *Daubert v. Merrell Dow Pharmaceuticals, Inc.*

---

### Daubert v. Merrell Dow Pharmaceuticals, Inc.*
*Supreme Court of the United States*
*Decided June 28, 1993*

Justice BLACKMUN delivered the opinion of the Court.
    [Petitioners, two minor children and their parents, alleged in their
suit against Merrell Dow Pharmaceuticals, Inc. (respondent) that the
children's serious birth defects had been caused by the mothers' prenatal ingestion of Bendectin, a prescription drug marketed by respondent.
The District Court found in favor of Merrell Dow based on a well-
credentialed expert's affidavit concluding, upon reviewing the extensive
published scientific literature on the subject, that maternal use of Bendectin has not been shown to be a risk factor for human birth defects.
Although petitioners had responded with the testimony of eight other
well-credentialed experts, who based their conclusion that Bendectin
can cause birth defects on animal studies, chemical structure analyses,
and the unpublished "reanalysis" of previously published human statistical studies, the court determined that this evidence did not meet the
applicable "general acceptance" standard for the admission of expert

---

*509 U.S. 579 (1993).

testimony. The Ninth Circuit Court of Appeals agreed and affirmed, citing *Frye* for the rule that expert opinion based on a scientific technique is inadmissible unless the technique is "generally accepted" as reliable in the relevant scientific community.]

In this case we are called upon to determine the standard for admitting expert scientific testimony in a federal trial. . . . In the 70 years since its formulation in the *Frye* case, the "general acceptance" test has been the dominant standard for determining the admissibility of novel scientific evidence at trial. Although under increasing attack of late, the rule continues to be followed by a majority of courts, including the Ninth Circuit.

The *Frye* test has its origin in a short and citation-free 1923 decision concerning the admissibility of evidence derived from a systolic blood pressure deception test, a crude precursor to the polygraph machine. In what has become a famous (perhaps infamous) passage, the then Court of Appeals for the District of Columbia described the device and its operation and declared:

> Just when a scientific principle or discovery crosses the line between the experimental and demonstrable stages is difficult to define. Somewhere in this twilight zone the evidential force of the principle must be recognized, and while courts will go a long way in admitting expert testimony deduced from a well-recognized scientific principle or discovery, *the thing from which the deduction is made must be sufficiently established to have gained general acceptance in the particular field in which it belongs.* 54 App. D.C. at 47 (emphasis added). . . .

The merits of the *Frye* test have been much debated, and scholarship on its proper scope and application is legion. Petitioners' primary attack, however, is not on the content but on the continuing authority of the rule. They contend that the *Frye* test was superseded by the adoption of the Federal Rules of Evidence. We agree.

We interpret the legislatively enacted Federal Rules of Evidence as we would any statute. Rule 402 provides the baseline: "All relevant evidence is admissible. . . ." "Relevant evidence" is defined as that which has "any tendency to make the existence of any fact that is of consequence to the determination of the action more probable or less probable than it would be without the evidence." Rule 401. The Rule's basic standard of relevance thus is a liberal one. . . .

Here there is a specific Rule that speaks to the contested issue. Rule 702, governing expert testimony, provides:

If scientific, technical, or other specialized knowledge will assist the trier of fact to understand the evidence or to determine a fact in issue, a witness qualified as an expert by knowledge, skill, experience, training, or education, may testify thereto in the form of an opinion or otherwise.

Nothing in the text of this Rule establishes "general acceptance" as an absolute prerequisite to admissibility. Nor does respondent present any clear indication that Rule 702 or the Rules as a whole were intended to incorporate a "general acceptance" standard. The drafting history makes no mention of *Frye,* and a rigid "general acceptance" requirement would be at odds with the "liberal thrust" of the Federal Rules. . . . Given the Rules' permissive backdrop and their inclusion of a specific rule on expert testimony that does not mention "general acceptance," the assertion that the Rules somehow assimilated *Frye* is unconvincing. *Frye* made "general acceptance" the exclusive test for admitting expert scientific testimony. That austere standard, absent from, and incompatible with, the Federal Rules of Evidence, should not be applied in federal trials.

That the *Frye* test was displaced by the Rules of Evidence does not mean, however, that the Rules themselves place no limits on the admissibility of purportedly scientific evidence. Nor is the trial judge disabled from screening such evidence. To the contrary, under the Rules the trial judge must ensure that any and all scientific testimony or evidence admitted is not only relevant, but reliable.

The primary locus of this obligation is Rule 702, which clearly contemplates some degree of regulation of the subjects and theories about which an expert may testify. "*If scientific,* technical, or other specialized *knowledge will assist the trier of fact* to understand the evidence or to determine a fact in issue" an expert "may testify *thereto."* (Emphasis added.) The subject of an expert's testimony must be "scientific. . . knowledge." The adjective "scientific" implies a grounding in the methods and procedures of science. Similarly, the word "knowledge" connotes more than subjective belief or unsupported speculation. The term "applies to any body of known facts or to any body of ideas inferred from such facts or accepted as truths on good grounds." (*Webster's* 1986, 1252.) Of course, it would be unreasonable to conclude that the subject of scientific testimony must be "known" to a certainty; arguably, there are no certainties in science. But, in order to qualify as "scientific knowledge," an inference or assertion must be derived by the scientific method. Proposed testimony must be supported by appropriate validation— i.e., "good grounds," based on what is known. In short, the requirement that an expert's testimony pertain to "scientific knowledge" establishes a standard of evidentiary reliability.

Rule 702 further requires that the evidence or testimony "assist the trier of fact to understand the evidence or to determine a fact in issue." This condition goes primarily to relevance, [which has been described as] . . . one of "fit." "Fit" is not always obvious, and scientific validity for one purpose is not necessarily scientific validity for other, unrelated purposes. . . . Rule 702's "helpfulness" standard requires a valid scientific connection to the pertinent inquiry as a precondition to admissibility.

That these requirements are embodied in Rule 702 is not surprising. Unlike an ordinary witness, an expert is permitted wide latitude to offer opinions, including those that are not based on firsthand knowledge or observation. Presumably, this relaxation of the usual requirement of firsthand knowledge . . . is premised on an assumption that the expert's opinion will have a reliable basis in the knowledge and experience of his discipline.

Faced with a proffer of expert scientific testimony, then, the trial judge must determine at the outset, pursuant to Rule 104(a), whether the expert is proposing to testify to (1) scientific knowledge that (2) will assist the trier of fact to understand or determine a fact in issue. This entails a preliminary assessment of whether the reasoning or methodology underlying the testimony is scientifically valid and of whether that reasoning or methodology properly can be applied to the facts in issue. We are confident that federal judges possess the capacity to undertake this review. . . . [S]ome general observations are appropriate.

Ordinarily, a key question to be answered in determining whether a theory or technique is scientific knowledge that will assist the trier of fact will be whether it can be (and has been) tested. . . .

Another pertinent consideration is whether the theory or technique has been subjected to peer review and publication. . . . [S]ubmission to the scrutiny of the scientific community is a component of "good science," in part because it increases the likelihood that substantive flaws in methodology will be detected. The fact of publication (or lack thereof) in a peer reviewed journal thus will be a relevant, though not dispositive, consideration in assessing the scientific validity of a particular technique or methodology on which an opinion is premised.

Additionally, in the case of a particular scientific technique, the court ordinarily should consider the known or potential rate of error, and the existence and maintenance of standards controlling the technique's operation.

Finally, "general acceptance" can yet have a bearing on the inquiry. A "reliability assessment does not require, although it does permit, explicit identification of a relevant scientific community and an express determination of a particular degree of acceptance within that community." United States v. Downing, 753 F.2d 1224, 1238 (3d Cir. 1985). Widespread acceptance can be an important factor in ruling particular evidence admissible, and "a known technique which has been able to attract only minimal support within the community," Downing, 753 F.2d, at 1238, may properly be viewed with skepticism. . . .

We conclude by briefly addressing what appear to be two underlying concerns of the parties and amici in this case. Respondent expresses apprehension that abandonment of "general acceptance" as the exclusive requirement for admission will result in a "free-for-all" in which befuddled juries are confounded by absurd and irrational pseudoscientific assertions. In this regard respondent seems to us to be overly pessimistic about the capabilities of the jury and of the adversary system generally. Vigorous cross-examination, presentation of contrary evidence, and careful instruction on the burden of proof are the traditional and appropriate means of attacking shaky but admissible evidence. . . .

Petitioners and, to a greater extent, their amici . . . suggest that recognition of a screening role for the judge that allows for the exclusion of "invalid" evidence will sanction a stifling and repressive scientific orthodoxy and will be inimical to the search for truth. It is true that open debate is an essential part of both legal and scientific analyses. Yet there are important differences between the quest for truth in the courtroom and the quest for truth in the laboratory. Scientific conclusions are subject to perpetual revision. Law, on the other hand, must resolve disputes finally and quickly. The scientific project is advanced by broad and wide-ranging consideration of a multitude of hypotheses, for those that are incorrect will eventually be shown to be so, and that in itself is an advance. Conjectures that are probably wrong are of little use, however, in the project of reaching a quick, final, and binding legal judgment—often of great consequence—about a particular set of events in the past. We recognize that, in practice, a gatekeeping role for the judge, no matter how flexible, inevitably on occasion will prevent the jury from learning of authentic insights and innovations. That, nevertheless, is the balance that is struck by Rules of Evidence designed not for the exhaustive search for cosmic understanding but for the particularized resolution of legal disputes. . . .

[T]he judgment of the Court of Appeals is vacated, and the case is remanded for further proceedings consistent with this opinion.

---

\*       \*       \*       \*       \*

The Supreme Court in *Daubert* left an important issue about admissibility unclear—whether the standards of reliability and relevancy apply only to the expert's methodology or whether they apply also to her conclusions. In other words, must the trial court blindly accept the anomalous conclusions of an expert who relies on valid studies? The Supreme Court in *General Electric Co. v. Joiner*, 522 U.S. 136 (1997), held that the trial court could critically examine whether the expert's conclusions were supported by the studies they cite (*id.* at 146): "[C]onclusions and methodology are not entirely distinct from one another. Trained experts commonly extrapolate from existing data. But . . . a district court [is not required] to admit opinion evidence which is connected to the existing data only by the *ipse dixit* of the expert. A court may conclude that there is simply too great an analytical gap between the data and the opinion proffered." Following *Joiner*, the Supreme Court in *Kumho Tire Co., Ltd. v. Carmichael*, 526 U.S. 137 (1999), held that the *Daubert* factors apply not only to scientific experts, but to all experts, such as engineers. The Court reasoned that no clear line divides scientific knowledge from technical or other specialized knowledge, and no convincing need exists to make such distinctions.

The Supreme Court has progressively tightened the permissive admissibility standard in the Federal Rules, giving trial judges considerable discretion to exclude both scientific methodologies and expert opinions of all kinds that fail to meet tests of reliability and relevance (Buckley and Haake 1998). The Court itself said that the law must make certain that an expert "employs in the courtroom the same level of intellectual rigor that characterizes the practice of an expert in the relevant field." *Kumho*, 526 U.S. at 152. The major criticism of the *Daubert* framework, however, is that judges do not possess adequate knowledge or scientific background to assess effectively the validity of theories and data offered by expert witnesses.

Has the Court reached the right balance with respect to the admissibility of scientific evidence? Some authors claim that judges permit the introduction of scientifically unfounded evidence (so-called junk science), with the effect that businesses are held liable for harms they did not create. Peter Huber, excerpted next, argues that trial lawyers have an incentive to introduce scientific evidence irrespective of its rigor, medical experts are willing to testify for a fee, and juries are prone to decide against defendants with "deep pockets." Think about the use of "science" in the silicone breast implant cases, where Dow Corning was held liable even though independent scientific reviews showed that implants do not cause autoimmune or connective tissue diseases (Angell 1997b; IOM 2000c).

## Galileo's Revenge: Junk Science in the Courtroom*
*Peter W. Huber*

INTRODUCTION

Ever wonder about Princess Di's recent affair with Elvis Presley? You can read all about it on the front page of the supermarket tabloid. Elsewhere on the page appear stories of bizarre accidents and fantastic misadventures. An impact with a car's steering wheel causes lung cancer. Breast cancer is triggered by a fall from a streetcar, a slip in a grocery store, an exploding hot-water heater, a blow from an umbrella handle, and a bump from a can of orange juice. Cancer is aggravated, if not actually caused, by lifting a forty-pound box of cheese. Everybody knows, of course, that such stories are fiction. Falls and bumps don't cause cancer.

Other stories tell how a spermicide used with most barrier contraceptives causes birth defects. We know it doesn't. The whooping cough vaccine causes permanent brain damage and death. That's not true either. The swine flu vaccine caused "serum sickness." It didn't. A certain model of luxury car accelerates at random, even as frantic drivers stand on the brakes. Not so. Incompetence by obstetricians is a leading cause of cerebral palsy. It isn't. The morning-sickness drug Bendectin caused an epidemic of birth defects. It didn't. Trace environmental pollutants cause "chemically induced AIDS." They don't.

How can anybody be absolutely, positively certain about these didn'ts, doesn'ts, and don'ts? No one can. But the science that refutes these claims is about as solid as science ever is.

And yet all of these bizarre and fantastic stories—Elvis and Di excepted—are drawn not from the tabloids but from legal reports. They are announced not in smudgy, badly typed cult newsletters but in calf-bound case reports; endorsed not by starry-robed astrologers but by black-robed judges; subscribed to not only by quacks one step ahead of the authorities but by the authorities themselves. They can be found on the dusty shelves of any major law library. The cancer-by-streetcar cases are decades old, but the others are recent.

When they learn of these legal frolics, most members of the mainstream scientific community are astounded, incredulous, and exasperated in about equal measure. . . . Maverick scientists shunned by their reputable colleagues have been embraced by lawyers. Eccentric theories that no respectable government agency would ever fund are rewarded munificently by the courts. Batteries of meaningless, high-tech tests that would amount to medical malpractice or insurance fraud if administered in a clinic for treatment are administered in court with complete impunity by fringe experts hired for litigation. The pursuit of truth, the whole truth, and nothing but the truth has given way to reams of meaningless data, fearful speculation, and fantastic conjecture. Courts resound with elaborate, systematized, jargon-filled, serious-sounding deceptions that fully deserve the contemptuous label used by trial lawyers themselves: *junk science.*

Junk science is the mirror image of real science, with much of the same form but none of the same substance. There is the astronomer, on the one hand, and the astrologist, on the other. The chemist is paired with the alchemist, the pharmacologist with the homeopathist. Take the serious sciences of allergy and immunology, brush away the detail and rigor, and you have the junk science of clinical ecology. The orthopedic surgeon is shadowed by the osteopath, the physical therapist by the chiropractor, the mathematician by the numerologist and the cabalist. Cautious and respectable surgeons are matched by some who cut and paste with gay abandon. Further out on the surgical fringe are outright charlatans, well documented in the credulous pulp press, who claim to operate with rusty knives but no anesthesia, who prey on cancer patients so desperate they will believe a palmed chicken liver is really a human tumor. Junk science cuts across chemistry and pharmacology, medicine and engineering. It is a hodgepodge of biased data, spurious inference, and logical legerdemain, patched together by researchers whose enthusiasm for discovery and diagnosis far outstrips their skill. It is a catalog of every conceivable kind of error: data dredging, wishful thinking, truculent dogmatism, and, now and again, outright fraud.

On the legal side, junk science is matched by what might be called liability science, a speculative theory that expects lawyers, judges, and juries to search for causes at the far fringes of science and beyond. The legal establishment has adjusted rules of evidence accordingly, so that almost any self-styled scientist, no matter how strange or iconoclastic his views, will be welcome to testify in court. The same scientific questions are litigated again and again, in one courtroom after the next, so that error is almost inevitable.

Junk science is impelled through our courts by a mix of opportunity and incentive. "Let-it-all-in" legal theory creates the opportunity. The incentive is money: the prospect that the Midas-like touch of a credulous jury will now and again transform scientific dust into gold. Ironically, the law's tolerance for pseudoscientific speculation has been rationalized in the name of science itself. The open-minded traditions of science demand that every claim be taken seriously, or at least that's what many judges have reasoned. A still riper irony is that in aspiring to correct scientific and medical error everywhere else, courts have become steadily more willing to tolerate quackery on the witness stand.

Experienced lawyers now recognize that anything is possible in this kind of system. The most fantastic verdict recorded so far was worthy of a tabloid: with the backing of expert testimony from a doctor and several police department officials, a soothsayer who decided she had lost her psychic powers following a CAT scan persuaded a Philadelphia jury to award her $1 million in damages. The trial judge threw out *that* verdict. But scientific frauds of similar character if lesser audacity are attempted almost daily in our courts, and many succeed. Most involve real, down-to-earth tragedies like birth defects, cancer, and car accidents. Many culminate in large awards. As the now dimly remembered cancer-by-streetcar cases illustrate, junk science is not an altogether new phenomenon in the courtroom. But its recent and rapid rise is unprecedented in the history of American jurisprudence. Junk science verdicts, once rare, are now common. Never before have so many lawyers grown so wealthy peddling such ambitious reports of the science of things that aren't so.

Yet among all the many refractory problems of our modern liability system, junk science is the most insidious and the least noted. . . . If the operator of a streetcar is to be blamed for cancer, serious science should be on hand to certify the connection. But often it isn't. The rule of law has drifted away from the rule of fact.

What is to be done . . . about accidents in court: how [do you] stop legions of case-hardened lawyers from attacking false causes, on behalf of false victims, on the basis of what nobody but a lawyer and his pocket expert call science[?] . . .

No one would suggest that junk science should generally be banned or its practitioners silenced. Freedom of speech includes the freedom to say silly and false things, even things that mislead, miseducate, or endanger. But our cherished freedom to say what we like on the front page of the *National Enquirer* need not imply the freedom to say similar things from a witness box in the solemnity of a courtroom. . . . It may be funny to see whimsical science in the astrology column next to the comics. It is considerably less funny when something masquerading as science is taken seriously in court, less funny still when millions of dollars change hands on the strength of arrant scientific nonsense, and not funny at all when such awards lead to the disappearance of valuable and perhaps even life-saving products and services.

---

*     *     *     *     *

Is there a better way to introduce scientific evidence into the courtroom? Can we ensure that experts do not become "guns for hire"? Trial judges have the power to appoint independent experts to evaluate evidence for the jury. Impartial experts could be chosen from a panel of scientists well regarded in their fields, without conflicts of interest, and independent from the parties to the case. Independent experts could then draw their conclusions from a wide breadth of peer-reviewed materials, applying scientifically sound principles to the facts of the case. Is this approach preferable to the adversarial method, where well-paid experts on both sides compete with one another?

## CONCLUSION

Part Two of the *Reader* has explored the major areas of public health law—constitutional powers, duties, and limits; administrative law; and tort litigation. Part Three examines the salient tensions and recurring themes in the theory and practice of public health — surveillance versus privacy; control of the informational environment versus free expression; immunization, screening, and treatment versus autonomy and bodily integrity; and civil confinement and criminal punishment versus personal liberty.

# Tensions and Recurring Themes

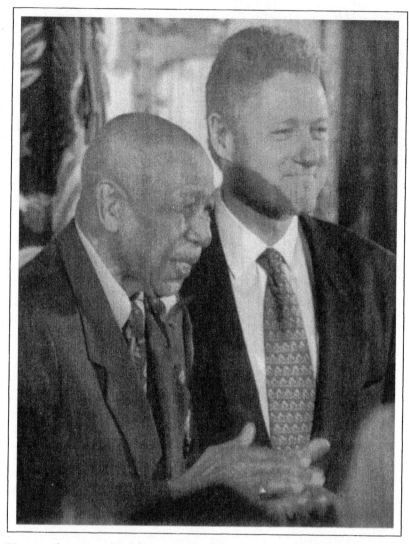

Herman Shaw, 94, a Tuskegee syphilis study victim, receives an official apology from President Clinton on May 16, 1997, in Washington, D.C. President Clinton's apology on behalf of the nation was addressed to all African Americans enrolled in the Tuskegee study whose syphilis went untreated by government doctors. (Greg Gibson, AP/Wide World Photos, 5/16/97.)

# TEN

# Surveillance and Public Health Research

*Privacy and the "Right to Know"*

To achieve collective benefits, public health authorities systematically collect, store, use, and disseminate vast amounts of personal information, commonly in electronic form. Public health authorities monitor health status to identify health problems; diagnose and investigate health hazards; conduct research to understand health problems and find innovative solutions; and disseminate information to inform, educate, and empower people in matters related to their health. These data provide the basic infrastructure necessary to effect many of the common goods of community health. These data are also often personally identifiable and sensitive. Data may reveal a person's lifestyle (e.g., sexual orientation), health status (e.g., mental illness, breast cancer, HIV), behaviors (e.g., unsafe sex or needle sharing), and familial health (e.g., genetics).

Society faces a hard choice between the collective benefits produced by public health data collection and individual interests in privacy. This chapter first explores this tension. The opening section describes the public health information infrastructure and the reasons many experts believe it is crumbling. Next, the chapter examines legal and ethical aspects of particular public health practices: reporting of injuries and diseases to state health departments, research on populations, and partner notification programs. Finally, the chapter presents a model public health privacy statute that seeks to reconcile the collective benefits of surveillance with individual interests in privacy.

## I. THE PUBLIC HEALTH
## INFORMATION INFRASTRUCTURE

The population faces numerous health threats, ranging from contaminated food and water to emerging infections and bioterrorism (see chapter 14). Public health agencies cannot avert these threats unless they have a system of early detection. Absent a strong public health information infrastructure, communities remain vulnerable to diseases and injuries, particularly those that are novel or not well understood. Unfortunately, the nation's capacity to detect health threats in a reliable and timely manner has deteriorated (Lewin Group 2000). In the following reading, influential public health practitioners explain the importance of surveillance and warn the public about its crumbling foundation (see further Osterholm, Birkhead, and Meriweather 1996).

---

### Infectious Disease Surveillance:
### A Crumbling Foundation*
*Ruth L. Berkelman, Ralph T. Bryan, Michael T. Osterholm,*
*James W. LeDuc, and James M. Hughes*

Our ability to detect and monitor infectious disease threats to health is in jeopardy. False perceptions that such threats had dwindled or disappeared led to complacency and decreased vigilance regarding infectious diseases, resulting in a weakening of surveillance—the foundation for control of infectious diseases. However, such infectious diseases as AIDS, influenza, and pneumonia are leading causes of death in the United States and the world. As microorganisms adapt to dramatic changes in our society and environment, we remain vulnerable to a wide array of new threats in the form of emerging, resurgent, and drug-resistant infections.

Surveillance has served as the basis for important public health responses to new threats: identifying contaminated food or other products,

---

*Reprinted from *Science* 264 (April 1994): 368–70 with permission. © 1994 American Association for the Advancement of Science.

determining the influenza virus strains to include in each year's vaccine, and monitoring the safety of our blood supply. Improved surveillance, including strengthened laboratories, is needed to assess the extent of illness and death associated with infectious diseases so that priorities can be assigned to control efforts. Surveillance is also critical in assessing the effectiveness of regulatory and advisory measures designed to safeguard public health, such as drinking water standards and guidelines for the prevention of infectious diseases in child care facilities.

Infectious disease surveillance in the United States relies heavily upon a national notifiable disease system. The legal authority for disease reporting rests with the states, which determine diseases or conditions to be reported by all physicians, laboratories, or others to local or state public health authorities. In turn, the states voluntarily report cases of infectious diseases to the CDC. Surveillance has encompassed not only the reporting and investigation of cases but also the submission of clinical specimens, when needed, for testing at local, state, or federal public health laboratories. This network has constituted the foundation for guiding communicable disease prevention and control activities. The system breaks down if any one step, such as appropriate diagnostic testing, reporting by physicians to public health agencies, or follow-up investigation, is not accomplished.

During the past decade, state and local support for infectious disease surveillance has diminished as a result of budget restrictions. . . . Targeted federal programs for prevention and control of AIDS, tuberculosis (TB), sexually transmitted diseases, and childhood vaccine-preventable diseases have been unable to rely on data from this crippled surveillance network and have developed independent, federally supported, surveillance systems to obtain data for their prevention and control activities. As an example, approximately 20 million federal dollars are spent annually on AIDS surveillance in the United States, providing valuable information to public health professionals, health care providers, policy-makers, and others.

As AIDS surveillance was being established, other parts of the surveillance system for communicable disease were failing. For example, federal spending on TB control had declined and the surveillance system for multidrug-resistant (MDR)-TB was discontinued in 1986. Consequently, a warning signal that prevention and control measures for MDR-TB needed to be enhanced or modified was absent in the late

1980s. This lack of early warning undoubtedly contributed to the more than $700 million in direct costs for TB treatment incurred in 1991 alone. Not until 1993, after MDR-TB became a public health crisis and federal dollars were allocated, was TB surveillance modified to reinstate collection of information on drug resistance. . . .

[The authors discuss large outbreaks of *Escherichia coli* due to contaminated food and *Cryptosporidium* from contaminated drinking water.]

That the United States . . . witnessed such severe epidemics as a result of these pathogens is not surprising. Both *E. coli* O157:H7 and *Cryptosporidium* were emerging as health threats while attention to public health functions required to detect and control infectious diseases was diminishing. Many factors were associated with the occurrence of each of these outbreaks; however, lack of prompt diagnosis and reporting likely contributed to morbidity, mortality, and economic costs. At the current level of disease surveillance, it may take thousands of cases for an outbreak causing diarrheal illness randomly in a large urban area to be detected by public health authorities. An even greater number of cases may be required for detection if a contaminated food product is widely dispersed across the United States.

In addition to strengthening domestic surveillance, it is necessary to establish effective global surveillance as international travel and commerce increase. The health of U.S. citizens is inextricably linked to the health of people in other parts of the world; microorganisms can and do cross borders easily and often without recognition. . . . [V]irology laboratories around the world are not fully prepared to recognize emerging viral diseases or to identify known viral pathogens not commonly occurring in their immediate geographic area. . . . Fewer than half of the surveyed laboratories had the ability to diagnose Japanese encephalitis (47%), hantaviruses (44%), Rift Valley fever virus (41%), or California encephalitis (18%). . . .

Surveillance needs may vary with the disease being monitored. Factors such as the frequency of the disease, the accuracy of diagnosis, the need for a rapid response, and the severity of the disease often determine what type of surveillance is most effective and efficient. Hence, the CDC strategy for improved surveillance emphasizes four complementary approaches to monitoring infectious diseases: (i) strengthening the national notifiable disease system, (ii) establishing sentinel surveillance networks, (iii) establishing population-based centers focused on epidemiology and prevention of emerging infections, and (iv) developing a system for enhanced global surveillance. . . .

The debate concerning health care reform is intensely focused on providing individual medical care; the debate has not adequately addressed the equally important topic of public health. Assuring effective surveillance has become even more important as new pathogens are recognized, as some diseases thought conquered reemerge, and as antibiotics become less effective. History has shown us repeatedly, in terms of both human suffering and economic loss, that the costs of preparedness through vigilance are far lower than those needed to respond to unanticipated public health crises.

## II. REPORTING INJURIES AND DISEASES

Because few resources are dedicated to public health surveillance, state and local governments rely heavily on clinical reports of disease and injury. Every state requires physicians and laboratories to report certain events that cause harm (e.g., child abuse and gunshot wounds) as well as specified infections (e.g., HIV) and diseases (e.g., hepatitis, rabies, and TB). Despite recent developments that may enhance the efficiency of public health surveillance (such as integrated public health surveillance teams and electronic hospital records review), clinical reporting remains a critical element in public health surveillance.

Reporting, although universally mandated, is highly controversial. Daniel Fox, president of the Milbank Memorial Fund and noted public health historian, explains that reporting statutes create tensions between physicians, whose primary role is to protect their patients' interests, and public health authorities, whose primary role is to protect the population's interests. In particular, physicians defend their confidential therapeutic relationships, whereas public health authorities insist on full reporting.

In the second reading, Sandra Roush and her colleagues from the Council of State and Territorial Epidemiologists (CSTE) explore the diversity in reporting requirements across the country. Such diversity is a prime example of how social values and priorities influence modern public health surveillance. Finally, the Supreme Court's decision in *Whalen v. Roe* describes a limited constitutional right to informational privacy relating to data reported to the health department.

## From TB to AIDS: Value Conflicts in Reporting Disease*
*Daniel M. Fox*

The AIDS epidemic has focused attention on the ethics as well as the effectiveness of the traditional public health responses to disease. These responses include surveillance, research, prevention, and treatment. Surveillance, which in the nineteenth century meant the observation of individuals for the development of the signs and symptoms of disease, now means "the continuing scrutiny of all aspects of occurrence and spread of a disease that are pertinent to effective control" (Last 1983, 101). The basic methods of surveillance are reporting and screening. When the AIDS epidemic began, public health professionals considered surveillance to be a complicated technical subject of little interest to the general public. Now, however, conflicts about policy for surveillance have become part of public debate.

The history of physicians' reports of cases to public health officials is usually presented as a struggle. On one side have been advocates of reporting, who justified it with arguments from science and the ethics of collective responsibility; on the other, private physicians who accorded higher priority to the privacy of their encounters with patients. . . . I regard the history of required reporting of disease as a political problem, as a series of accommodations among people with different beliefs about the public interest, patients' interests, and their own self-interest.

Required reporting in general—for example, compulsory submission to government agencies of information about business transactions, income, births, and deaths as well as about disease—is part of the elaboration of the modern bureaucratic state. By the late nineteenth century, advocates of compulsory reporting of disease in the United States and Europe had four principal goals. They wanted to gather data for epidemiological analysis, to identify patients in order to treat them, to warn anyone who might be infected and, most important, to establish a new relationship between practicing physicians and public officials who applied the findings of laboratory science.

The initiation of compulsory notification for any disease in a particular country, state, or city was almost never a direct response to

*Reprinted from *Hastings Center Report* 11 (December 1986): 11–16.

particular scientific advances. Public health officials usually described recent scientific advances in order to justify mandatory reporting. But arguments from science were erratically and belatedly persuasive. Britain, for instance, did not require notification for smallpox until 1899, a century after Jenner's successful experiments with a vaccine.

The reporting of syphilis was required in the Scandinavian countries in the 1870s, but nowhere else. Even though tuberculosis was the major cause of death in Europe and the United States in the nineteenth century, and was a great economic threat because it was most virulent among males in their thirties, reporting was not required in most jurisdictions until a generation after Robert Koch isolated the bacillus. . . .

The results of political controversies about compulsory reporting often contradicted conventional assumptions about national differences in health policy. Britain, for example, did not make TB reportable until 1912, and did not unambiguously mandate the reporting of syphilis until World War II. Robert Koch, among others, was astonished to discover that, at the turn of the century, New York City's regulations requiring notification of cases of TB were more rigorously enforced than those in Prussia.

## COMPULSORY NOTIFICATION IN NEW YORK CITY

The early history of compulsory notification in New York is the best documented example of the centrality of politics in disease reporting. In the closing years of the nineteenth century, most foreign and domestic students of public affairs regarded American municipal government as a conspicuous failure. New York was dominated by Tammany Hall, which was criticized as a venal political machine by almost everyone except the 80 percent of New Yorkers who were immigrants or first-generation Americans. Yet Koch and other medical visitors to New York City were astonished by the extent to which physicians complied with regulations requiring them to report cases of tuberculosis to the city's health department and were willing to have the department's laboratory test samples of sputum.

This extraordinary compliance began when compulsory notification for TB occurred in New York in the mid-1890s because the dominant person in the health department, Hermann N. Biggs, had a precise agenda, extraordinary political talent, and uncommon energy. For Biggs, medical research and education, public health, and private practice were a continuum. . . .

Unlike health officers elsewhere in the United States who were pioneers in compulsory reporting, Biggs exchanged epidemiological accuracy and the ability to treat or at least to track all of the patients with reportable diseases for physicians' support. The regulations he promulgated guaranteed that reports would remain confidential. More important, Biggs condoned selective reporting. He muted health department criticism of physicians for underreporting and rarely invoked the penalties for noncompliance. Selective reporting, self-policed by the medical profession, was, Biggs believed, more effective in the long run than actions that would polarize public health officials and private practitioners. Biggs valued accurate epidemiological data and prompt treatment, but he cared even more about creating a hierarchical medical profession unified by a belief in progress through science.

Almost twenty years after TB became reportable in New York, Biggs (1912) decided to mandate the reporting of venereal disease. In a report to the Board of Health in December 1911, he declared: "The moral and social aspects of the problem do not primarily concern the sanitary authorities." Physicians' reports should, he continued, be "treated as absolutely confidential." Moreover, since his goal was merely "the fullest information obtainable," the regulations he proposed "required" that physicians report cases they diagnosed in institutions but merely "requested" reports "concerning private patients under their care." Biggs had used the same strategy in the regulations for reporting TB in the 1890s: first requesting reports of private cases and then requiring them three years later, after he had more leverage on the medical profession. In 1911, as in the 1890s, moreover, Biggs offered physicians the incentive of free diagnostic services. . . .

## THREATS TO THE UNITY OF HEALTH POLICY

By 1915, many private physicians and public health officials were uncomfortable with the agenda and political strategy advocated by Biggs and officials who shared his views in a few other states—Massachusetts, California, and Michigan, for example. Professional unity about health policy in general was threatened after about 1910 from three directions: the social hygiene movement, conflict over state legislation to create health insurance, and the professionalization of public health.

Many public health officials and physicians active in the social hygiene movement now asserted that the goals of public health and private medicine conflicted. In 1911, for instance, Prince Morrow, a physician prominent in the campaign against venereal disease, said in defense of compulsory reporting of syphilis that the "progress of preventive medicine" was the "history of the conflict between so-called rights of the individual and the higher rights of the community" (Morrow 1911, 8). . . .

Since World War II, and particularly in the last twenty years, there have been enormous changes in both the organization of medical care and the definition and scope of public health practice. For a variety of reasons, physicians became more specialized, more accepting—however grudgingly—of hierarchy and accountability, and more resigned to record-keeping and regulation.

During the same years, moreover, public health practice changed considerably. . . . [P]ublic employees became prominent in conducting and applying biomedical research for the first time since Biggs's generation. . . . Monitoring the incidence and prevalence of disease, not identifying sick individuals, was now taken to be the purpose of reporting and other surveillance techniques. . . .

## THE IMPACT OF AIDS

Instead of unifying public health and private medicine, the AIDS epidemic has highlighted many of the flaws in our health policy, including unresolved issues about the reporting of cases of disease. . . . [H]igh compliance of physicians with reporting requirements has been overshadowed by unprecedented controversy about how case reports should or could be used. . . .

Four points of view about the potential use of case reports for purposes other than epidemiological analysis have emerged: (1) a defense of traditional standards of public health practice; (2) concern that this tradition may be overwhelmed by external pressures; (3) attempts to reassert a definition of surveillance as the observation of particular individuals; and (4) the assertion by many gay men that discussions of the confidentiality of reports miss the real point, which is protecting their anonymity.

Officials of several public health agencies, assuring me that there is no cause to fear that traditional standards of confidentiality will be violated, described the tenacity with which the names of individuals are protected. . . . [P]ublic health officials, [however], fear that the tradition of maintaining confidential reports may not withstand external pressures. Some are worried about threats to confidentiality as a result of the intense media fascination with AIDS; the stigmatization of homosexuals and drug users; and the strong desire of employers, the military, and insurance companies to reduce their investment in persons who have, or may develop, AIDS. . . .

Controversies about disease reporting in the present as in the past must be understood as political conflicts; that is, conflicts about power and about values. The critical issues have never been scientific or technological. Debates about reporting have always been about ideology, about the distribution of authority within the medical profession, about the relationship between medical and general politics, and about competing social values.

---

\*     \*     \*     \*     \*

The tension between reporting and privacy discussed by Fox is powerfully illustrated by the modern policy debates around named HIV reporting. The CDC (1999c) recommends named HIV reporting to improve monitoring of the epidemic. Many persons, however, oppose HIV reporting, expressing deep concern about government's collecting the names of persons living with HIV. These advocates prefer a "unique identifier" system that does not disclose patient names. For a discussion of the public health and civil liberties perspective, *compare* Gostin, Ward, and Baker (1997) and Gostin and Hodge (1998a) *with* ACLU (1998).

---

## Mandatory Reporting of Diseases and Conditions by Health Care Providers and Laboratories\*
*Sandra Roush, Guthrie Birkhead, Denise Koo, Angela Cobb, and David Fleming*

Public health surveillance systems in the United States were designed for the reporting of infectious diseases of public health interest, and health care professionals (usually physicians and nurses) have been the primary source of disease reporting. Recently, laboratories have also become an important source of reporting for public health surveillance. Together, health care provider reporting and laboratory reporting may ensure more complete and timely reporting for diseases and conditions recommended to be under national surveillance. The list of diseases and

---

\*Reprinted from *Journal of the American Medical Association* 282 (July 14, 1999): 164–70.

conditions that are recommended for national surveillance is designed
to reflect the current needs and priorities for public health surveillance
at any given time. . . .

[The authors explain the purpose of a survey to assess the state and
territorial public health reporting requirements for health care professionals and laboratories for diseases and conditions that are recommended for national surveillance.]

Epidemiologists from each of the 50 states and from New York City,
Puerto Rico, and Guam responded to the survey. . . . Of the 58 diseases
and conditions recommended for national reporting, 35 (60%) were reportable in greater than 90% of the states and territories, 15 (26%)
were reportable in 75% to 90% of the states and territories, and 8
(14%) were reportable in less than 75% of the states and territories.
Nineteen of the infectious diseases (AIDS, botulism, cholera, diphtheria, gonorrhea, hepatitis A, hepatitis B, malaria, measles, pertussis, poliomyelitis [paralytic], human rabies, rubella, salmonella, shigella,
syphilis, tetanus, tuberculosis, and typhoid fever) were reportable in all
of the states and territories that responded to this survey. . . . [Thus,]
only 19 (33%) of the 58 diseases and conditions on the list for national
surveillance were actually reportable in each of the 53 responding states
and territories. [The authors further explain why they believe many
states do not require reporting of all of the diseases on the list of national surveillance. Additional survey results are available on the Internet (http://www.cste.org).]

In the United States, the authority to require notification of cases
of diseases resides in the respective state legislatures. The states exercise their authority to require reporting by enacting legislation; some
state statutes delegate the authority to enumerate the health conditions that are reportable to state or local agencies. Subsequent reporting of morbidity data by the state or territorial health department
to CDC is voluntary.

Because of each state's autonomy with regard to morbidity reporting,
the list of diseases and conditions that are reported varies by state. In addition to the variation among states for the conditions and diseases to
be reported, the time frames for reporting, agencies receiving reports,
persons required to report, and conditions under which reports are required also may differ among states. In many states, local health departments provide epidemiologic services; as a consequence, health care
professionals in many states are encouraged by their public health officials to report diseases directly to local health departments rather than

to the state health department. Health care professionals are encouraged to determine the specific requirements in their area by contacting their state health department.

Standardized case definitions for the diseases under national surveillance have been created to provide uniform criteria for reporting cases. Although the public health case definitions are useful for surveillance, they are not designed to influence clinical treatment or to delay the reporting of pending case confirmation. Case definitions for the diseases under national surveillance were first developed and approved by CDC and CSTE in 1989 and were published in the MMWR (*Morbidity and Mortality Weekly Report*) in 1990. The most recent revisions to the case definitions are available at http://www.cdc.gov. The CDC and CSTE also have initiated development of standardized case definitions for injury, chronic, environmental, occupational, and other health conditions.

Historically in the United States, infectious disease surveillance has relied primarily on case reports from physicians and other health care professionals. Although these diseases are usually underreported (reporting is estimated at 6%–90% for many of the diseases under national surveillance), if the reporting is consistent over time, these data are a good source of temporal and geographic trends and characteristics of the persons experiencing morbidity. For diseases or other health conditions for which there is a substantial laboratory component included in case diagnosis or definition, laboratory reporting is a useful mechanism to supplement reporting from physicians by clinicians.

Although reporting by clinicians to public health authorities allows immediate public health response, including case investigation, contact prophylaxis, and outbreak control, other methods of surveillance are also necessary to meet the changing needs of public health assessment. Some of these other methods are sentinel surveillance and secondary analysis of hospital discharge or other administrative data sets, prevalence surveys, and vital records. These methods may be used in combination to improve the comprehensiveness of data collection and to provide more complete information to assess local, state, or national goals for public health. . . .

The CDC coordinates the states' and territories' surveillance data, providing weekly reports in the MMWR and annually in the MMWR Summary of Notifiable Diseases, which are available on the Internet (http://www.cdc.gov). . . . Surveillance summaries for injury, hazardous substances and emergency events, infant mortality, childhood lead poisonings, low birth weight, neural tube defects, occupational asthma, occupational hazards, silicosis, and smoking illustrate that other mechanisms for surveillance and data collection must be flexible and appropriate to the specific public health issue. . . .

Public health has expanded from its traditional base in infectious disease control, and as the scope of public health expands, the list of diseases and conditions of public health interest will vary between jurisdictions and over time. In the future, greater emphasis should be placed on gathering data electronically from existing sources, including clinical laboratories and computerized medical records. Those concerned about public health will increasingly be required to make the best use of limited resources for surveillance to meet the challenges of a changing medical care system using new information technology.

*    *    *    *    *

Although public health surveillance achieves many common goods, it also invades individual interests in privacy. As the technology of surveillance becomes more advanced, the public becomes more concerned about how electronic personal information will be used and who will be able to access the information. *See generally* Bartnicki v. Vopper, 121 S. Ct. 1753 (2001).

The Supreme Court, in the foundational case of *Whalen v. Roe*, proclaimed a narrow constitutional right to health informational privacy. The Court upheld a New York law that required reporting the names and addresses of all persons who have obtained, pursuant to a doctor's prescription, certain drugs for which there is both a lawful and an unlawful market. The Court, however, noted the strong security protections surrounding the health department's collection and storage of these data.

## Whalen v. Roe*

*Supreme Court of the United States*
*Decided February 22, 1977*

Justice STEVENS delivered the opinion of the Court.

The constitutional question presented is whether the State of New York may record, in a centralized computer file, the names and addresses of all

*429 U.S. 589 (1977).

persons who have obtained, pursuant to a doctor's prescription, certain drugs for which there is both a lawful and an unlawful market. . . .

In response to a concern that such drugs were being diverted into unlawful channels, in 1970 the New York Legislature created a special commission to evaluate the State's drug-control laws. The commission found the existing laws deficient in several respects. There was no effective way to prevent the use of stolen or revised prescriptions, to prevent unscrupulous pharmacists from repeatedly refilling prescriptions, to prevent users from obtaining prescriptions from more than one doctor, or to prevent doctors from over-prescribing, either by authorizing an excessive amount in one prescription or by giving one patient multiple prescriptions. . . .

[The Court describes the New York statute, which classified drugs according to their potential for abuse, and the filing requirements that compelled physicians to file prescription forms for potentially addictive drugs with the State Department of Health.]

With an exception for emergencies, the Act requires that all prescriptions for Schedule II drugs [i.e., the most dangerous and addictive drugs] be prepared by the physician in triplicate on an official form. The completed form identifies the prescribing physician; the dispensing pharmacy; the drug and dosage; and the name, address, and age of the patient. One copy of the form is retained by the physician, the second by the pharmacist, and the third is forwarded to the New York State Department of Health in Albany. . . .

[A]bout 100,000 Schedule II prescription forms are delivered to a receiving room at the Department of Health in Albany each month. They are sorted, coded, and logged and then taken to another room where the data on the forms is recorded on magnetic tapes for processing by a computer. Thereafter, the forms are returned to the receiving room to be retained in a vault for a five-year period, and then destroyed as required by the statute. The receiving room is surrounded by a locked wire fence and protected by an alarm system. The computer tapes containing the prescription data are kept in a locked cabinet. When the tapes are used, the computer is run "off-line," which means that no terminal outside of the computer room can read or record any information. Public disclosure of the identity of patients is expressly prohibited by the statute and by a Department of Health regulation. Willful violation of these prohibitions is a crime punishable by up to one year in prison and a $2,000 fine.

A few days before the Act became effective, this litigation was commenced by a group of patients regularly receiving prescriptions for Schedule II drugs, by doctors who prescribe such drugs, and by two associations of physicians. After various preliminary proceedings, a three-judge District Court conducted a one-day trial. Appellees offered evidence tending to prove that persons in need of treatment with Schedule II drugs will from time to time decline such treatment because of their fear that the misuse of the computerized data will cause them to be stigmatized as "drug addicts." . . .

Appellees contend that the statute invades a constitutionally protected "zone of privacy." The cases sometimes characterized as protecting "privacy" have in fact involved at least two different kinds of interests. One is the individual interest in avoiding disclosure of personal matters, and another is the interest in independence in making certain kinds of important decisions. Appellees argue that both of these interests are impaired by this statute. The mere existence in readily available form of the information about patients' use of Schedule II drugs creates a genuine concern that the information will become publicly known and that it will adversely affect their reputations. This concern makes some patients reluctant to use, and some doctors reluctant to prescribe, such drugs even when their use is medically indicated. It follows, they argue, that the making of decisions about matters vital to the care of their health is inevitably affected by the statute. Thus, the statute threatens to impair both their interest in the nondisclosure of private information and also their interest in making important decisions independently. We are persuaded, however, that the New York program does not, on its face, pose a sufficiently grievous threat to either interest to establish a constitutional violation.

Public disclosure of patient information can come about in three ways. Health Department employees may violate the statute by failing, either deliberately or negligently, to maintain proper security. A patient or a doctor may be accused of a violation and the stored data may be offered in evidence in a judicial proceeding. Or, thirdly, a doctor, a pharmacist, or the patient may voluntarily reveal information on a prescription form.

The third possibility existed under the prior law and is entirely unrelated to the existence of the computerized data bank. Neither of the other two possibilities provides a proper ground for attacking the statute as invalid on its face. There is no support in the record, or in the experience of the two States that New York has emulated, for an assumption that the security provisions of the statute will be administered improperly.

And the remote possibility that judicial supervision of the evidentiary use of particular items of stored information will provide inadequate protection against unwarranted disclosures is surely not a sufficient reason for invalidating the entire patient-identification program.

Even without public disclosure, it is, of course, true that private information must be disclosed to the authorized employees of the New York Department of Health. Such disclosures, however, are not significantly different from those that were required under the prior law. Nor are they meaningfully distinguishable from a host of other unpleasant invasions of privacy that are associated with many facets of health care. Unquestionably, some individuals' concern for their own privacy may lead them to avoid or to postpone needed medical attention. Nevertheless, disclosures of private medical information to doctors, to hospital personnel, to insurance companies, and to public health agencies are often an essential part of modern medical practice even when the disclosure may reflect unfavorably on the character of the patient. Requiring such disclosures to representatives of the State having responsibility for the health of the community, does not automatically amount to an impermissible invasion of privacy.

Appellees also argue, however, that even if unwarranted disclosures do not actually occur, the knowledge that the information is readily available in a computerized file creates a genuine concern that causes some persons to decline needed medication. The record supports the conclusion that some use of Schedule II drugs has been discouraged by that concern; it also is clear, however, that about 100,000 prescriptions for such drugs were being filled each month prior to the entry of the District Court's injunction. Clearly, therefore, the statute did not deprive the public of access to the drugs. A final word about issues we have not decided. We are not unaware of the threat to privacy implicit in the accumulation of vast amounts of personal information in computerized data banks or other massive government files. . . . The right to collect and use such data for public purposes is typically accompanied by a concomitant statutory or regulatory duty to avoid unwarranted disclosures. Recognizing that in some circumstances that duty arguably has its roots in the Constitution, nevertheless New York's statutory scheme, and its implementing administrative procedures, evidence a proper concern with, and protection of, the individual's interest in privacy. We therefore need not, and do not, decide any question which might be presented by the unwarranted disclosure of accumulated private data whether intentional or unintentional or by a system that did not contain comparable security provisions. We simply hold that this record does not establish an invasion of any right or liberty protected by the Fourteenth Amendment.

Justice BRENNAN, concurring.

The New York statute under attack requires doctors to disclose to the State information about prescriptions for certain drugs with a high potential for abuse, and provides for the storage of that information in a central computer file. The Court recognizes that an individual's "interest in avoiding disclosure of personal matters" is an aspect of the right of privacy, but holds that in this case, any such interest has not been seriously enough invaded by the State to require a showing that its program was indispensable to the State's effort to control drug abuse.

The information disclosed by the physician under this program is made available only to a small number of public health officials with a legitimate interest in the information. As the record makes clear, New York has long required doctors to make this information available to its officials on request, and that practice is not challenged here. Such limited reporting requirements in the medical field are familiar ante, and are not generally regarded as an invasion of privacy. Broad dissemination by state officials of such information, however, would clearly implicate constitutionally protected privacy rights, and would presumably be justified only by compelling state interests.

What is more troubling about this scheme, however, is the central computer storage of the data thus collected. Obviously, as the State argues, collection and storage of data by the State that is in itself legitimate is not rendered unconstitutional simply because new technology makes the State's operations more efficient. However, as the example of the Fourth Amendment shows, the Constitution puts limits not only on the type of information the State may gather, but also on the means it may use to gather it. The central storage and easy accessibility of computerized data vastly increase the potential for abuse of that information, and I am not prepared to say that future developments will not demonstrate the necessity of some curb on such technology.

---

## III. PUBLIC HEALTH RESEARCH

Public health authorities collect data not only for the purposes of surveillance, but also for research. Ethical controversies often have arisen out of the conduct of public health researchers. Allan M. Brandt, a professor of the history of medicine at Harvard Medical School, insightfully examines perhaps the most infamous example of public health research abuse: the Tuskegee syphilis study.

### Racism and Research: The Case
### of the Tuskegee Syphilis Study*
*Allan M. Brandt*

In 1932 the U.S. Public Health Service (USPHS) initiated an experiment in Macon County, Alabama, to determine the natural course of untreated, latent syphilis in black males. The test comprised 400 syphilitic men, as well as 200 uninfected men who served as controls. The first published report of the study appeared in 1936 with subsequent papers issued every four to six years, through the 1960s. When penicillin became widely available by the early 1950s as the preferred treatment for syphilis, the men did not receive therapy. In fact on several occasions, the USPHS actually sought to prevent treatment. Moreover, a committee at the federally operated Centers for Disease Control [(CDC)] decided in 1969 that the study should be continued. Only in 1972, when accounts of the study first appeared in the national press, did the Department of Health, Education and Welfare (HEW) halt the experiment. At that time seventy-four of the test subjects were still alive; at least twenty-eight, but perhaps more than 100, had died directly from advanced syphilitic lesions. In August 1972, HEW appointed an investigatory panel which issued a report the following year. The panel found the study to have been "ethically unjustified," and argued that penicillin should have been provided to the men. . . .

Despite the media attention which the study received, the HEW *Final Report,* and the criticism expressed by several professional organizations, the experiment has been largely misunderstood. The most basic questions of *how* the study was undertaken in the first place and *why* it continued for forty years were never addressed by the HEW investigation. Moreover, the panel misconstrued the nature of the experiment, failing to consult important documents available at the National Archives which bear significantly on its ethical assessment. Only

---

*Reprinted from *Hastings Center Report* 8 (December 1978): 21–29.

by examining the specific ways in which values are engaged in scientific research can the study be understood. . . .

## THE ORIGINS OF THE EXPERIMENT

In 1929, under a grant from the Julius Rosenwald Fund, the USPHS conducted studies in the rural South to determine the prevalence of syphilis among blacks and explore the possibilities for mass treatment. The USPHS found Macon County, Alabama, in which the town of Tuskegee is located, to have the highest syphilis rate of the six counties surveyed. The Rosenwald Study concluded that mass treatment could be successfully implemented among rural blacks. Although it is doubtful that the necessary funds would have been allocated even in the best economic conditions, after the economy collapsed in 1929, the findings were ignored. It is, however, ironic that the Tuskegee Study came to be based on findings of the Rosenwald Study that demonstrated the possibilities of mass treatment.

Three years later, in 1932, Dr. Taliaferro Clark, Chief of the USPHS Venereal Disease Division and author of the Rosenwald Study report, decided that conditions in Macon County merited renewed attention. Clark believed the high prevalence of syphilis offered an "unusual opportunity" for observation. From its inception, the USPHS regarded the Tuskegee Study as a classic "study in nature," rather than an experiment. As long as syphilis was so prevalent in Macon and most of the blacks went untreated throughout life, it seemed only natural to Clark that it would be valuable to observe the consequences. He described it as a "ready-made situation." Surgeon General H. S. Cumming wrote to R. R. Moton, Director of the Tuskegee Institute:

> The recent syphilis control demonstration carried out in Macon County, with the financial assistance of the Julius Rosenwald Fund, revealed the presence of an unusually high rate in this county and, what is more remarkable, the fact that 99 per cent of this group was entirely without previous treatment. This combination, together with the expected cooperation of your hospital, offers an unparalleled opportunity for carrying on this piece of scientific research which probably cannot be duplicated anywhere else in the world (September 20, 1932).

Although no formal protocol appears to have been written, several letters of Clark and Cumming suggest what the USPHS hoped to find. Clark indicated that it would be important to see how disease affected the daily lives of the men. It also seems that the USPHS believed the experiment might demonstrate that antisyphilitic treatment was unnecessary. As

Cumming noted: "It is expected the results of this study may have a marked bearing on the treatment, or conversely the non-necessity of treatment, of cases of latent syphilis" (September 20, 1932). . . .

Every major textbook of syphilis at the time of the Tuskegee Study's inception strongly advocated treating syphilis even in its latent stages, which follow the initial inflammatory reaction. . . . [U]ntreated syphilis could lead to cardiovascular disease, insanity, and premature death. "Another compelling reason for treatment," noted Moore (1933, 236) [a leading venereologist], "exists in the fact that every patient with latent syphilis may be, and perhaps is, infectious for others." In 1932, the year in which the Tuskegee Study began, the USPHS sponsored and published a paper by Moore and six other syphilis experts that strongly argued for treating latent syphilis. . . .

[T]he suppositions that conditions in Tuskegee existed "naturally" and that the men would not be treated anyway provided the experiment's rationale. In turn, these two assumptions rested on the prevailing medical attitudes concerning blacks, sex, and disease. For example, Clark explained the prevalence of venereal disease in Macon County by emphasizing promiscuity among blacks. . . .

The doctors who devised and directed the Tuskegee Study accepted the mainstream assumptions regarding blacks and venereal disease. The premise that blacks, promiscuous and lustful, would not seek or continue treatment, shaped the study. A test of untreated syphilis seemed "natural" because the USPHS presumed the men would never be treated; the Tuskegee Study made that a self-fulfilling prophecy.

## SELECTING THE SUBJECTS

Clark sent Dr. Raymond Vonderlehr to Tuskegee in September 1932 to assemble a sample of men with latent syphilis for the experiment. The basic design of the study called for the selection of syphilitic black males between the ages of twenty-five and sixty, a thorough physical examination including x-rays, and finally, a spinal tap to determine the incidence of neuro-syphilis. They had no intention of providing any treatment for the infected men. The USPHS originally scheduled the whole experiment to last six months; it seemed to be both a simple and inexpensive project.

The task of collecting the sample, however, proved to be more difficult than the USPHS had supposed. Vonderlehr canvassed the largely illiterate, poverty-stricken population of sharecroppers and tenant farmers in search of test subjects. . . . Vonderlehr found that only the offer of treatment elicited the cooperation of the men. They were told they were ill and were promised free care. . . . The USPHS did not tell the men that they were participants in an experiment; on the contrary, the subjects believed they were being treated for "bad blood"—the rural South's colloquialism for syphilis. They thought they were participating in a public health demonstration similar to the one that had been conducted by the Julius Rosenwald Fund in Tuskegee several years earlier. In the end, the men were so eager for medical care that the number of defaulters in the experiment proved to be insignificant.

To preserve the subjects' interest, Vonderlehr gave most of the men mercurial ointment, a noneffective drug, while some of the younger men apparently received inadequate dosages of neoarsphenamine. This required Vonderlehr to write frequently to Clark requesting supplies. He feared the experiment would fail if the men were not offered treatment. . . . The readiness of the test subjects to participate of course contradicted the notion that blacks would not seek or continue therapy.

The final procedure of the experiment was to be a spinal tap to test for evidence of neuro-syphilis. The USPHS presented this purely diagnostic exam, which often entails considerable pain and complications, to the men as a "special treatment." . . . The letter to the subjects announcing the spinal tap read:

> Some time ago you were given a thorough examination and since that time we hope you have gotten a great deal of treatment for bad blood. You will now be given your last chance to get a second examination. This examination is a very special one and after it is finished you will be given a special treatment if it is believed you are in a condition to stand it. . . .
> REMEMBER THIS IS YOUR LAST CHANCE FOR SPECIAL FREE TREATMENT. BE SURE TO MEET THE NURSE (Macon County Health Department, "Letter to Subjects").

The HEW investigation did not uncover this crucial fact: the men participated in the study under the guise of treatment.

Despite the fact that their assumption regarding prevalence and black attitudes toward treatment had proved wrong, the USPHS decided in the summer of 1933 to continue the study. Once again, it seemed only "natural" to pursue the research since the sample already existed, and with a depressed economy, the cost of treatment appeared prohibitive—although there is no indication it was ever considered. . . . "As I see it," [said] Dr. O. C. Wenger [chief of the federally operated venereal disease clinic in Hot Springs, Arkansas], "we have no further interest in these patients *until they die*" (July 21,

1933). Apparently, the physicians engaged in the experiment believed that only autopsies could scientifically confirm the findings of the study. . . . Bringing the men to autopsy required the USPHS to devise a further series of deceptions and inducements. Wenger warned Vonderlehr that the men must not realize that they would be autopsied:

> There is one danger in the latter plan and that is if the colored population become aware that accepting free hospital care means a post-mortem, every darkey will leave Macon County and it will hurt [Dr. Eugene] Dibble's hospital (July 21, 1933).

"Naturally," responded Vonderlehr, "it is not my intention to let it be generally known that the main object of the present activities is the bringing of the men to necropsy" (July 27, 1933). The subjects' trust in the USPHS made the plan viable. . . .

The USPHS offered several inducements to maintain contact and to procure the continued cooperation of the men. Eunice Rivers, a black nurse, was hired to follow their health and to secure approval for autopsies. She gave the men noneffective medicines—"spring tonic" and aspirin—as well as transportation and hot meals on the days of their examinations. More important, Nurse Rivers provided continuity to the project over the entire forty-year period. By supplying "medicinals," the USPHS was able to continue to deceive the participants, who believed that they were receiving therapy from the government doctors. Deceit was integral to the study. . . . In fact, after the first six months of the study, the USPHS had furnished no treatment whatsoever.

Finally, because it proved difficult to persuade the men to come to the hospital when they became severely ill, the USPHS promised to cover their burial expenses. The Milbank Memorial Fund provided approximately $50 per man for this purpose beginning in 1935. This was a particularly strong inducement as funeral rites constituted an important component of the cultural life of rural blacks. One report of the study concluded, "Without this suasion it would, we believe, have been impossible to secure the cooperation of the group—and their families" (Schuman et al. 1955, 555).

Reports of the study's findings, which appeared regularly in the medical press beginning in 1936, consistently cited the ravages of untreated syphilis. . . . [The author discusses medical reports from 1936 to 1975 showing that morbidity and mortality among the untreated group were much higher than in the control group.]

During the forty years of the experiment the USPHS had sought on several occasions to ensure that the subjects did not receive treatment from other sources. To this end, Vonderlehr met with groups of local black doctors in 1934, to ask their cooperation in not treating the men. Lists of subjects were distributed to Macon County physicians along with letters requesting them to refer these men back to the USPHS if they sought care. The USPHS warned the Alabama Health Department not to treat the test subjects when they took a mobile VD unit into Tuskegee in the early 1940s. In 1941, the Army drafted several subjects and told them to begin antisyphilitic treatment immediately. The USPHS supplied the draft board with a list of 256 names they desired to have excluded from treatment, and the board complied.

In spite of these efforts, by the early 1950s many of the men had secured some treatment on their own. By 1952, almost 30 percent of the test subjects had received some penicillin, although only 7.5 percent had received what could be considered adequate doses. Vonderlehr wrote to one of the participating physicians, "I hope that the availability of antibiotics has not interfered too much with this project" (February 5, 1952).

When the USPHS evaluated the status of the study in the 1960s they continued to rationalize the racial aspects of the experiment. . . . A group of physicians [met] at the CDC in 1969 to decide whether or not to terminate the study. Although one doctor argued that the study should be stopped and the men treated, the consensus was to continue. . . . When the first accounts of the experiment appeared in the national press in July 1972, data were still being collected and autopsies performed.

## THE HEW *FINAL REPORT*

HEW finally formed the Tuskegee Syphilis Study Ad Hoc Advisory Panel on August 28, 1972, in response to criticism that the press descriptions of the experiment had triggered. . . . By focusing on the issues of penicillin therapy and informed consent, the *Final Report* and the investigation betrayed a basic misunderstanding of the experiment's purposes and design. The HEW report implied that the failure to provide penicillin constituted the study's major ethical misjudgment; implicit was the assumption that no adequate therapy existed prior to penicillin. Nonetheless medical authorities firmly believed in the efficacy of arsenotherapy for treating syphilis at the time of the experiment's inception in 1932. The panel further failed to recognize that the entire study had been predicated on nontreatment. Provision of effective medication would have violated the rationale of the experiment—to study the natural course of the disease until death. On several occasions, in fact, the

USPHS had prevented the men from receiving proper treatment. Indeed, there is no evidence that the USPHS ever considered providing penicillin.

The other focus of the *Final Report*—informed consent—also served to obscure the historical facts of the experiment. In light of the deceptions and exploitations which the experiment perpetrated, it is an understatement to declare, as the *Report* did, that the experiment was "ethically unjustified," because it failed to obtain informed consent from the subjects. The *Final Report*'s statement, "Submitting voluntarily is not informed consent," indicated that the panel believed that the men had volunteered *for the experiment.* The records in the National Archives make clear that the men did not submit voluntarily to an experiment; they were told and they believed that they were getting free treatment from expert government doctors for a serious disease. The failure of the HEW *Final Report* to expose this critical fact—that the USPHS lied to the subjects—calls into question the thoroughness and credibility of their investigation.

Failure to place the study in a historical context also made it impossible for the investigation to deal with the essentially racist nature of the experiment. The panel treated the study as an aberration, well-intentioned but misguided. Moreover, concern that the *Final Report* might be viewed as a critique of human experimentation in general seems to have severely limited the scope of the inquiry. The *Final Report* is quick to remind the reader on two occasions: "The position of the Panel must not be construed to be a general repudiation of scientific research with human subjects." The *Report* assures us that a better designed experiment could have been justified. . . .

The HEW *Final Report* ignores many of the essential ethical issues which the study poses. The Tuskegee Study reveals the persistence of beliefs within the medical profession about the nature of blacks, sex, and disease—beliefs that had tragic repercussions long after their alleged "scientific" bases were known to be incorrect. Most strikingly, the entire health of a community was jeopardized by leaving a communicable disease untreated. There can be little doubt that the Tuskegee researchers regarded their subjects as less than human. As a result, the ethical canons of experimenting on human subjects were completely disregarded.

The study also raises significant questions about professional self-regulation and scientific bureaucracy. Once the USPHS decided to extend the experiment in the summer of 1933, it was unlikely that the test would be halted short of the men's deaths. The experiment was widely reported for forty years without evoking any significant protest within the medical community. Nor did any bureaucratic mechanism exist within the government for the periodic reassessment of the Tuskegee experiment's ethics and scientific value. The USPHS sent physicians to Tuskegee every several years to check on the study's progress, but never subjected the morality or usefulness of the experiment to serious scrutiny. Only the press accounts of 1972 finally punctured the continued rationalizations of the USPHS and brought the study to an end. Even the HEW investigation was compromised by fear that it would be considered a threat to future human experimentation.

In retrospect the Tuskegee Study revealed more about the pathology of racism than it did about the pathology of syphilis; more about the nature of scientific inquiry than the nature of the disease process. . . . As this history of the study suggests, the notion that science is a value-free discipline must be rejected. The need for greater vigilance in assessing the specific ways in which social values and attitudes affect professional behavior is clearly indicated.

---

\*     \*     \*     \*     \*

The Tuskegee syphilis study may be the most notorious example of disreputable public health research in modern America, but it is not the only example. During the Cold War, vulnerable human subjects were exposed to radiation without their knowledge or consent (Advisory Committee on Human Radiation Experiments 1996). More recently, the CDC sponsored a study in inner-city Los Angeles that administered an unlicensed measles vaccine to predominantly African-American and Latino children. The children's parents were not notified that the vaccine had not received FDA approval (Simmons 1996).

Controversy has also swirled around international collaborative research conducted in resource-poor countries (Peckham and Newell 2000). In 1997, for example, federally supported investigators conducted trials in Africa and Asia to test the efficacy of a low-dose regimen of zidovudine (AZT) in pregnant women. The hypothesis was that low doses, which were more affordable, would reduce vertical transmission of HIV infection (i.e., from mother to baby). The trials employed placebo control groups, despite the fact that AZT had already been shown to significantly reduce the rate of vertical transmission and is recommended in the United States for all HIV-infected pregnant women (Lurie and Wolfe 1997).

Marcia Angell (1997a, 847), then editor of the *New England Journal of Medicine,* harshly criticized the study: "The justifications are reminiscent of those for the Tuskegee study. Women in the Third World would not receive antiretroviral treatment anyway, so the investigators are simply observing what would happen to the subjects' infants if there were no study. And a placebo-controlled study is the fastest, most efficient way to obtain unambiguous information that will be of greatest value in the Third World." Harold Varmus and David Satcher (1997, 1003), then heads of the agencies conducting the trials (the NIH and CDC, respectively), responded vigorously: "[Critics] allude inappropriately to the infamous Tuskegee study, which did not test an intervention. The Tuskegee study ultimately deprived people of a known, effective, affordable intervention. To claim that countries seeking help in stemming the tide of maternal-infant HIV transmission by seeking usable interventions have followed that path trivializes the suffering of the men in the Tuskegee study and shows a serious lack of understanding of today's trials."

The central ethical issue is whether trials in developing countries should meet the standards applicable in the United States. On the one hand, it appears inequitable to use lower ethical standards for poor, vulnerable communities than are used in developed countries. If the trial would not have been ethical in the United States, why would it be ethical in Africa and Asia? On the other hand, failure to conduct such trials could jeopardize the health and lives of countless people in resource-poor countries. Individuals in these countries simply cannot afford the expensive treatment regime that is the standard of care in the United States.

## IV. PARTNER NOTIFICATION

Communicable or sexually transmitted diseases pose risks to sexual partners, family members, and other persons who may become exposed to infection. If the risk is significant, an intriguing dilemma exists: whether to safeguard individual privacy or disclose the risk. This tension between privacy and the duty to protect persons at risk is particularly pertinent in partner notification. Partner notification is a complex concept that has at least two distinct, if at times overlapping, meanings (Gostin and Hodge 1998b): (1) *duty to warn*—the power or duty of private health care professionals to inform their patients' sexual or other partners of foreseeable risks; and (2) *contact tracing*—the statutory power of public health agencies to identify and locate sexual partners and other "contacts" at risk of infection, and to notify them of the risk. In this section, Ronald Bayer, a prominent ethicist from the Mailman School of Public Health at Columbia University, and Kathleen Toomey, a well-known state health officer from Georgia, discuss these "two faces" of partner notification.

## HIV Prevention and the Two Faces of Partner Notification*
*Ronald Bayer and Kathleen E. Toomey*

As public health officials confronted the AIDS epidemic in the early 1980s they came to recognize the crucial importance of confidentiality. Only if those at risk for HIV could be convinced that their clinical encounters would not be disclosed without their consent could they be encouraged to undergo counseling and testing. Thus, the CDC, the Surgeon General, the Institute of Medicine, and the Presidential Commission on the HIV Epidemic all came to stress a common point: that the protection of the public's health was not compromised by the protection of confidentiality. On the contrary, the protection of confidentiality was a precondition for the achievement of public health goals.

Although the protection of confidentiality was supported by public health officials, gay rights organizations, and civil liberties groups, the best strategy for reaching those unknowingly placed at risk for infection or those who might inadvertently place others at risk was the subject of profound disagreement. . . . [D]eep and sometimes bitter disputes arose over partner notification in the epidemic's first decade.

Disagreements over the scope and limits of the principle of confidentiality, deep distrust over the motives of public health officials, doubts about the relevance and potential efficacy of traditional public health approaches to sexually transmitted diseases in dealing with

*Reprinted from *American Journal of Public Health* 82 (August 1992): 1158–64.

AIDS, and the enduring suspicions of those who viewed government agencies as a source of endangerment rather than protection were all involved in the controversy. Each of these factors helped to shape the context within which a profound confusion emerged between two very different approaches to informing unsuspecting third parties about their potential exposure to medical risk. . . .

The first approach, involving the moral "duty to warn," arose out of the clinical setting in which the physician knew the identity of the person deemed to be at risk. This approach provided a warrant for disclosure to endangered persons without the consent of the patient and could involve the revelation of the identity of the "threatening" party (the index patient). The second approach, that of contact tracing, emerged from sexually transmitted disease (STD) control programs in which the clinician typically did not know the identity of those who might have been exposed. This approach was formally predicated upon the voluntary cooperation of the patient in providing the names of contacts, never involved the disclosure of the identity of the index patient, and entailed the protection of the absolute confidentiality of the entire process of notification. . . .

## THE TRADITION OF CONTACT TRACING

Clinicians in STD control programs often did not have knowledge of a patient's background or family relationships. To elicit the names of sexual contacts, it was therefore necessary to obtain the cooperation of the index patient. Although considerable pressure might be applied, and indeed there are undocumented reports that on some occasions STD workers threatened to withhold treatment from those who would not provide the names of contacts, typically the patient's willingness to cooperate dictated the ultimate success of the partner-locating effort. To facilitate such cooperation, STD programs promised that the identity of the index patient would never be made available to contacts who were named. The index patient maintained ultimate control over the process, retaining the ability to withhold or provide names. Thus, the tradition of contact tracing was predicated on the voluntary cooperation of index patients and on a striking commitment to the protection of their anonymity. There were, quite obviously, circumstances when the identity of the index patient could be deduced even if he or she was not named, the paradigmatic case being the monogamous partner who was informed that he or she had been exposed to an STD. Yet even in such situations the two central principles of contact tracing remained uncompromised. The public health worker would not confirm the identity of the obvious source of exposure. Even when the index patients themselves requested that their identity be revealed to contacts, no exceptions were to be made.

Despite the four decades of experience with contact tracing, all efforts to undertake such public health interventions in the context of AIDS met with fierce resistance in the first years of the epidemic. Opposition by gay leaders and civil liberties groups had a profound impact on the response of public health officials, especially in states with relatively large numbers of AIDS cases. . . .

Underlying this debate was the fact that in the first years of the AIDS epidemic, no therapy could be offered to asymptomatic infected individuals. Thus, the role of contact tracing in the context of HIV infection differed radically from its role in the context of other STDs. In the latter case, effective treatments could be offered to notified partners. Once cured, such individuals would no longer pose a threat of transmission. In the case of HIV, nothing could be offered other than information about possible exposure to HIV. For public health officials, who saw in such information an opportunity to target efforts to foster behavioral changes among individuals still engaging in high-risk behavior that could place both the individual contacted and future partners at risk, that was reason enough to undertake the process. For opponents of contact tracing, the very effort to reach out to such individuals represented a profound intrusion on privacy with little or no compensating benefit. The task of behavioral change, they asserted, could be achieved more effectively and efficiently through general education.

By the late 1980s, the debate over contact tracing had shifted from one centered on the ethical issues of privacy to one focused on efficacy. The debate was fueled by questions that had begun to surface about the utility of contact tracing in the control of syphilis in populations where individuals had large numbers of sexual partners, many of whom were anonymous. This transformation reflected a maturing of the discussion. Early misapprehensions about the extent to which public health officials typically relied on overt coercion in the process, and the degree to which confidentiality might be compromised, had by decade's end all but vanished. With such political concerns allayed, many gay leaders had come to recognize that partner notification, in fact, could be a "useful tool" in efforts to control AIDS. . . .

## THE DUTY TO WARN

As physicians were called upon to treat patients with infectious diseases, it was inevitable that they would be confronted by the question of whether the duty to protect the privileged communications within the clinical relationship took priority over the obligation to protect others from their patients' communicable conditions. A misreading of a number of early 20th century cases has led some commentators to conclude that state courts had established an affirmative duty to breach confidentiality to protect known third parties. Indeed, it was such a misreading that permitted the California Supreme Court to claim the authority of precedent when in 1974 it crafted a doctrine that represented the most striking judicial challenge to the professional discretion of physicians when faced with patients who might endanger third parties. The "protective privilege ends where the public peril begins," wrote the majority in *Tarasoff v. Regents of California*, 551 P.2d 332 (Cal. 1976). . . .

[*Editor's note:* In *Tarasoff* (posted on the *Reader* web site), the California Supreme Court held that mental health professionals have a duty to warn identifiable third parties of threats of violence by the professional's patients. The case involved the murder of Tatiana Tarasoff, who had a prior casual relationship with Prosenjit Poddar, a mentally deranged patient. In therapy sessions Poddar indicated to his psychotherapist, Dr. Lawrence Moore, his intent to kill a girl. Although Poddar did not specifically name Tarasoff, it was evident to Dr. Moore that she was the intended victim. Dr. Moore did not warn Tarasoff or her parents, but instead asked the police to pick up Poddar. Although the police detained Poddar initially, he was later released and advised to stay away from Tarasoff. Two months later, Poddar murdered Tarasoff. Tarasoff's parents later sued Dr. Moore on the theory that he had a duty to warn their daughter of the risk Poddar presented.]

At the root of the *Tarasoff* decision was an ethical judgment that, although confidentiality was crucial for individual patients' autonomy, the protection of third parties vulnerable to potentially serious harm must be given priority. As a matter of moral principle, that determination provoked widespread support. What remained a matter of great controversy, however, was the question of whether such a determination represented wise public policy. Would the recognition of a legal duty to warn or protect so subvert the trust necessary to the therapeutic relationship that patients with violent fantasies would be constrained from talking about them with their therapists? Would the reduction in candor ultimately harm the public good by limiting the capacity of therapists to help their patients control their dangerous behaviors?

The *Tarasoff* doctrine and its ethical underpinnings provided the backdrop to the disputes that would surface as physicians confronted the dilemma of how to respond to HIV-infected patients who refused to inform their needle-sharing or sexual partners of their exposure when the clinician knew the identity of the endangered party. For some the dilemma arose solely in the context of partners who quite obviously had no reason to suspect that they had been placed at risk, the paradigmatic case being the female partner of a bisexual man. Other physicians extended their concern to those who might have reason to know but might nevertheless be ignorant of the risk to which they had been exposed, for example, the gay male partner in a long-standing, apparently monogamous relationship. The choices to be made would be all the more difficult given the extraordinary efforts that had been made to protect the confidentiality and rights of those infected with HIV. . . .

As public health officials began to consider the issues posed by the warning of third parties discovered during the clinical work of physicians to be at risk, they sought to chart a response that was cognizant of both the centrality of confidentiality in the effort to control the spread of HIV infection and the importance of ensuring that known parties were informed of their possible exposure to HIV. . . . [P]ublic health officials argued for a "privilege to disclose," thus freeing physicians from liability for either breaching confidentiality or not warning those who were at risk. In so arguing, these officials were reasserting the principle that had guided public policy in the era before *Tarasoff* and that historically had guided physician behavior.

The doctrine of the privilege to disclose was a political compromise designed to meet the concerns of a number of constituencies, not all of whom shared assumptions about the appropriate role of physicians in protecting vulnerable third parties from HIV infection. For all clinicians, the doctrine offered the freedom to make complex ethical judgments without the imposition of state mandates. For clinicians committed to warning as many unsuspecting partners as possible, it offered the opportunity to act on their professional obligations without being burdened by the dictates of the state. For those who believed that breaches of confidentiality were acceptable only in the rarest of circumstances, the privilege to disclose permitted a principled recognition that disclosure could be justified without the dangers associated with an overbroad commitment to notification.

CONCLUSIONS

From the perspective of the ethics of the clinical relationship, those who may have been placed at risk unknowingly have a moral right to such information [regarding their potential infection]. They are entitled to such information so that they may take steps to protect themselves, so that they can seek HIV testing and clinical evaluation, so that they may commence treatment if necessary, and so that they may avoid the inadvertent transmission of HIV. The moral claim of those who have unknowingly been placed at risk entails the correlative moral duty of the clinician to ensure that the unsuspecting party is informed. Neither the principle of confidentiality nor the value attached to professional autonomy is an absolute.

If the duty to warn poses difficult ethical questions, contact tracing does not. Contact tracing typically entails neither disclosure without the consent of the infected patient nor breaches of confidentiality. In fact, it can be argued that public health departments have a moral responsibility to undertake efforts modeled on the tradition of contact tracing programs that can inform individuals at risk about matters crucial to their lives and to the lives of their sexual and needle-sharing partners without recourse to mandatory measures.

But such a moral injunction may create difficult choices for policymakers, who must try to balance these activities with other moral claims on limited resources. Whatever the strengths of contact tracing, it is but one clement in a much broader array of educational and programmatic efforts to limit the spread of HIV infection. What proportions of the overall prevention efforts should be devoted to this labor-intensive and inevitably costly strategy? How are limited resources to be allocated among alternative strategies for achieving behavioral change? To these questions there can be no universal response, one that is applicable to all locales with their differing patterns of HIV infection. Targeted programmatic reviews based on the local epidemiological conditions and resource availability will be required. But what an advance it will represent to face the question of partner notification without the misconception that bedeviled discussions during the first decade of the AIDS epidemic.

---

\*     \*     \*     \*     \*

Bayer and Toomey examine partner notification in terms of the duties of private health care professionals and governmental health officials.

There is, of course, another potential duty that is equally contested. That duty is the one placed on contagious persons themselves to disclose the risk to their sexual or needle-sharing partners. Many people claim a "right to know" the serologic status of their partners. Armed with this knowledge, individuals can make informed decisions about engaging in intimate relationships and protecting themselves against infection.

Bioethicists urge persons with HIV or other serious infections to inform their partners (Bayer 1996). They reason that in engaging in intimate behavior, infected individuals owe a duty to their partners to apprise them of the risks. However, many gay men question this conventional position (Ainslie 1999). For them, persons with HIV and those uninfected together assume the risk of disease transmission. Rather than impose a stigmatizing duty to disclose on those who are HIV positive, they claim that everyone should engage in safer sex practices. An issue in this debate is, should it matter if, as a consequence of informing a partner, the infected person herself is placed at risk? Karen Rothenberg and Stephen J. Paskey (1995) argue that many women are subject to physical and sexual abuse if they reveal their HIV status.

## V. RECONCILING PUBLIC GOODS AND INDIVIDUAL INTERESTS IN PRIVACY

The Health Insurance Portability and Accountability Act of 1996, Pub. L. No. 104-191, 110 Stat. 1936 (also known as the Kennedy-Kassebaum Act or HIPAA), encouraged the development of electronic patient records. As part of this initiative, Congress recognized the need for national health information privacy safeguards. Under section 264 of HIPAA, Congress created a self-imposed deadline of August 21, 1999, for enacting comprehensive health information privacy legislation. HIPAA required the Secretary of the Department of Health and Human Services (DHHS) to promulgate privacy regulations if Congress failed to act by the deadline. The Secretary issued a proposed rule in November 1999 (64 Fed. Reg. 59,918) and a final rule late in President Clinton's term in office (45 C.F.R. pt. 160–64). President Bush set April 14, 2001, as the "effective date" for the rule, beginning a phase-in period requiring full compliance by April 14, 2003 (66 Fed. Reg. 12,434 (Feb. 26, 2001)). (To review the final rule, see www.aspe.hhs.gov/admnsimp.) Notably, DHHS regulations protect health care information but leave public health data to be protected under state law. As a result, the department asked the Center for Law and the Public's Health at Georgetown and Johns Hopkins universities to draft a model public health information privacy law with the assisstance of an expert national panel. The full text of the model law can be found at www.critpath.org/msphpa/privacy.htm. In the following selection, Lawrence O. Gostin, James G. Hodge, and Ronald O. Valdiserri explain the purposes and terms of the model law.

---

### Informational Privacy and the Public's Health:
### The Model State Public Health Privacy Act*
*Lawrence O. Gostin, James G. Hodge, Jr., and Ronald O. Valdiserri*

Assessing populational health is a core function of state and local public health departments which requires the acquisition, use, and storage of health-related information about individuals. . . . The accumulation and exchange of these personal data within an increasingly automated public health information infrastructure promises significant public health benefits. Widespread transmission of electronic public health data can more effectively identify, track, and evaluate health threats in the population. Well-planned surveillance helps identify health problems, target interventions, and influence funding decisions. Databases of health information facilitate existing and future epidemiologic investigations and research studies. These essential public health functions rely on the quality and reliability of health information.

Although the ability of public health agencies to utilize health data serves important public health purposes, it also raises fundamental privacy concerns. As identifiable health data are increasingly gathered, stored, and exchanged, people lose control over the use of their personal information. Many Americans distrust government agencies and believe the simple collection of personal data without their explicit permission is morally wrong. If public health authorities disclose intimate information, individuals may suffer embarrassment, stigma, and discrimination in employment, insurance, and government programs. Privacy is important not only because of its intrinsic value, but also because of its importance in facilitating health seeking behaviors. Persons

---

*Reprinted from *American Journal of Public Health* 91 (September 2001):1388–92. © 2001 by the American Public Health Association.

may avoid clinical tests and treatments, withdraw from research, or provide inaccurate or incomplete health information if they fear invasions of privacy. . . .

Current state laws differ significantly in the degree of privacy protections, give varying rights to access identifiable data, and allow multiple exceptions to disclosure prohibitions outside public health agencies. . . . What is absent from current law and policy, and what we hope to supply, is a rational approach that reconciles individual privacy interests with collective public health interests in identifiable health data (i.e., any health-related information which reveals, or could reveal under certain circumstances, the identity of the individual who is the subject of the information). Civil libertarians and consumers see informational privacy as a fundamental right and have vociferously asserted the importance of stronger legal safeguards. Public health professionals, on the other hand, have just as strongly asserted the need to use data to achieve important public health purposes. To reconcile these two divergent approaches, the Georgetown/Johns Hopkins Program on Law and Public Health convened a multi-disciplinary team of privacy, public health, and legislative experts to propose a model public health information privacy statute (Model Act). The Model Act would provide, for the first time, strong and consistent privacy safeguards for public health data, while still preserving the ability of state and local health departments to act for the common good. CDC (1999c, 21) recommends that states consider adopting the model legislation to "strengthen the current level of protection of public health data."

## RECONCILING PUBLIC HEALTH AND PRIVACY INTERESTS

The Model Act's approach is to maximize privacy safeguards where they matter most to patients and facilitate data uses where . . . necessary to promote the public's health. This accommodation between privacy and public health balances individual and collective interests.

Consider the sequence of events when government collects public health data through, for example, reporting or other forms of surveillance [see Figure 10 in the companion text (p. 140)]. First, the agency *collects* the data, typically after the patient has given informed consent (usually to a medical care provider) to provide a biologic sample (e.g., blood or urine) or health-related behavioral information (e.g., sexual history or drug use practices). Providing there is a strong public health interest, most people believe that patients should forgo this privacy invasion for the collective good. Next, the agency *uses* the data strictly within the confines of the health department. Again, providing the agency has a strong public health interest and the data are shared only with agency officials who have a need to know, data uses should prevail over privacy. The reason for this conclusion is that when public health authorities acquire and use data strictly within the agency, public health benefits are at their highest and privacy risks are at their lowest. The agency needs the freedom to use the data to monitor and prevent health risks. . . .

Finally, the agency may be asked or, under unusual circumstances, may seek to *disclose* personally identifiable information to persons outside the agency—e.g., to employers, insurers, commercial marketers, family, or friends. These kinds of disclosures are not very important for the public's health, but they do place patients at considerable risk of embarrassment, stigma, and discrimination. For these reasons, the law ought to provide maximum privacy protection. The Model Act's approach, therefore, is to give government flexibility to acquire and use data strictly within the mission of the public health agency. However, the Model Act affords public health authorities very little discretion to release personally identifiable data outside the agency and imposes serious penalties for disclosures without the patient's informed consent.

## THE MODEL STATE PUBLIC HEALTH PRIVACY ACT

The Model Act is based on several core assumptions. . . .

*All identifiable health information deserves legal protection.* The Model Act safeguards all personally identifiable data regardless of their source or holder. Thus, the Act applies to all "protected health information" held by public health agencies. This includes any public health information, whether oral, written, electronic, or visual, that relates to an individual's past, present, or future physical or mental health status, condition, treatment, service, products purchased, or provision of care. This broad definition of protected health information recognizes that any identifiable data (e.g., HIV, STD, or immunization status) can be sensitive.

*Non-identifiable health information requires no protection.* The definition of "protected health information" specifically incorporates another core assumption: non-identifiable health data do not merit privacy protection. Where health data are truly non-identifiable (although difficult to assess), individual privacy interests are not implicated. . . .

*Disclosures must be strictly limited.* While the Act affords public health agencies the power to acquire and use health data for important public health purposes, it grants very little authority to disclose identifiable data outside the public health system. The Act clarifies that protected health information is not subject to public review, and may not be disclosed without the specific, informed consent of the individual (or the individual's lawful representative) who is the subject of the information, except under narrow circumstances. . . .

[The authors describe the circumstances where disclosures are permitted without informed consent: directly to the individual, to appropriate federal agencies, to health care personnel in a medical emergency, pursuant to a court order, to agencies performing health oversight functions, and to identify a deceased individual.]

Finally, the Model Act permits the exchange of data among public health agencies within the state and outside the state. These information exchanges are viewed as data acquisitions or uses, not disclosures. As such, public health agencies may exchange identifiable health data with other state or local agencies provided the exchanges are necessary for the public's health. . . .

FAIR INFORMATION PRACTICES

Safeguarding privacy requires data holders to engage in a range of fair information practices. These practices assure strong security and privacy of public health information, but do not unreasonably burden public health authorities. The Act incorporates the following fair information practices:

*Justifying the need for data collection.* Acquiring identifiable data is not an inherent good. Rather, public health authorities must substantiate the need for identifiable data. . . . [T]he Model Act affirms that public health agencies shall only acquire identifiable health information which (a) relates directly to a legitimate public health purpose and (b) is reasonably likely to achieve such purpose. When information is no longer needed to fulfill the purpose for which it is acquired, it must be expunged or made non-identifiable.

*Informing data subjects.* The Act acknowledges that individuals are entitled to know how information about them is being used. Secretive acquisitions of identifiable data are prohibited. Prior to acquiring such data, public health agencies must provide public notice concerning their intentions to acquire the data and the purposes for which the data will be used. Individuals are entitled to view records of disclosures of their protected health information which public health agencies are required to maintain.

*Access to one's own data.* Subject to reasonable limitations, individuals are entitled to access, inspect, and copy their health data. Public health agencies are required to explain any code, abbreviation, notation, or other marks appearing in the information for the individual's benefit, as well as ensure the accuracy of such data and amend any errors.

*Assuring privacy and security.* Public health agencies have a duty to acquire, use, store, and disclose protected health information in a careful manner with strong privacy and security safeguards. Specific privacy and security protections are administered by a designated health information officer in each public health agency and enforced through significant administrative, criminal, and civil penalties. These protections apply to identifiable health data, regardless of their holder. The Act contains additional provisions which help ensure the right to privacy. For example, the Act: (a) requires an affirmative statement of privacy protections to accompany the disclosure of protected health information, (b) imposes a duty to uphold privacy and security standards, and (c) applies criminal and civil sanctions for unlawful disclosures—whether these disclosures are made by public health officials or by secondary holders of the data.

## CONCLUSION

Though not perfect, the Act provides a balance between the social good of data collection (recognizing its substantial value to community health) and the individual good of privacy (recognizing the normative value of respect for persons). . . . States that adopt the Act or laws consistent with its structure can stabilize and modernize public health information practices. If the Act serves as a model across multiple jurisdictions, it could reduce variability of existing protections among states, allow for the responsible exchange of health data within a national public health information infrastructure, and ultimately improve public health outcomes.

---

\*     \*     \*     \*     \*

This chapter has explored the tension between personal interests in privacy and communal interests in data collection. This tension is apparent in many surveillance and public health research activities. Powerful ethical issues arise as to which value should prevail, and why.

The conflict between surveillance and privacy is just one of the many recurrent tensions in public health. Another, equally divisive conflict is between health promotion and health communication on the one hand, and autonomy and free expression on the other. That is the topic of the next chapter.

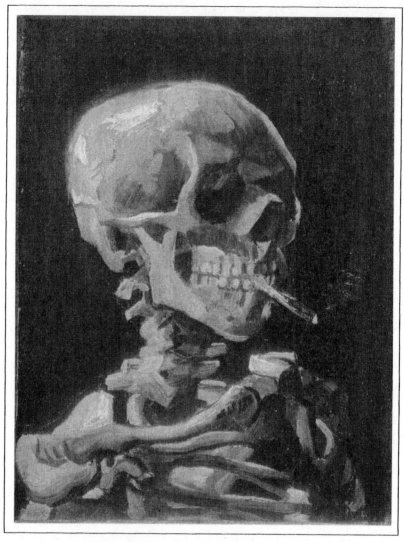

Vincent Van Gogh painted *Skull of a Skeleton with a Burning Cigarette* in an art class in Antwerp during the winter of 1885–1886. Though Van Gogh likely painted this image in jest, the painting eerily depicts the effects of smoking on the public's health. (Amsterdam, Van Gogh Museum [Vincent Van Gogh Foundation].)

# ELEVEN

# Health Promotion

*Education, Persuasion,
and Free Expression*

Public health authorities recognize behavior as an important determinant of health in the community. This idea is reflected mostly in modern discourse about the roles of smoking, diet, and sedentary lifestyle in the development of chronic disease, but the influence of behavior in transmitting infection (e.g., sexual or needle-sharing behavior) or causing injury (e.g., automobiles and firearms) is also well recognized. Researchers seek to identify effective techniques for changing people's behavior to achieve reductions in chronic and infectious diseases, as well as injuries. Public health assessments and interventions occur at the point of human conduct, whether at the individual, group, or organizational level.

Human behavior is highly complex, influenced by numerous social and environmental factors (Institute of Medicine 2001), but information is a prerequisite for change. The population must at least be aware of the health consequences of risk behaviors to make informed decisions. The citizenry is inundated with messages about health and behavior by the media, businesses, religious and charitable organizations, family, and peers. Perhaps the most important goal of health promotion is to alter the informational environment so that the public can hear messages conducive to their health and avoid messages that encourage risk behavior.

As Figure 14 suggests, public health authorities have many tools at their disposal to construct a favorable informational environment, even though, in practice, they may not be particularly adept or successful. Government can add its voice to the marketplace of ideas by delivering

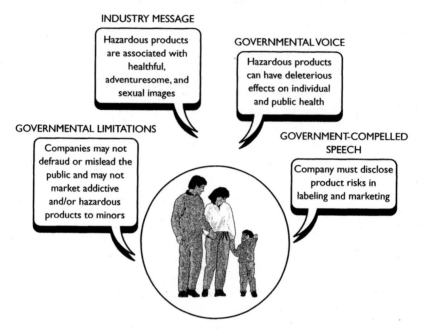

Figure 14.   A governmental role in health promotion and education.

health messages directly or providing incentives for others to do so. Government can also constrain the speech of others by limiting advertising and promotions of hazardous products. Finally, government can compel businesses to reveal health and safety risks through disclosure and labeling requirements.

The readings in this chapter discuss the goals and techniques of health promotion. (Readers are referred to other helpful resources: Callahan 2000; Watson and Platt 2000; Bayer and Moreno 1986; Doxiadis 1991.) Section I, "An Ethic for Health Promotion," provides theoretical perspectives. The reading explains the meanings of, and government influences on, social norms. Health promotion, as we will see, is not a matter of pure science or reason, but involves important values. Section II, "Health Communication Campaigns," offers a closer examination of ethical aspects of government communication. Here, the appropriateness of government speech itself is the concern. The selection describes the justifications for health communications, as well as the morally troubling aspects. Section III, "Commercial Speech," examines government's role in suppressing private messages that encourage unhealthy behavior. The Supreme Court cases examine the protection afforded to advertising and promotions in a constitutional democracy. The final section, "Compelled Commercial Speech," discusses government-imposed health and safety disclosures. Public health authorities frequently require businesses to provide instructions for the safe use of products and labels warning consumers of potential hazards.

## I. AN ETHIC FOR HEALTH PROMOTION

Not long ago, the media revealed that Barry McCaffrey (the "Drug Czar"), of the National Office of Drug Control Policy in the Clinton administration, had been reading advance scripts of prime-time television programs. McCaffrey made "recommendations" about the programmatic content, urging broadcasters to filter out messages that tacitly condone drug use and reinforce messages that discourage drug use. Broadcasters who complied were relieved of regulatory burdens (e.g, they were exempt from the obligation to run antidrug public service advertisements). Consumers were never informed that the scripts had been filtered in advance by federal officials or that broadcasters had altered images and content (Lacey and Carter 2000).

What is wrong with this story? From a public health perspective, perhaps nothing. Assuming that illicit drug use presents a health hazard and that controlling the informational environment reduces the risk, this curtailment of expressive freedom has much in common with many other forms of health promotion. Public health authorities are passionately concerned with health messages. They understand that behavior is responsible for a sizable burden of injury and disease in the population, and information is an important influence on how people behave.

Health promotion is thought to be a benign activity. After all, most people believe that government ought to inform the polity about behaviors that cause injury and disease. And the public is prepared to give its government the benefit of the doubt when the state acts benevolently to promote healthy communities. But public officials can go only so far in a constitutional democracy. The public is likely to bristle at government efforts to prescribe social orthodoxies, particularly if officials deceive them (Lessig 1995; Sunstein 1996b). What is wrong with the Drug Czar's censorship of television programming? Some might say that government's good intentions do not excuse deceit, that is, altering messages or images without the public's knowledge.

In 1999 the U.S. Postal Service reproduced a pose of famous abstract expressionist Jackson Pollack for a postage stamp, but the image was cleansed by removing the cigarette from Pollack's mouth (Knight 1999) (see photograph on page 149 of the companion text). When Mark Yudof (1983) wrote his influential book on government speech, he used as an example the former Soviet Union news image of the May Day parade. Each year the same photograph was published in the newspapers, but certain public officials were added or deleted from the image, depending on whether they were currently favored or disfavored by the Kremlin. In each case, the government presumably felt it was acting for the public's good, but failed to fully inform the community or seek its consent.

Government can deceive in much more subtle ways, and, given the government's good intentions, it is not at all clear when the state goes "too far" in health promotion. What if public health officials act as if there were sound scientific support underlying the health message, but the data are inconclusive or nonexistent? What if government knowingly exaggerates the risk or underestimates the extent of the behavioral change necessary to convince the public to follow public health advice?

Health promotion activities can also become controversial if government associates behaviors with unattractive characteristics, causing stigma and embarrassment. Suppose that government implies or suggests that smoking, having unsafe sex, or eating high-fat foods is immoral, irresponsible, or unattractive. Individuals who engage in those behaviors may be blamed for their illnesses and risk losing social sympathy and support. They also may come to have a lower self-image and suffer psychological harm. (For a discussion on the relationship between stigmatization of sexual behaviors and public health efforts relating to AIDS, see Allen 2000).

An introductory reading by David R. Buchanan, of the University of Massachusetts School of Public Health and Health Sciences, asks an important question: What are the goals of health promotion and the most appropriate means of achieving them? He sees the goals as prolonging life and reducing mortality rates, and the means as finding more effective ways to change people's behavior. But at what cost? Buchanan sets out to explain why a science of health promotion is neither imminent nor estimable. He argues that health promotion is inescapably a moral and political endeavor, and the goals more befitting the realization of human well-being are to promote self-knowledge, individual autonomy, integrity, and responsibility through putting into

practice more democratic processes of self-direction and mutual support in civil society.

---

## Disquietudes*
David R. Buchanan

The common theme [in modern health promotion activities] is that science and technology will provide the tools to address our nation's
health problems and that politics and morality stand in the way of taking full advantage of these advances. To prevent drug abuse, the executive office proposes to implement a well-financed national media campaign, broadcasting skillfully constructed messages that use the most
effective techniques known to the communication sciences. To prevent
AIDS, a panel of experts from the NIH recommends stepped up public
distribution of sterile syringes and more sex education programs in
schools. To reduce obesity (a risk factor for heart disease, the leading
cause of death in the nation), researchers have developed new drugs
with greater power to control appetite. In short, applied scientific research offers the best prospect for remedying public health problems. It
is a tantalizing picture and one that I think fairly represents the consensus of official opinion on how to improve the nation's health. . . .

What are we to make of these [claims]? How are we to think about
improving the health and well-being of individuals and communities?
Do the results of scientific research offer the best guide to better living?
Are moral apprehensions archaic and unfortunate obstacles? Does it
matter whether we lose weight through pills, or through diet and exercise? Or whether teenage drug use is reduced through the same techniques that are used to induce them to start smoking or drink beer?
How might these different ways of promoting health make a difference
in terms of the quality of outcomes? . . .

PURPOSES

Thinking in the field of health promotion is currently framed by the
scientific terminology of morbidity and mortality rates, risk factors,
randomized control trials, independent and dependent variables, null

---

*Reprinted from *An Ethic for Health Promotion: Rethinking the Sources of Human
Well-Being* (Oxford: Oxford University Press, 2000), 1–22.

hypotheses, cost-benefit analyses, and effective behavior change techniques. [I] recommend a new direction marked by the concepts of well-being, integrity, virtues, autonomy, responsibility, civility, caring, and solidarity. These concepts better reflect the larger aims of the field and the direction advocated here. . . .

[I am] critical of the unstinting institutional commitment to the positivist (experimental) paradigm of scientific research for determining the causes of "lifestyle" diseases and for developing interventions to prevent them. . . . Many people practice a far different approach to health promotion that cannot be squared with the technical scientific framework; their work affirms the values of autonomy, justice, caring, and solidarity over the pursuit of more effective behavior change techniques. . . . Instead of scientific reasoning, the alternative proposed here is based on practical reasoning. Instead of seeking the power to change people's behavior, it recommends seeking common understandings with community members about the good life for human beings. Instead of pursuing the development of a science of health promotion, it recommends an ethical and political process of improving institutional practices in order to foster individual and community well-being. . . .

The field of health promotion needs to revive and reorient its practices toward having people together as citizens and community members to decide for themselves the kinds of lives they think are most worth living, rather than continuing to develop the "technologies of prevention." Explaining the shortcomings of the current approach and establishing the foundations for an alternative approach will take us into complex philosophical issues, but we ignore them at our peril. . . . [T]he problem is probably even greater for behavioral scientists in the health field, due to their proximity, allegiance, and perhaps envy of the successes of medical science. But greater familiarity with the ethical and epistemological assumptions underlying current practices and with the merits of an alternative approach is essential in order to establish a more propitious and principled ethic for health promotion.

## CHALLENGES

A key tenet of the field of health promotion today is that health problems are attributable to the prevalence and distribution of identifiable risk factors and that the most fruitful approach for identifying suspect risk factors is scientific research. The scientific method is regarded as having indisputable superiority in determining the causes of these problems. The purpose of such research is to identify the underlying social and psychological factors that cause people to behave in ways that compromise their health (i.e., to start smoking, to take drugs, to overeat, to commit violent acts, etc.). In light of the significant accomplishments of science, from heart bypass surgery to landing men on the moon, one might expect similarly striking progress through these methods in identifying the causes of and solutions to contemporary health problems.

But the current program of health promotion research has not produced a cogent response to questions about causation. . . . [B]ecause health has both physical and social dimensions, understanding the nature of modern ailments presents new problems that are not readily amenable to scientific analysis. For now, in surveying the field, it is simply an indisputable fact that studies of behavioral health problems have not been able to produce results even remotely comparable to those found in biomedical research. . . .

Two additional considerations provide further support for reconsidering the current direction of the field. First, a growing mass of evidence shows that the most carefully designed scientific interventions intended to reduce modern health problems have not proven successful. Carefully controlled, scientifically designed health promotion interventions . . . have produced little evidence of success. . . .

Finally, in direct contrast, there are ample indications that the most beneficial responses to these problems have come from people acting on their own without recourse to scientifically designed interventions. The most effective treatment for alcohol abuse is Alcoholics Anonymous (AA). The most effective treatment for substance abuse is an analogous 12-step program based on the AA model. Likewise, we know that 90% of people who quit smoking successfully do so on their own without the assistance of professional interventions. . . . These observations have led me to the conclusion that it is time to consider a new direction for the field.

## IS THE QUEST FOR A SCIENCE OF HEALTH
## PROMOTION CONTRIBUTING TO THE PROBLEM?

In health promotion, research is instrumental to the extent that it focuses on identifying the causes of behavior—ascertained, through rigorous adherence to well-known and well-defined research methods—and disregards questions about what makes human behavior good. Reflecting the pressures for precision, quantification, and efficiency maximization of these times, the nation's public health goals and objectives are now defined in terms of reducing morbidity and mortality rates. The leading causes of morbidity and mortality are now most influenced by smoking, a poor diet, and lack of exercise. Therefore, health promotion research and practice focus virtually exclusively on developing more effective and efficient means to accomplish these behavioral change objectives. These narrow objectives are indicative of the failure to think through the ends of health promotion.

To press the point about the need for reviving the exercise of practical reason—the type of thinking that asks, "Are the postulated ends worth pursuing, in light of the means they seem to require? Are the institution's values, as presently formulated, worthy of realization? What costs are imposed on *other* ends and *other* values?"—let me be heretical: I do not think that lowering heart disease rates is the most important goal of health promotion. On the contrary, I think most people are drawn to the field because they want to be part of forging social and political conditions in which we all can live together decently. Nonsmoking, a strict diet, and regular exercise are really rather trivial parts of any broader understanding of social well-being, but that is where all of the field's resources are now directed. . . .

I have three concerns. First, on some level, people who smoke, drink, eat a fatty diet, get pregnant as teenagers, take drugs, or fail to exercise do not share the goals of eliminating smoking, drug-taking, eating red meat, physical inactivity, premarital sex, and so on. They do not share or agree with our vision of how we think they ought to live. However when we in the field of health promotion try to rationalize our efforts, we are saying that we think we know how people should live their lives better than they do themselves. And the best way to accomplish our goals is to develop and to wield effective techniques to change their behavior. (To anticipate ready objections, I take up the question of voluntary consent below.) Second . . . research protocols . . . designed to uncover the same power to effectively control human behavior . . . pose serious threats to human autonomy, dignity, and responsibility. If autonomy, dignity, and responsibility are intrinsic to human well-being, then the current direction of the field is self-defeating. Third, health promotion research is not now aimed at clarifying normative values, which might prove helpful in assisting people to exercise better judgment. The origins of contemporary health problems, I believe, do indeed lie in disturbances in people's values and judgments about their immediate felt desires. But the scientific method of testing hypotheses is incapable of answering questions about which values should matter to us and why, about the kinds of lives most worth living and the kind of society we should work toward creating together. . . .

Let me be clear: I think hypothesis testing works remarkably well in the natural sciences, such as physics, chemistry, and medicine. . . . I think experimental research designs are effective in discovering and demonstrating causal relationships in the natural world, including, notably, the physiological processes of the human body. Just as the natural sciences are not wholly subsumed by experimental methods (for example, research in geology and ecology), not all research in health promotion involves experimental research designs. In practice, a great deal of research in the field involves simple empiricism. Researchers simply count things (no matter how sophisticated the statistical techniques) and try to see what goes together with what ("correlations"). . . .

Although correlational and quasi-experimental research designs are common, the experimental method of hypothesis testing is a tremendously powerful ideal that guides the bulk of day-to-day research activities in public health. . . . Randomized control trials are the highest standard against which all other types of research are compared and the endpoint toward which all health research is expected to progress. . . . [T]he commitment to this particular method has displaced other types of research in ways that are ultimately debilitating to the field. . . .

Based on what the positivist, hypothesis-testing methodology can and cannot do, instead of strengthening our collective capacity to think more clearly, carefully, and conscientiously about values that matter, the instrumental orientation of health promotion today is headed in the opposite direction. If the field achieved its own stated objectives to gain the power to effectively change human behavior, it would further erode the grounds of human dignity, the individual sense of responsibility, and the most basic understandings of ethical human relationships. We believe human beings have dignity and deserve to be treated with respect because we believe human beings have autonomy, that is, because we believe human beings have a capacity for free choice unlike any other creature on earth. It is autonomy per se which affords humankind its peculiar dignity. Moreover, our entire understanding of the concept of responsibility is anchored in understandings of human beings as free and autonomous agents. If people did not have the capacity to make free choices, then we could not hold them responsible for their actions.

So, in health promotion, whenever we treat people as if we know what they need better than they do themselves and whenever we assume that their behavior is caused or conditioned by antecedent factors (which tacitly sanctions the right to intervene, since they are evidently not fully responsible for the choices they make), we treat them as a means to serve our ends. . . .

But I have another, deeper concern. The issue involves the relationship between means and ends. When one thinks about the world in instrumental terms, means and ends tend to be viewed as independent of one another in the following sense. One can define and characterize the goal independently of the means used to achieve it. Weight loss, for example, can be defined and measured regardless of whether the means used to achieve it are a sensible diet and exercise, diet pills, liposuction, or colon staples. From an instrumental perspective, different means are regarded as interchangeable techniques, and barring side effects, the outcomes are considered independent of the means used to produce them. . . . Since the results are not defined in terms of the methods, the most important question from an instrumental perspective, and the one that is currently absorbing the preponderance of the field's resources, is determining which means are most effective.

But when one is concerned with normative questions in the social world, ends cannot be characterized independently of the means. . . . The product is defined, at least in part, through the process by which it is achieved. In the concept of virtue, [something] can be both a cause and a constituent element of the ends being sought.

The different ways of thinking about health and well-being—instrumentally versus practically—lie at the bottom of nagging intuitions that there are important differences in terms of the quality of outcomes depending on how we get there. It does make a difference, for example, whether young people consciously and deliberately choose not to use drugs, or whether their attitudes are effectively altered through "indirect influence techniques" and "conditioning in low thought situations." Likewise, people may lose weight by taking pills, but they will not gain the dignity and self-respect that comes through exercising self-control. As the field heads down the path of technical efficiency, we are in danger of losing sight of how different means affect the quality of outcomes. To promote well-being, the means must be consonant with the ends to be achieved. We cannot promote integrity, autonomy, responsibility, caring, trust, or justice through the exercise of power—through the development of more effective techniques—no matter how strictly protocols for obtaining voluntary consent are enforced.

Fortunately, there is a tradition in health education that has worked to strengthen individual autonomy and social solidarity through practices centered on caring and fulfilling our collective responsibility for creating more humane living conditions for all people. Change and growth are possible when community members connect with one another as human beings in caring relationships characterized by trust and mutual support. It is a type of health promotion practice that is fully accountable, yet not dependent on exercising instrumental power to accomplish predetermined outcome objectives. It is based on the knowledge that, with a modicum of trust and institutional support, many good things can happen—many we may never have even considered before listening to, learning from, and engaging with fellow community members.

## II. HEALTH COMMUNICATION CAMPAIGNS

Government messages about health and behavior are pervasive, delivered through mass media technologies: radio and television (paid and public-service advertisements), newspapers and magazines (press releases and briefings), telephone lines ("800" number hotlines and "broadcast" and "auto-response" faxes), and the Internet (web sites). Government also subsidizes educational messages through grants and contracts with private and voluntary organizations. Government selects the funding recipient and the messages that the organization will convey. For a systematic description and analysis of health communication campaigns, see Rice and Atkin (2000) and Bennett and Calman (1999).

Health education is often a preferred public health strategy and, in many ways, it is unobjectionable. In health communication campaigns, government persuades individuals to alter risk behaviors. By imparting knowledge, government helps inform the polity about activities that promote health and well-being. When government speaks, citizens may choose to listen and adhere, or they are free to reject health messages. The selection that follows acknowledges the good that can come from health information but also discusses the intrusion on personal sovereignty and the attribution of personal responsibility inherent in mass communication campaigns. (As for the role of fear in health education, see Soames [1988].)

Ruth R. Faden, director of the Phoebe R. Berman Bioethics Institute at Johns Hopkins, discusses the morally relevant attributes of health communication campaigns. Although she recognizes the coercive aspects,

Faden explains why many government health messages are ethically acceptable. See further Guttman (2000), Guttman and Ressler (2001), Resnik (2001), and Wikler and Beauchamp (1995).

### Ethical Issues in Government-Sponsored
### Public Health Campaigns*
*Ruth R. Faden*

[P]ublic health campaigns have been the subject of two major criticisms. First, they have been accused of being ineffective or at least not cost-effective. Second, they have been accused of being a kind of governmental red herring—of being token efforts used by the government to avoid having to confront the true, but politically problematic, causes of ill health. In addition to these two major concerns, questions have been raised about the extent to which health campaigns interfere with free choice and about the general propriety of governmental attempts to direct social values and lifestyles.

In the case of public health campaigns, and probably in the case of all health promotion strategies, each of these sets of concerns—about efficacy, about justice, and about autonomy—are inextricably interrelated. In some cases, there is almost a hydraulic relationship between these problems. The more one is improved, the more others are exacerbated. For example, if public health campaigns are made more effective, some concerns about injustice may be removed. However, the more effective public health campaigns become, the more one becomes concerned about governmental interferences with autonomy. . . .

EFFICACY OF HEALTH COMMUNICATION CAMPAIGNS

There are many problems in evaluating the cost and effectiveness of public health campaigns (Aldana 2001). One problem is deciding what counts as a successful campaign, that is, deciding what the criteria for success ought to be. For example, should success be defined in terms of behavior change or attitude change? How much change must be achieved before the campaign can be called a success?

---

*Reprinted from *Health Education Quarterly* 14 (Spring 1987): 33–34.

Another problem is deciding what counts as a public campaign, for purposes of evaluation. For example, one of the earliest, if not the first, public health campaigns conducted in the U.S. was launched by Cotton Mather in 1721. Mather used pamphleteering and rhetoric to persuade the citizens of Boston to accept inoculation at the outbreak of a smallpox epidemic. While this kind of personal crusading is not usually what we have in mind when we think of public health campaigns, it is true that until fairly recently public health campaigns were dominated by private citizens organized into special interest, voluntary organizations. Voluntary organizations still play a central role in public health campaigns. In many areas such as smoking and nutrition, it has been very difficult to tease apart the effects of campaigns sponsored by the government from the effects of campaigns sponsored by voluntary organizations. Particularly in the modern, television era of medical campaigning, it is by no means obvious what effects to attribute to government interventions, nor is it necessarily obvious which government interventions count as health media campaigns.

Another problem in making judgments about the efficacy of health and other public service campaigns is that while many such campaigns have been mounted, a considerable number have not been reported in the public literature, and as a result, little is known about them. Most of the campaigns about which we do know something have had no formal evaluation; campaigns which have been evaluated have often suffered from inadequate evaluation methodology. As a result, much of what is thought about the effectiveness of these campaigns is based on anecdotal comment and gut reaction, rather than empirically reliable data. . . .

Although there have been notable failures of specific, individual campaigns in the past, recently researchers have pointed to the successful effects of health campaigns when taken cumulatively and over time. . . . Increasingly, researchers are becoming optimistic about the potential for success of well-designed and properly implemented public health campaigns. . . .

At least two factors interact to permit recent projects to be comparatively more successful—adequate resources and skillful application of behavioral science theory and research. In terms of resources, it is generally acknowledged that for media campaigns to work it is usually necessary that: (1) they be continued for long periods of time (years, not months); (2) the main points of the message be presented repeatedly, but in novel and different ways; (3) multimedia be used, and that (4) mass media be augmented by more personal interventions and the organization of community resources at the local level. . . .

## AUTONOMY AND HEALTH CAMPAIGNS

One of the consequences of any strategy for increasing the effectiveness of health campaigns—whether it is the sophisticated application of behavioral science theory or an increase in expenditures—is that the very fact that the strategy is now more effective may serve to raise other concerns about the propriety of the campaign. Here we must face the somewhat awkward realization that we are not altogether certain that all government-sponsored health campaigns ought to succeed. For at least some campaigns, there are real questions about the conditions under which such programs should be permitted.

The central issue here is the compatibility of government-sponsored health campaigns with respect for individual autonomy and related values. A thorough analysis of the compatibility of government-sponsored health campaigns with autonomy would probably involve developing a theory of individual autonomy and, if not a theory of the state, at least some strong presuppositions about the nature of government in the liberal state. . . .

*Persuasion* can be defined as the intentional and successful attempt to induce a person(s), through appeals to reason, to freely accept—as his or her own—the beliefs, attitudes, values, intentions, or actions advocated by the influence agent. In persuasion, the influence agent must bring to the persuadee's attention reasons for acceptance of the desired perspective. In paradigmatic cases of persuasion, these reasons are conveyed through written or spoken language, by use of structured argument and reasoning. However, reasons can also be conveyed through nonverbal communication—through, for example, visual evidence— and by artful questioning and structured listening.

One central feature of persuasion is that the reasons that comprise the persuasive appeal exist independent of the persuader. If the influence agent creates or in some way has control over the contingencies that the agent offers as "reasons," the influence is no longer strictly persuasive, but rather manipulative or even coercive. . . .

*Manipulation of information* is a deliberate act that successfully influences a person(s) by nonpersuasively altering the person's understanding of the situation, thereby modifying perceptions of the available options. The influence agent does not change the person's actual options; only the person's perception is modified as a result of the manipulation. Thus, informational manipulation affects what a person believes. Manipulation of information compromises autonomy to the extent that it renders people ignorant, thereby causally constraining relevant aspects of their decisions. Manipulation by deception is the most common form of manipulation of information. Deception includes such strategies as lying, withholding of information, and misleading exaggeration where people are led to believe what is false. Deception may also be effected through nonverbal communications, which make use of certain ordinary expectations to cause the manipulee to infer certain informational relationships or beliefs. . . . Also qualifying as informational manipulations are such interventions as: (1) intentionally overwhelming a person with excessive information so as to induce confusion and a reduction of understanding, (2) intentionally provoking or taking advantage of fear, anxiety, pain, or other negative affective or cognitive states known to compromise a person's ability to process information effectively, and (3) intentionally presenting information in a way that leads the manipulatee to draw certain predictable and misleading influences. . . .

Questions concerning psychological and informational manipulation have been raised much more frequently about commercial campaigns (advertising) than about public service campaigns. In advertising, the central issue thus far has been deception. Assuring so-called "truth in advertising" is a major focus of the Federal Trade Commission. . . . By contrast, health campaigns are rarely (if ever) deceptive, at least in any ordinary or straightforward, intentional sense. If there are any autonomy-related problems with health campaigns, they are apt to be much more subtle and to derive largely from the potential for skillful application of psychological theory. It is often difficult in practice to distinguish between persuasion and certain forms of psychological and informational manipulation. Many social influence attempts, including many health campaigns, contain elements of both persuasion and manipulation. . . .

To the extent that [some] health campaigns . . . involve elements of psychological or informational manipulation, in the strictest sense they violate the principle of respect for individual autonomy. However, merely because violations are involved . . . it does not necessarily follow that the campaign is morally unacceptable. The campaign may still be morally justifiable, depending on the seriousness of the violation and on the moral importance of the warrant for conducting the campaign and using the specific strategies that are disrespectful of autonomy.

## JUSTICE, AUTONOMY, AND HEALTH CAMPAIGNS

Many different kinds of justifications can and have been offered for government health promotion efforts generally, and health campaigns in particular. . . . First, it can be argued that the government has a basic responsibility to protect and promote the nation's health—the public health—independent of the preference structure of individual citizens. This position places an intrinsic value on the public's health as expressed through such aggregate indicators as national life expectancy and morbidity data. Second, there is the closely related argument that at least the majority of citizens desire certain kinds of health promotion or protection that can only be achieved through collective state action. Applying this collective efficiency position to health campaigns, it can be argued that the majority of individuals want to have healthier lifestyles but they do not have the resources either to educate themselves or to modify unhealthful habits on their own. A third argument grounds government intervention by appeal to broadly construed third party or state interests. A prime example here is cost containment. Health promotion programs are justified to the extent that they reduce health care costs or sick day losses. The fourth argument justifies government lifestyle programs to the extent that the targeted lifestyle behavior has the effect of harming innocent others.

These four arguments are by no means mutually exclusive. They can obviously be used in concert to justify the same health campaign: Antismoking campaigns are paradigmatic examples of state health promotion efforts that can plausibly appeal to all four arguments for their justification. Nevertheless, each of these justifications will not strike every critic as equally compelling. . . . [T]here is a close correspondence between one's position on the justifiability of state-sponsored lifestyle campaigns, what one would count as an acceptable justification, and one's views about how government should function in the liberal state. . . .

Similarly, objections can and have been raised against the public health justification. One can deny that there is any basic or important value to the nation's health, apart from or independent of the value each citizen places on his or her own health. Someone holding this position may interpret an appeal to the state's obligation to protect the public health as a thinly disguised instance of unjustifiable state paternalism when a lifestyle program disregards the value or preference structures of the individual citizens who are its targets.

Objections can also be mounted against the "social harm, cost containment" justification and "the harm to others" justification. Objections to these positions often reflect empirical and moral disputes about the magnitude and acceptability of the harm at issue, as well as disputes about the limits of government in the liberal state to provide harm protection and to make acceptable tradeoffs between highly valued social goods.

There is a direct relationship between the warrants for a particular health campaign and the extent to which it is morally acceptable for the campaign to violate the principle of respect for autonomy. If one finds the justification for conducting a specific state-financed health campaign to be very morally compelling, one would be more likely to view as ethical the campaign's including elements that violate respect for autonomy. . . .

When people oppose government health campaigns on the grounds that the government ought not to interfere with or attempt to shape existing patterns of health behaviors and lifestyles, a standard response is that, if the government does not get into the business of shaping health attitudes and behavior, those attitudes and behavior will be left to be shaped entirely by the short-term contingencies of our market economy. The argument here is that through extensive advertising efforts industry shapes the public's preferences and affects secular trends in the direction of increasing consumption of unhealthful products. Thus, a major justification for government media campaigns is that they are needed to counter commercial advertising. From this perspective, government campaigns serve an essential function as corrective advertising for the harmful activities of the private sector. However, those who reject this justification for government media campaigns counter with the argument that if the government is convinced that an industry is marketing an unhealthful product, instead of engaging in counter-advertising, the government should ban all promotional advertising of the product. Better yet, the government should either set standards that make the product healthful, or if that is not possible, make the product illegal. . . .

Implicit in this position is a different set of assumptions about the role of government from that underlying the current federal position on deregulation. Particularly as regards matters of health and safety, collective efficiency arguments favor strong intervention by [federal] agencies. . . .

[E]ven for those health problems where there is a preferable, alternative solution (for example, through regulatory or legislative engineering or through technological change), there still may be an appropriate role for health campaigns. This role involves the little discussed function of health media campaigns to create a constituency for regulation or legislation, that is, to create the public climate needed to make these options politically possible. I am, of course, talking here about the long-term, cumulative effects of sustained public campaigning. For example, the current legislative interest in restricting public smoking areas would likely not have been possible without a background of favorable public opinion. Of course, there is no way to determine exactly how important health campaigns have been to the development of this climate. It is very difficult to distinguish the effect of public service media campaigns from the complexity of social forces which contribute to shifts in public opinion and popular cultural values. However, it is likely that the anti-smoking campaigning of the past 20 years has contributed significantly to the current climate of increasing hostility toward smoking. . . .

Real questions remain about whether health campaigns should be conducted for the explicit purpose of modifying public or legislative opinion over time. There are problems about the use of governmental funds to conduct interventions that may influence the legislative process, however subtly or indirectly. Nevertheless, I see this long-term effect of changing public opinion and perceptions about health practices as one of the more viable justifications for continued federal support of health media campaigns.

---

## III. COMMERCIAL SPEECH

Public health officials' attempts to control the informational environment, of course, are not confined to health education campaigns. Most people understand that government messages have a paltry effect on public attitudes and behaviors. There are just too many voices in the market for government to dominate or, sometimes, even to have a discernible influence. The business community has a particularly potent voice in the market of ideas. Corporations have a profit incentive to influence consumers to buy their products. For example, manufacturers of hazardous products (e.g., cigarettes, alcoholic beverages, and firearms) spend billions of dollars on advertisements and promotions. Public health officials cannot hope to compete with these private purveyors of information. Consequently, restraint of commercial speech is one of the most important health promotion strategies.

For most of the nation's history, the Supreme Court declined to protect commercial speech under the First Amendment of the Constitution. However, in the mid-1970s the Court began to protect advertisements and promotions of products. Bigelow v. Virginia, 421 U.S. 809 (1975). The early commercial speech cases involved instances where the message itself had public health value: abortion referral services, advertisements for contraceptives, or the price of pharmaceuticals.

Nominally, commercial speech operates as a category of "lower-value" expression, deserving of less constitutional protection than social or political discourse. In reality, though, the level of scrutiny for commercial speech has changed over the years and is still in transition. This section explores the evolution of the commercial speech doctrine from the mid-1970s to the present day. Before discussing the constitutional safeguards, however, it is necessary to understand what the Court means by "commercial speech."

Commercial speech is an expression related solely to the economic interests of the speaker and its audience that does no more than propose a commercial transaction. Virginia State Bd. of Pharmacy v. Virginia Citizens Consumer Council, Inc., 425 U.S. 748 (1976). The three attributes of commercial speech are that it (1) identifies a specific product (i.e., offers a product for sale), (2) is a form of advertising (i.e., is designed to attract public attention to, or patronage for, a product or service, by paid announcements proclaiming its qualities or advantages), and (3) confers economic benefits (i.e., the speaker stands to profit financially).

These criteria appear to be clear but raise perplexing issues about the boundaries between political and commercial speech. For example, in *Bad Frog Brewery, Inc. v. New York State Liquor Auth.*, 134 F.3d 87 (2d Cir. 1998), the Court of Appeals found that a beer label displaying a frog giving an insulting gesture was commercial speech, but not more fully protected social commentary or political speech.

Consider the two editorial-style advertisements ("advertorials") shown in Figures 15 and 16, paid for by tobacco manufacturers, that appeared in the *New York Times*. Should these advertorials be classified as commercial or political speech, and why?

Both advertisements express an opinion on a matter of public interest rather than proposing a commercial transaction. Most people recognize

# CAN WE REALLY MAKE THE UNDERAGE SMOKING PROBLEM SMALLER BY MAKING THE FEDERAL BUREAUCRACY BIGGER?

The President's new anti-smoking proposal is intended to reduce underage smoking. But in the process, it will balloon the Federal bureaucracy, which will gain unprecedented control over virtually every aspect of the tobacco industry.

Americans have had enough of rampant Government regulation. They've had enough of seeing their taxpayer dollars spent on measures that, either directly or indirectly, restrict the rights of adults to make decisions for themselves.

We all agree we must do something to keep cigarettes out of the hands of children under the age of eighteen. But the answer isn't more bureaucracy. A proven solution is to teach young people how to resist peer pressure and to enforce the existing laws in 50 states denying children access to cigarettes.

This message is brought to you in the interest of an informed debate by the R.J. Reynolds Tobacco Company. To recieve a free 12-page brochure and Youth Education Kit, call 1-800-366-8441.

Figure 15. "Can we really make the underage smoking problem smaller by making the federal bureaucracy bigger?" (*Source: New York Times*, September 26, 1995, A17.)

the first advertorial as political speech because the industry is expressing its viewpoint on a matter of public policy. The second advertisement may be regarded as morally reprehensible because the industry seems to intentionally twist scientific facts. However, would it be a mistake to suppress statements that cast doubt on scientific orthodoxies of the day? Are scientific "truths" so stable and certain?

Once the Supreme Court finds that a message is "commercial" in nature, it has to decide whether the government may suppress it to

# Of cigarettes and science.

This is the way science is supposed to work.

A scientist observes a certain set of facts. To explain these facts, the scientist comes up with a theory.

Then, to check the validity of the theory, the scientist performs an experiment. If the experiment yields positive results, and is duplicated by other scientists, then the theory is supported. If the experiment produces negative results, the theory is re-examined, modified or discarded.

But, to a scientist, both positive and negative results should be important. Because both produce valuable learning.

Now let's talk about cigarettes.

You probably know about research that links smoking to certain diseases. Coronary heart disease is one of them.

Much of this evidence consists of studies that show a statistical association between smoking and the disease.

But statistics themselves cannot explain *why* smoking and heart disease are associated. Thus, scientists have developed a theory: that heart disease is *caused* by smoking. Then they performed various experiments to check this theory.

We would like to tell you about one of the most important of these experiments.

## A little-known study

It was called the Multiple Risk Factor Intervention Trial (MR FIT).

In the words of the *Wall Street Journal,* it was "one of the largest medical experiments ever attempted." Funded by the Federal government, it cost $115,000,000 and took 10 years, ending in 1982.

The subjects were over 12,000 men who were thought to have a high risk of heart disease because of three risk factors that are statistically associated with this disease: smoking, high blood pressure and high cholesterol levels.

Half of the men received no special medical intervention. The other half received medical treatment that consistently reduced all three risk factors, compared with the first group.

It was assumed that the group with lower risk factors would, over time, suffer significantly fewer deaths from heart disease than the higher risk factor group.

But that is not the way it turned out.

After 10 years, there was no statistically significant difference between the two groups in the number of heart disease deaths.

## The theory persists

We at R.J. Reynolds do not claim this study proves that smoking doesn't cause heart disease. But we do wish to make a point.

Despite the results of MR FIT and other experiments like it, many scientists have not abandoned or modified their original theory, or re-examined its assumptions.

They continue to believe these factors cause heart disease. But it is important to label their belief accurately. It is an opinion. A judgment. But *not* scientific fact.

We believe in science. That is why we continue to provide funding for independent research into smoking and health.

But we do *not* believe there should be one set of scientific principles for the whole world, and a different set for experiments involving cigarettes. Science is science. Proof is proof. That is why the controversy over smoking and health remains an open one.

Figure 16. "Of cigarettes and science." (*Source: New York Times,* March 19, 1985, A26.)

achieve a public good. In 1980 the Court articulated a four-part test to determine the constitutional protection that should be afforded to commercial speech. The criteria laid down in *Central Hudson Gas & Electric Corp. v. Public Service Comm'n,* 447 U.S. 557, 566 (1980) (posted on the *Reader* web site), are still used by the Court today: "For commercial speech to come within [the First Amendment], it at least must concern lawful activity and not be misleading. Next, we ask whether the asserted governmental interest is substantial. If both inquiries yield positive answers, we must determine whether the regulation directly advances the governmental interest asserted, and whether it is not more extensive than is necessary to serve that interest."

In the years following *Central Hudson,* the Supreme Court took a permissive approach to government regulation of commercial speech. In 1986, for example, the Court upheld a ban on the advertising of casino gambling directed at residents of Puerto Rico. The Court said that Puerto Rico had a substantial state interest and a reasonable belief that advertising would increase casino gambling. *Posadas de Puerto Rico Ass'n v. Tourism Co. of Puerto Rico,* 478 U.S. 328 (1986).

Chief Justice Rehnquist in *Posadas* made an argument, now discredited, that the greater power to completely ban a product necessarily includes the lesser power to regulate advertising of that product: "It would surely . . . be a strange constitutional doctrine which would concede to the legislature the authority to totally ban a product or activity, but deny to the legislature the authority to forbid the stimulation of demand for the product or activity." 478 U.S. at 345–46. This "greater includes the lesser" theory would give public health authorities virtually plenary authority to suppress advertising of tobacco, alcoholic beverages, and gambling. However, is Justice Rehnquist correct in assuming that speech restrictions *are* the lesser included power? Arguably, product prohibitions on health or safety grounds would be less offensive to the Constitution than speech prohibitions.

The Supreme Court's permissive approach to regulation of commercial speech evolved into "close scrutiny" in the mid-1990s. In *Rubin v. Coors Brewing Co.,* 514 U.S. 476 (1995) (reproduced on the *Reader* web site), the Court insisted that government must have a clear and consistent policy when regulating commercial speech. The Court invalidated a federal law prohibiting manufacturers from displaying alcohol content on beer labels. *Accord,* Greater New Orleans Broadcasting Ass'n v. United States, 527 U.S. 173, 174 (1999) (Congress's policy on gambling, which proscribed private casino advertising but promoted gambling on certain Native American land and in state-run lotteries, was "so pierced by exemptions and inconsistency that the Government cannot hope to exonerate it").

In *44 Liquormart, Inc. v. Rhode Island,* the Court insisted further that the government affirmatively demonstrate a relationship between commercial speech regulation and the attainment of an important health objective. Justice Steven's plurality opinion emphasizes the "special dangers that attend complete bans on truthful, nonmisleading commercial speech." 517 U.S. 484, 502 (1996).

---

**44 Liquormart, Inc. v. Rhode Island***
*Supreme Court of the United States*
*Decided May 13, 1996*

Justice STEVENS delivered the opinion of the Court.

Last Term we held that a federal law abridging a brewer's right to provide the public with accurate information about the alcoholic content of malt beverages is unconstitutional. Rubin v. Coors Brewing Co., 514 U.S. 476, 491 (1995). We now hold that Rhode Island's statutory prohibition against advertisements that provide the public with accurate information about retail prices of alcoholic beverages is also invalid. Our holding rests on the conclusion that such an advertising ban is an abridgment of speech protected by the First Amendment.

In 1956, the Rhode Island Legislature enacted two separate prohibitions against advertising the retail price of alcoholic beverages. The first applies to vendors licensed in Rhode Island as well as to out-of-state manufacturers, wholesalers, and shippers. It prohibits them from "advertising in any manner whatsoever" the price of any alcoholic beverage offered for sale in the State; the only exception is for price tags or signs displayed with the merchandise within licensed premises and not visible from the street. The second statute applies to the Rhode Island news media. It contains a categorical prohibition against the

---

*517 U.S. 484 (1996).

publication or broadcast of any advertisements—even those referring to sales in other States—that "make reference to the price of any alcoholic beverages.". . . .

Advertising has been a part of our culture throughout our history. Even in colonial days, the public relied on "commercial speech" for vital information about the market. . . . In accord with the role that commercial messages have long played, the law has developed to ensure that advertising provides consumers with accurate information about the availability of goods and services. In the early years, the common law, and later, statutes, served the consumers' interest in the receipt of accurate information in the commercial market by prohibiting fraudulent and misleading advertising. It was not until the 1970's, however, that this Court held that the First Amendment protected the dissemination of truthful and nonmisleading commercial messages about lawful products and services.

In *Bigelow v. Virginia*, 421 U.S. 809 (1975), we held that it was error to assume that commercial speech was entitled to no First Amendment protection or that it was without value in the marketplace of ideas. The following Term in *Virginia Bd. of Pharmacy v. Virginia Citizens Consumer Council, Inc.*, 425 U.S. 748 (1976), we expanded on our holding in *Bigelow* and held that the State's blanket ban on advertising the price of prescription drugs violated the First Amendment.

*Virginia Bd. of Pharmacy* reflected the conclusion that the same interest that supports regulation of potentially misleading advertising, namely, the public's interest in receiving accurate commercial information, also supports an interpretation of the First Amendment that provides constitutional protection for the dissemination of accurate and nonmisleading commercial messages. . . . The opinion further explained that a State's paternalistic assumption that the public will use truthful, nonmisleading commercial information unwisely cannot justify a decision to suppress it. . . . On the basis of these principles, our early cases uniformly struck down several broadly based bans on truthful, nonmisleading commercial speech, each of which served ends unrelated to consumer protection. . . .

At the same time, our early cases recognized that the State may regulate some types of commercial advertising more freely than other forms of protected speech. Specifically, we explained that the State may require commercial messages to "appear in such a form, or include such additional information, warnings, and disclaimers, as are necessary to prevent its being deceptive," *Virginia Bd. of Pharmacy*, 425 U.S., at

772, and that it may restrict some forms of aggressive sales practices that have the potential to exert "undue influence" over consumers, see *Bates v. State Bar of Ariz.,* 433 U.S. 350, 366 (1977).

*Virginia Bd. of Pharmacy* attributed the State's authority to impose these regulations in part to certain "commonsense differences" that exist between commercial messages and other types of protected expression. Our opinion noted that the greater "objectivity" of commercial speech justifies affording the State more freedom to distinguish false commercial advertisements from true ones, and that the greater "hardiness" of commercial speech, inspired as it is by the profit motive, likely diminishes the chilling effect that may attend its regulation. . . .

In *Central Hudson Gas & Electric Corp. v. Public Service Comm'n,* 447 U.S. 557 (1980), we took stock of our developing commercial speech jurisprudence. In that case, we considered a regulation "completely" banning all promotional advertising by electric utilities. Our decision acknowledged the special features of commercial speech but identified the serious First Amendment concerns that attend blanket advertising prohibitions that do not protect consumers from commercial harms. . . .

As our review of the case law reveals, Rhode Island errs in concluding that all commercial speech regulations are subject to a similar form of constitutional review simply because they target a similar category of expression. The mere fact that messages propose commercial transactions does not in and of itself dictate the constitutional analysis that should apply to decisions to suppress them.

When a State regulates commercial messages to protect consumers from misleading, deceptive, or aggressive sales practices, or requires the disclosure of beneficial consumer information, the purpose of its regulation is consistent with the reasons for according constitutional protection to commercial speech and therefore justifies less than strict review. However, when a State entirely prohibits the dissemination of truthful, nonmisleading commercial messages for reasons unrelated to the preservation of a fair bargaining process, there is far less reason to depart from the rigorous review that the First Amendment generally demands. . . .

Our commercial speech cases have recognized the dangers that attend governmental attempts to single out certain messages for suppression. . . . The special dangers that attend complete bans on truthful, nonmisleading commercial speech cannot be explained away by appeals to the "commonsense distinctions" that exist between commercial and noncommercial speech. *Virginia Bd. of Pharmacy,* 425 U.S. at 771. Regulations that suppress the truth are no less troubling because they target objectively verifiable information, nor are they less effective because they aim at durable messages. As a result, neither the "greater objectivity" nor the "greater hardiness" of truthful, nonmisleading commercial speech justifies reviewing its complete suppression with added deference.

It is the State's interest in protecting consumers from "commercial harms" that provides "the typical reason why commercial speech can be subject to greater governmental regulation than noncommercial speech." Cincinnati v. Discovery Network, Inc., 507 U.S. 410, 426 (1993). . . . Precisely because bans against truthful, nonmisleading commercial speech rarely seek to protect consumers from either deception or overreaching, they usually rest solely on the offensive assumption that the public will respond "irrationally" to the truth. Linmark Assoc., Inc. v. Willingboro, 431 U.S. 85, 96 (1977). The First Amendment directs us to be especially skeptical of regulations that seek to keep people in the dark for what the government perceives to be their own good. That teaching applies equally to state attempts to deprive consumers of accurate information about their chosen products. . . .

[The Court finds that Rhode Island does not provide sufficient evidence correlating the advertising of alcohol prices with increases in alcohol consumption.]

The State also cannot satisfy the requirement that its restriction on speech be no more extensive than necessary. It is perfectly obvious that alternative forms of regulation that would not involve any restriction on speech would be more likely to achieve the State's goal of promoting temperance. . . .

As a result, even under the less than strict standard that generally applies in commercial speech cases, the State has failed to establish a "reasonable fit" between its abridgment of speech and its temperance goal. Board of Trustees of State Univ. of N.Y. v. Fox, 492 U.S. 469, 480 (1989). . . . It necessarily follows that the price advertising ban cannot survive the more stringent constitutional review that *Central Hudson* itself concluded was appropriate for the complete suppression of truthful, nonmisleading commercial speech.

The State responds by arguing that it merely exercised appropriate "legislative judgment" in determining that a price advertising ban would best promote temperance. Relying on the *Central Hudson* analysis set forth in *Posadas* . . . Rhode Island first argues that, be-cause expert opinions as to the effectiveness of the price advertising ban "go both ways,". . . the ban constituted a "reasonable choice" by the legislature. The State next contends that precedent requires us to give particular deference to that legislative choice because the State could, if it chose, ban the sale of alcoholic beverages outright. Finally, the State argues that deference is appropriate because alcoholic bever-ages are so-called "vice" products. . . .

The State's first argument fails to justify the speech prohibition at issue. Our commercial speech cases recognize some room for the exer-cise of legislative judgment. However, Rhode Island errs in concluding that . . . *Posadas* establish the degree of deference that its decision to impose a price advertising ban warrants. . . .

[In] *Posadas* . . . a five-Member majority held that, under the *Cen-tral Hudson* test, it was "up to the legislature" to choose to reduce gam-bling by suppressing in-state casino advertising rather than engaging in educational speech. Rhode Island argues that this logic demonstrates the constitutionality of its own decision to ban price advertising in lieu of raising taxes or employing some other less speech-restrictive means of promoting temperance.

The reasoning in *Posadas* does support the State's argument, but, on re-flection, we are now persuaded that *Posadas* erroneously performed the First Amendment analysis. The casino advertising ban was designed to keep truthful, nonmisleading speech from members of the public for fear that they would be more likely to gamble if they received it. As a result, the advertising ban served to shield the State's antigambling policy from the public scrutiny that more direct, nonspeech regulation would draw. Given our longstanding hostility to commercial speech regulation of this type, *Posadas* clearly erred in concluding that it was "up to the legisla-ture" to choose suppression over a less speech-restrictive policy. . . . In-stead, in keeping with our prior holdings, we conclude that a state legis-lature does not have the broad discretion to suppress truthful, nonmisleading information for paternalistic purposes that the *Posadas* majority was willing to tolerate. As we explained in *Virginia Bd. of Phar-macy,* "[i]t is precisely this kind of choice, between the dangers of sup-pressing information, and the dangers of its misuse if it is freely available, that the First Amendment makes for us." 425 U.S. at 770.

We also cannot accept the State's second contention, which is premised entirely on the "greater-includes-the-lesser" reasoning endorsed toward the end of the majority's opinion in *Posadas*. There, the majority stated that "the greater power to completely ban casino gambling necessarily includes the lesser power to ban advertising of casino gambling." 478 U.S. at 345–46. It went on to state that "because the government could have enacted a wholesale prohibition of [casino gambling] it is permissible for the government to take the less intrusive step of allowing the conduct, but reducing the demand through restrictions on advertising." *Id.* at 346. . . . On the basis of these statements, the State reasons that its undisputed authority to ban alcoholic beverages must include the power to restrict advertisements offering them for sale. . . .

Although we do not dispute the proposition that greater powers include lesser ones, we fail to see how that syllogism requires the conclusion that the State's power to regulate commercial activity is "greater" than its power to ban truthful, nonmisleading commercial speech. Contrary to the assumption made in *Posadas*, we think it quite clear that banning speech may sometimes prove far more intrusive than banning conduct. As a venerable proverb teaches, it may prove more injurious to prevent people from teaching others how to fish than to prevent fish from being sold. . . . In short, we reject the assumption that words are necessarily less vital to freedom than actions, or that logic somehow proves that the power to prohibit an activity is necessarily "greater" than the power to suppress speech about it. . . .

Thus, just as it is perfectly clear that Rhode Island could not ban all obscene liquor ads except those that advocated temperance, we think it equally clear that its power to ban the sale of liquor entirely does not include a power to censor all advertisements that contain accurate and nonmisleading information about the price of the product. As the entire Court apparently now agrees, the statements in the *Posadas* opinion on which Rhode Island relies are no longer persuasive.

Finally, we find unpersuasive the State's contention that, under *Posadas*, the price advertising ban should be upheld because it targets commercial speech that pertains to a "vice" activity. . . . [T]he scope of any "vice" exception to the protection afforded by the First Amendment would be difficult, if not impossible, to define. Almost any product that poses some threat to public health or public morals might reasonably be characterized by a state legislature as relating to "vice activity." Such characterization, however, is anomalous when applied to products such as alcoholic beverages, lottery tickets, or playing cards, that may be lawfully purchased on the open market. The recognition of such an exception would also have the unfortunate consequence of either allowing state legislatures to justify censorship by the simple expedient of placing the "vice" label on selected lawful activities, or requiring the federal courts to establish a federal common law of vice. For these reasons, a "vice" label that is unaccompanied by a corresponding prohibition against the commercial behavior at issue fails to provide a principled justification for the regulation of commercial speech about that activity. . . .

Because Rhode Island has failed to carry its heavy burden of justifying its complete ban on price advertising, we conclude that R.I. GEN. LAWS §§ 3-8-7 and 3-8-8.1 (1989), as well as Regulation 32 of the Rhode Island Liquor Control Administration, abridge speech in violation of the First Amendment as made applicable to the States by the Due Process Clause of the Fourteenth Amendment. The judgment of the Court of Appeals is therefore reversed.

---

\*      \*      \*      \*      \*

None of the opinions in *44 Liquormart* garnered a majority of the Court. Justice Stevens's plurality opinion argued that the government must provide scientific evidence demonstrating that the advertising regulation would significantly reduce demand for a hazardous product or service. However, Justice O'Connor, writing for four members of the Court, pointedly declined to adopt Justice Stevens's approach. In *Greater New Orleans Broadcasting*, 527 U.S. at 189, the Court said it was not necessary on the facts of the case to resolve the dispute within the Court about the need for the state to produce evidence.

The Supreme Court continued its more demanding inquiry of the regulation of commercial speech in 2001. In *Rubin, 44 Liquormart*, and *Greater New Orleans Broadcasting*, the Court signaled that it will not tolerate restrictions on truthful information that consumers wish to know. This was the context in which the Supreme Court reviewed Massachusetts regulations that prohibited advertising of tobacco products within 1,000 feet of a public playground or school, either outdoors or at the point of sale below five feet from the floor of a retail establishment. The Court held that these regulations, as they apply to cigarettes, were preempted by the Federal Cigarette Labeling and Advertising Act (FCLAA) (see chapter 6). Consequently, the Court had no need to examine whether the cigarette regulations violated the First Amendment. Smokeless tobacco and cigars, however, are outside the FCLAA's scope, setting the stage for a major First Amendment ruling on tobacco advertising.

## Lorillard Tobacco Co. v. Reilly*
*Supreme Court of the United States*
*Decided June 28, 2001*

Justice O'CONNOR delivered the opinion of the Court.

[In January 1999 the attorney general of Massachusetts promulgated comprehensive regulations governing the advertising and sale of cigarettes, smokeless tobacco, and cigars. Petitioners, a group of cigarette, smokeless tobacco, and cigar manufacturers and retailers, filed suit in federal district court claiming that the regulations violate the First Amendment. The smokeless tobacco and cigar petitioners raise First Amendment challenges to the State's outdoor and point-of-sale advertising regulations. In addition, petitioners claim that certain sales practice regulations for tobacco products violate the First Amendment.]

Petitioners urge us to reject the *Central Hudson* analysis and apply strict scrutiny. . . . Admittedly, several Members of the Court have expressed doubts about the *Central Hudson* analysis and whether it should apply in particular cases. But here, as in *Greater New Orleans,* we see "no need to break new ground. *Central Hudson,* as applied in our more recent commercial speech cases, provides an adequate basis for decision." 527 U.S. 173, 184 (1999).

Only the last two steps of *Central Hudson*'s four-part analysis are at issue here. The Attorney General has assumed for purposes of summary judgment that petitioners' speech is entitled to First Amendment protection. With respect to the second step, none of the petitioners contests the importance of the State's interest in preventing the use of tobacco products by minors.

[The Court first analyzes smokeless tobacco and cigar petitioners' challenge to the State's outdoor advertising regulations.] The outdoor advertising regulations prohibit smokeless tobacco or cigar advertising within a 1,000-foot radius of a school or playground. . . . The smokeless tobacco and cigar petitioners contend that the Attorney General's regulations do not satisfy *Central Hudson*'s third step [which requires that the regulation directly advance the governmental interest asserted]. They maintain that although the Attorney General may have identified a problem with underage cigarette smoking, he has not identified an

---

*121 S. Ct 2404 (2001).

equally severe problem with respect to underage use of smokeless tobacco or cigars. . . . The cigar petitioners catalogue a list of differences
between cigars and other tobacco products, including the characteristics of the products and marketing strategies. The petitioners finally
contend that the Attorney General cannot prove that advertising has a
causal link to tobacco use such that limiting advertising will materially
alleviate any problem of underage use of their products.

In previous cases, we have acknowledged the theory that product advertising stimulates demand for products, while suppressed advertising
may have the opposite effect. The Attorney General cites numerous
studies to support this theory in the case of tobacco products. [He] relies in part on evidence gathered by the Food and Drug Administration
(FDA) in its attempt to regulate the advertising of cigarettes and smokeless tobacco. [Editor's note: See chapter 8 for more on the FDA's efforts.] . . . In its rulemaking proceeding, the FDA considered several
studies of tobacco advertising and trends in the use of various tobacco
products. The Surgeon General's report (1994) and the Institute of
Medicine's report (1994) found that "there is sufficient evidence to
conclude that advertising and labeling play a significant and important
contributory role in a young person's decision to use cigarettes or
smokeless tobacco products." 60 Fed. Reg. 41,332 (1995). . . .

The FDA also made specific findings with respect to smokeless tobacco. The FDA concluded that "the recent and very large increase in
the use of smokeless tobacco products by young people and the addictive nature of these products has persuaded the agency that these products must be included in any regulatory approach that is designed to
help prevent future generations of young people from becoming ad-
dicted to nicotine-containing tobacco products." *Id.* at 41,318 . . . Researchers tracked a dramatic shift in patterns of smokeless tobacco use
from older to younger users over the past 30 years. In particular, the
smokeless tobacco industry boosted sales tenfold in the 1970s and
1980s by targeting young males. Another study documented the targeting of youth through smokeless tobacco sales and advertising techniques.

The Attorney General [also] presents . . . evidence with respect to cigars. . . . The National Cancer Institute (1998) concluded that the rate of
cigar use by minors is increasing and that, in some States, the cigar use
rates are higher than the smokeless tobacco use rates for minors. In its
Report to Congress, the FTC (1999, 9) concluded that "substantial numbers of adolescents are trying cigars." Studies have also demonstrated a

link between advertising and demand for cigars. After Congress recognized the power of images in advertising and banned cigarette advertising in electronic media, television advertising of small cigars "increased dramatically in 1972 and 1973," "filled the void left by cigarette advertisers," and "sales . . . soared" (National Cancer Institute 1998, 24). . . . In the 1990s, cigar advertising campaigns triggered a boost in sales.

Our review of the record reveals that the Attorney General has provided ample documentation of the problem with underage use of smokeless tobacco and cigars. In addition, we disagree with petitioners' claim that there is no evidence that preventing targeted campaigns and limiting youth exposure to advertising will decrease underage use of smokeless tobacco and cigars. On this record and in the posture of summary judgment, we are unable to conclude that the Attorney General's decision to regulate advertising of smokeless tobacco and cigars in an effort to combat the use of tobacco products by minors was based on mere "speculation [and] conjecture." Edenfield v. Fane, 507 U.S. 761, 770 (1993).

Whatever the strength of the Attorney General's evidence to justify the outdoor advertising regulations, however, we conclude that the regulations do not satisfy the fourth step of the *Central Hudson* analysis. The final step of the *Central Hudson* analysis requires . . . a reasonable fit between the means and ends of the regulatory scheme. The Attorney General's regulations do not meet this standard. The broad sweep of the regulations indicates that the Attorney General did not "carefully calculate the costs and benefits associated with the burden on speech imposed" by the regulations. Cincinnati v. Discovery Network, Inc., 507 U.S. 410, 417 (1993). . . .

In the District Court, petitioners maintained that this prohibition would prevent advertising in 87% to 91% of Boston, Worcester, and Springfield, Massachusetts. The 87% to 91% figure appears to include not only the effect of the regulations, but also the limitations imposed by other generally applicable zoning restrictions. The Attorney General disputed petitioners' figures but "conceded that the reach of the regulations is substantial." Consolidated Cigar Corp. v. Reilly, 218 F.3d 30, 50 (2000). . . .

The substantial geographical reach of the Attorney General's outdoor advertising regulations is compounded by other factors. "Outdoor" advertising includes not only advertising located outside an establishment, but also advertising inside a store if that advertising is visible from outside the store. The regulations restrict advertisements of any size and the term advertisement also includes oral statements.

In some geographical areas, these regulations would constitute nearly a complete ban on the communication of truthful information about smokeless tobacco and cigars to adult consumers. The breadth and scope of the regulations, and the process by which the Attorney General adopted the regulations, do not demonstrate a careful calculation of the speech interests involved.

First, the Attorney General did not seem to consider the impact of the 1,000-foot restriction on commercial speech in major metropolitan areas. The Attorney General apparently selected the 1,000-foot distance based on the FDA's decision to impose an identical 1,000-foot restriction when it attempted to regulate cigarette and smokeless tobacco advertising. But the FDA's 1,000-foot regulation was not an adequate basis for the Attorney General to tailor the Massachusetts regulations. The degree to which speech is suppressed—or alternative avenues for speech remain available—under a particular regulatory scheme tends to be case specific. And a case specific analysis makes sense, for although a State or locality may have common interests and concerns about underage smoking and the effects of tobacco advertisements, the impact of a restriction on speech will undoubtedly vary from place to place. The FDA's regulations would have had widely disparate effects nationwide. Even in Massachusetts, the effect of the Attorney General's speech regulations will vary based on whether a locale is rural, suburban, or urban. The uniformly broad sweep of the geographical limitation demonstrates a lack of tailoring.

In addition, the range of communications restricted seems unduly broad. For instance, it is not clear from the regulatory scheme why a ban on oral communications is necessary to further the State's interest. Apparently that restriction means that a retailer is unable to answer inquiries about its tobacco products if that communication occurs outdoors. Similarly, a ban on all signs of any size seems ill suited to target the problem of highly visible billboards, as opposed to smaller signs. To the extent that studies have identified particular advertising and promotion practices that appeal to youth, tailoring would involve targeting those practices while permitting others. As crafted, the regulations make no distinction among practices on this basis. . . .

The State's interest in preventing underage tobacco use is substantial, and even compelling, but it is no less true that the sale and use of tobacco products by adults is a legal activity. We must consider that tobacco retailers and manufacturers have an interest in conveying truthful information about their products to adults, and adults have a corresponding interest in receiving truthful information about tobacco products. . . .

368 Tensions and Recurring Themes

In some instances, Massachusetts' outdoor advertising regulations would impose particularly onerous burdens on speech. For example, we disagree with the Court of Appeals' conclusion that because cigar manufacturers and retailers conduct a limited amount of advertising in comparison to other tobacco products, "the relative lack of cigar advertising also means that the burden imposed on cigar advertisers is correspondingly small." *Consolidated Cigar Corp.,* 218 F.3d at 49. If some retailers have relatively small advertising budgets, and use few avenues of communication, then the Attorney General's outdoor advertising regulations potentially place a greater, not lesser, burden on those retailers' speech. Furthermore, to the extent that cigar products and cigar advertising differ from that of other tobacco products, that difference should inform the inquiry into what speech restrictions are necessary.

In addition, a retailer in Massachusetts may have no means of communicating to passersby on the street that it sells tobacco products because alternative forms of advertisement, like newspapers, do not allow that retailer to propose an instant transaction in the way that onsite advertising does. The ban on any indoor advertising that is visible from the outside also presents problems in establishments like convenience stores, which have unique security concerns that counsel in favor of full visibility of the store from the outside. It is these sorts of considerations that the Attorney General failed to incorporate into the regulatory scheme.

We conclude that the Attorney General has failed to show that the outdoor advertising regulations for smokeless tobacco and cigars are not more extensive than necessary to advance the State's substantial interest in preventing underage tobacco use. . . .

Massachusetts has also restricted indoor, point-of-sale advertising for smokeless tobacco and cigars. Advertising cannot be "placed lower than five feet from the floor of any retail establishment which is located within a one thousand foot radius of" any school or playground. 940 Code of Mass. Regs. §§ 21.04(5)(b), 22.06(5)(b) (2000). . . .

We conclude that the point-of-sale advertising regulations fail both the third and fourth steps of the *Central Hudson* analysis. . . . [T]he State's goal is to prevent minors from using tobacco products and to curb demand for that activity by limiting youth exposure to advertising. The 5-foot rule does not seem to advance that goal. Not all children are less than 5 feet tall, and those who are certainly have the ability to look up and take in their surroundings. . . . Massachusetts may wish to target tobacco advertisements and displays that entice children, much like floor-level candy displays in a convenience store, but the blanket height restriction does not constitute a reasonable fit with that goal. . . .

The Attorney General also promulgated a number of regulations that restrict sales practices by cigarette, smokeless tobacco, and cigar manufacturers and retailers. Among other restrictions, the regulations bar the use of self-service displays and require that tobacco products be placed out of the reach of all consumers in a location accessible only to salespersons. . . . As we read the regulations, they basically require tobacco retailers to place tobacco products behind counters and require customers to have contact with a salesperson before they are able to handle a tobacco product.

The cigarette and smokeless tobacco petitioners contend that "the same First Amendment principles that require invalidation of the outdoor and indoor advertising restrictions require invalidation of the display regulations at issue in this case." Brief for Petitioners Lorillard Tobacco Co. et al. in No. 00-596, at 46, n. 7. . . . We reject these contentions. Assuming that petitioners have a cognizable speech interest in a particular means of displaying their products, these regulations withstand First Amendment scrutiny.

Massachusetts' sales practices provisions regulate conduct that may have a communicative component, but Massachusetts seeks to regulate the placement of tobacco products for reasons unrelated to the communication of ideas. [According to *United States v. O'Brien,* 391 U.S. 367 (1968), non–content-based government regulation of communicative conduct is valid if (1) it furthers an important government interest, (2) it is unrelated to the suppression of free expression, and (3) the incidental restriction is no greater than essential to the furtherance of that interest.] . . .

Unattended displays of tobacco products present an opportunity for access without the proper age verification required by law. Thus, the State prohibits self-service and other displays that would allow an individual to obtain tobacco products without direct contact with a salesperson. It is clear that the regulations leave open ample channels of communication. The regulations do not significantly impede adult access to tobacco products. Moreover, retailers have other means of exercising any cognizable speech interest in the presentation of their products. We presume that vendors may place empty tobacco packaging on open display, and display actual tobacco products so long as that display is only accessible to sales personnel. As for cigars, there is no indication in the regulations that a customer is unable to examine a cigar prior to purchase, so long as that examination takes place through a salesperson. . . .

We conclude that the sales practices regulations withstand First Amendment scrutiny. The means chosen by the State are narrowly tailored to prevent access to tobacco products by minors, are unrelated to expression, and leave open alternative avenues for vendors to convey information about products and for would-be customers to inspect products before purchase.

---

## IV. COMPELLED COMMERCIAL SPEECH

Public health agencies are not concerned merely with what businesses say, but also with what they fail to say. If industry does not provide accurate explanations of product content, instructions for safe use, and potential hazards, it places consumers at risk. Consequently, the government compels a great deal of speech for public health or consumer protection purposes. First, government requires businesses to *label* their products by specifying the content or ingredients (e.g., foods and cosmetics), the potential adverse effects (e.g., pharmaceuticals and vaccines), and the hazards (e.g., "warnings" on packages of cigarettes, alcoholic beverages, or pesticides). Second, government provides a *right to know* for consumers (e.g., performance of managed care organizations), workers (e.g., health and safety risks), and the public (e.g., hazardous chemicals in drinking water). Third, government mandates *counteradvertising* whereby industry or the media must provide health education as a counterbalance to advertisements of hazardous products (e.g., forced dissemination of antidrinking or antismoking messages). (For a discussion of government-compelled health and safety disclosures, see Graham [2000] and Sage [1999].)

Government health and safety disclosure laws require businesses to provide more consumer information. The First Amendment, however, bestows a right not only to speak freely, but also to refrain from speaking at all. United States v. United Foods, Inc., 121 S. Ct. 2334 (2001). The compelled commercial speech doctrine protects individuals from being forced to enunciate views that are opposed to their conscience or beliefs. In *44 Liquormart*, we saw that the Court fully protects the right to express truthful, nonmisleading commercial messages about lawful products. It is likely that the Court would support a corollary principle— that government has constitutional power to compel businesses to make accurate, nondeceptive disclosures for health, safety, or consumer protection purposes. On this theory, would government labeling rules regarding content or ingredients, approved uses, potential adverse effects, or hazard warnings be constitutionally permissible? What if the substance to be disclosed is not known to be a health risk? Consider the controversial subject of mandatory disclosure of Bovine Growth Hormone in dairy products (Greenberg and Graham 2000).

---

### International Dairy Foods Association v. Amestoy*
*Court of Appeals for the Second Circuit*
*Decided August 8, 1996*

Circuit Judge ALTIMARI delivered the opinion of the court.

Plaintiffs-appellants [a group of dairy manufacturers] appeal from a decision of the district court denying their motion for a preliminary injunction. The dairy manufacturers challenged the constitutionality of VT. STAT. ANN. tit. 6, § 2754(c), which requires dairy manufacturers to identify products which were, or might have been, derived from dairy cows treated with a synthetic growth hormone used to increase milk production. The dairy manufacturers alleged that the statute violate[s] the . . . Constitution's First Amendment. . . . Because we find that the district court abused its discretion in failing to grant preliminary injunctive relief to the dairy manufacturers on First Amendment grounds, we reverse and remand.

### BACKGROUND

In 1993, the federal Food and Drug Administration (FDA) approved the use of recombinant Bovine Somatotropin (rBST) (also known as recombinant Bovine Growth Hormone (rGBH)), a synthetic growth hormone that increases milk production by cows. It is undisputed that the dairy products derived from herds treated with rBST are indistinguishable from products derived from untreated herds; consequently, the FDA declined to require the labeling of products derived from cows receiving the supplemental hormone.

In April 1994, defendant-appellee the State of Vermont (Vermont) enacted a statute requiring that "[i]f rBST has been used in the production

---

*92 F.3d 67 (2d Cir. 1996).

of milk or a milk product for retail sale in this state, the retail milk or milk product shall be labeled as such." *Id.* at § 2754(c). Vermont's Commissioner of Agriculture (Commissioner) subsequently promulgated regulations giving those dairy manufacturers who use rBST four labeling options. . . .

## DISCUSSION

### Irreparable Harm

Focusing principally on the economic impact of the labeling regulation, the district court found that appellants had not demonstrated irreparable harm to any right protected by the First Amendment. We disagree. . . . Because the statute at issue requires appellants to make an involuntary statement whenever they offer their products for sale, we find that the statute causes the dairy manufacturers irreparable harm. . . . to the[ir] constitutional right *not* to speak. . . .

### Likelihood of Success on the Merits

It is not enough for appellants to show, as they have, that they were irreparably harmed by the statute; because the dairy manufacturers challenge government action taken in the public interest, they must also show a likelihood of success on the merits. We find that such success is likely. In *Central Hudson,* the Supreme Court articulated a four-part analysis for determining whether a government restriction on commercial speech is permissible. We need not address the controversy concerning the nature of the speech in question—commercial or political—because we find that Vermont fails to meet the less stringent constitutional requirements applicable to compelled commercial speech. Under *Central Hudson,* we must determine: (1) whether the expression concerns lawful activity and is not misleading; (2) whether the government's interest is substantial; (3) whether the labeling law directly serves the asserted interest; and (4) whether the labeling law is no more extensive than necessary. . . .

In our view, Vermont has failed to establish the second prong of the *Central Hudson* test, namely that its interest is substantial. In making this determination, we rely only upon those interests set forth by Vermont before the district court. . . . As the district court made clear, Vermont "does not claim that health or safety concerns prompted the passage of the Vermont Labeling Law," but instead defends the statute on the basis of "strong consumer interest and the public's 'right to know.' . . ." 898 F.

Supp. 246, 249 (D. Vt. 1995). These interests are insufficient to justify compromising protected constitutional rights.

Vermont's failure to defend its constitutional intrusion on the ground that it negatively impacts public health is easily understood. After exhaustive studies, the FDA has "concluded that rBST has no appreciable effect on the composition of milk produced by treated cows, and that there are no human safety or health concerns associated with food products derived from cows treated with rBST." *Id.* at 248. Because bovine somatotropin ("BST") appears naturally in cows, and because there are no BST receptors in a cow's mammary glands, only trace amounts of BST can be detected in milk, whether or not the cows received the supplement. Moreover, it is undisputed that neither consumers nor scientists can distinguish rBST-derived milk from milk produced by an untreated cow. Indeed, the already extensive record in this case contains no scientific evidence from which an objective observer could conclude that rBST has any impact at all on dairy products. It is thus plain that Vermont could not justify the statute on the basis of "real" harms.

We do not doubt that Vermont's asserted interest, the demand of its citizenry for such information, is genuine; reluctantly, however, we conclude that it is inadequate. We are aware of no case in which consumer interest alone was sufficient to justify requiring a product's manufacturers to publish the functional equivalent of a warning about a production method that has no discernible impact on a final product. . . .

Although the Court is sympathetic to the Vermont consumers who wish to know which products may derive from rBST-treated herds, their desire is insufficient to permit Vermont to compel the dairy manufacturers to speak against their will. Were consumer interest alone sufficient, there is no end to the information that states could require manufacturers to disclose about their production methods. . . . Because appellants have demonstrated both irreparable harm and a likelihood of success on the merits, the judgment of the district court is reversed, and the case is remanded for entry of an appropriate injunction.

LEVAL, Circuit Judge, dissenting:

The policy of the First Amendment, in its application to commercial speech, is to favor the flow of accurate, relevant information. The majority's invocation of the First Amendment to invalidate a state law requiring disclosure of information consumers reasonably desire stands the Amendment on its ear. In my view, the district court correctly found that plaintiffs were unlikely to succeed in proving Vermont's law unconstitutional. . . .

[T]he majority oddly concludes that Vermont's sole interest in requiring disclosure of rBST use is to gratify "consumer curiosity," and that this alone "is not a strong enough state interest to sustain the compulsion of even an accurate factual statement." Maj. Op. at 12. The majority seeks to justify its conclusion in three ways.

First, it simply disregards the evidence of Vermont's true interests and the district court's findings recognizing those interests. Nowhere does the majority opinion discuss or even mention the evidence or findings regarding the people of Vermont's concerns about human health, cow health, biotechnology, and the survival of small dairy farms.

Second, the majority distorts the meaning of the district court opinion. It relies substantially on Judge Murtha's statement that Vermont "does not claim that health or safety concerns prompted the passage of the Vermont Labeling Law," but "bases its justification . . . on strong consumer interest and the public's 'right to know.'" 898 F. Supp. at 249; Maj. Op. at 10. The majority takes this passage out of context. . . . In the light of the district judge's further explicit findings, it is clear that his statement could not mean what the majority concludes. More likely, what Judge Murtha meant was that Vermont does not claim to *know* whether rBST is harmful. . . .

Third, the majority suggests that, because the FDA has not found health risks in this new procedure, health worries could not be considered "real" or "cognizable." Maj. Op. at 11–12. . . . I find this proposition alarming and dangerous; at the very least, it is extraordinarily unrealistic. Genetic and biotechnological manipulation of basic food products is new and controversial. Although I have no reason to doubt that the FDA's studies of rBST have been thorough, they could not cover *long-term* effects of rBST on humans. Furthermore, there are many possible reasons why a government agency might fail to find real health risks, including inadequate time and budget for testing, insufficient advancement of scientific techniques, insufficiently large sampling populations, pressures from industry, and simple human error. To suggest that a government agency's failure to find a health risk in a short-term study of a new genetic technology should bar a state from requiring simple disclosure of the use of that technology where its citizens are concerned about such health risks would be unreasonable and dangerous. . . .

In short, the majority has no valid basis for its conclusion that Vermont's regulation advances no interest other than the gratification of consumer curiosity, and involves neither health concerns nor other substantial interests. . . .

Notwithstanding their self-righteous references to free expression, the true objective of the milk producers is concealment. . . . The question is simply whether the First Amendment prohibits government from requiring disclosure of truthful relevant information to consumers. . . . The milk producers' invocation of the First Amendment for the purpose of concealing their use of rBST in milk production is entitled to scant recognition. They invoke the Amendment's protection to accomplish exactly what the Amendment opposes. And the majority's ruling deprives Vermont of the right to protect its consumers by requiring truthful disclosure on a subject of legitimate public concern. . . .

---

\*     \*     \*     \*     \*

The Second Circuit Court of Appeals appears to argue that the power to compel truthful speech is constitutionally permissible only if government has a strong public health interest; satisfying consumer curiosity is an insufficient governmental objective. Suppose consumers feel strongly that they do not wish to buy genetically modified foods, but they cannot produce conclusive evidence of adverse effects of genetically modified foods on human health or the environment. Should government have the power to compel manufacturers or grocery stores to disclose which foods have been genetically modified?

## CONCLUSION

This chapter discussed government attempts to regulate by controlling the informational environment—government speech, restraints on commercial speech, and mandatory disclosures. The following chapters discuss more direct public health regulation. Chapter 12 explores the use of government power to prevent infectious diseases through compulsory immunization, screening, and medical treatment.

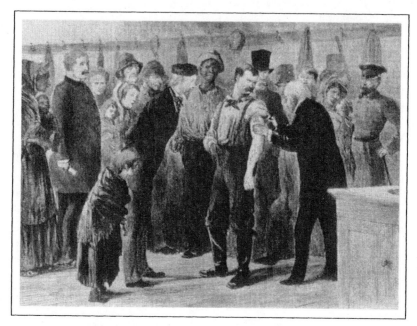

This drawing, entitled "Vaccinating the Poor," depicts the once-common practice involving mass vaccination, probably for smallpox, of indigent persons in the community.

# TWELVE

# Biological Interventions to Control Infectious Disease

*Immunization, Screening, and Treatment*

This chapter and the next examine the most ancient and enduring threats to health in the population—infectious diseases. The effects of epidemics in society are as destructive as those of war (Garrett 2000; Levy and Sidel 1997). For example, the estimated 45 million deaths from AIDS in the world exceed the combatants killed in World War I, World War II, Korea, and Vietnam combined (Gellman 2000a). Not surprisingly, the United States classified HIV/AIDS as a national security threat in 2000, reasoning that it would result in destabilization of strategic regions such as Africa and Asia (Gellman 2000b).

For most of history, society's only response to epidemics has been crude separation of persons with disease. But in more recent history, science has developed the biological means to help prevent, detect, and intervene in epidemics. (For a review of the major trends in dealing with infectious diseases during the twentieth century, see CDC [1999a], posted on the *Reader* web site.) The three major biological approaches are vaccination to prevent outbreaks, screening to identify persons who are infectious, and treatment to alleviate symptoms and reduce infectiousness. The readings in this chapter discuss these biological approaches; the readings in chapter 13 discuss deprivations of liberty as a method of disease control— civil confinement (isolation and quarantine) and criminal punishment.

The value of biological approaches to infectious diseases cannot be exaggerated. Vaccination programs, for example, have eradicated (e.g., smallpox) or significantly reduced the incidence of diseases (e.g., polio) that have decimated populations (John 2000). Antibiotics have been just as important as vaccinations, offering a means to medically treat a wide variety of infectious conditions and reduce contagiousness. Medical treatments for syphilis, tuberculosis (TB), and, more recently, HIV/AIDS have transformed our approach to these and other communicable diseases.

Despite the undoubted value of biological approaches, they are neither sufficient nor unambiguously beneficial. Social, economic, and environmental factors are just as important in the prevalence and control of contagious diseases. For example, René and Jean Dubois (1987) sought to demonstrate that improved sanitation, diet, and general economic and social conditions were instrumental in reducing the burden of TB in the mid-twentieth century. Other scholars have drawn attention to the importance of "ecological" factors such as the physical and social environment in controlling infectious diseases (see chapter 14). Overreliance on biological approaches can reduce the salience of social, behavioral, and economic interventions. Sometimes treatment is regarded as a "magic bullet," stifling other kinds of public health innovation (Brandt 1987).

Biological approaches, although often successful, have distinct limitations. Vaccinations can cause infection or other adverse events in previously healthy patients. For example, the swine flu vaccination program was discontinued in the mid-1970s because it was thought to be associated with Guillain-Barré syndrome (Dowdle 1997). Antibiotics can be prescribed or used in such inconsistent ways that pathogens become resistant. Resistance to medication is one of the most important problems facing medicine today (see chapter 14).

Biological approaches can also be intrusive. Vaccination, screening, or treatment imposed without consent invades personal autonomy and bodily integrity. As a result, some people oppose mandatory therapeutic interventions on grounds of conscience, principle, or religion. Even if treatments for diseases such as TB are beneficial and reduce transmission, individuals claim the freedom to make therapeutic decisions for themselves.

Finally, biological approaches pose social risks—invasions of privacy, stigma, and discrimination. For example, screening reveals intimate personal information that can be used to deny individuals employment or insurance. Additionally, when screening is targeted primarily against vulnerable or disfavored populations, it can appear unfair or raise important questions of equity and justice.

The readings in this chapter explore the multiple benefits and burdens of biological approaches. When health care or public health professionals act to prevent, identify, or treat an infectious disease, undoubtedly they can improve the health and well-being of individuals and populations. At the same time, however, biological approaches often reduce the resources, or political will, available for broader social, behavioral, and economic interventions. Biological approaches, moreover, can diminish individual freedoms and pose risks of privacy invasion and discrimination. These trade-offs—between therapeutic benefits and social risks—are discussed in this chapter's readings.

## I. COMPULSORY VACCINATION: IMMUNIZING THE POPULATION AGAINST DISEASE

Vaccinations are among the most cost-effective and widely used public health interventions (McDonnel and Askari 1997). For a discussion of the remarkable improvements in the population's health that are attributable to vaccination policy in the twentieth century, see CDC (1999b), posted on the *Reader* web site. The rate of complete immunization of school-age children in the United States (more than 95 percent) is as high or higher than in most other developed countries. Vaccination rates for preschool children are also improving (CDC 2001, 2000a). As a result, common childhood illnesses, such as measles, pertussis, and polio, which once accounted for a substantial proportion of child morbidity and mortality, have been substantially reduced (NVAC 1999).

All states, as a condition of school entry, require proof of vaccination against a number of diseases on the immunization schedule, such as diphtheria, measles, and rubella. (For a list of currently recommended vaccines, see ACIP [1999], updated at http://www.cdc.gov.) State statutes also often require schools to maintain immunization records and report information to health authorities (Gostin and Lazzarini 1995).

Although the exact provisions differ from state to state, all school immunization laws grant exemptions for children with medical contraindications to immunization. Thus, if a physician certifies that the child is susceptible to adverse effects from the vaccine, the child is exempt. Forty-eight states grant religious exemptions for persons who have sincere religious beliefs in opposition to immunization. (Only Mississippi and West Virginia compel children to accede to vaccination against the religious beliefs of their parents.) A minority of states also grant exemptions for parents who profess philosophical convictions in opposition to immunization. In practice, legal exemptions for vaccinations constitute only a small percentage of total school entrants. However, disease outbreaks in religious communities that have not been vaccinated do occur (Salmon et al. 1999; Novotny et al. 1988). Table 6 documents school vaccination

## TABLE 6
### SCHOOL IMMUNIZATION LAWS AMONG STATES

| State | Statutory Source(s) | DPT | MMR | Polio | Hib† | Hep B | Var | Religious Exemptions | Philosophical Exemptions |
|---|---|---|---|---|---|---|---|---|---|
| Alabama | Ala. Code § 16-30-1 | ✓ | ✓ | ✓ | | | | § 16-30-3 | N |
| Alaska | Alaska Stat. § 14.30.125 | ✓ | ✓ | ✓ | | | | § 14.07.125 | N |
| Arizona | Ariz. Rev. Stat. Ann. § 15-872 | ✓ | ✓ | ✓ | ✓ | ✓ | | § 15-873 | Y |
| Arkansas | Ark. Code Ann. § 6-18-702 | ✓ | ✓MR | ✓ | | | ✓ | § 6-18-702 | N |
| California | Cal. Health & Safety Code § 120325 | ✓ | ✓ | ✓ | | ✓ | ✓ | § 120365 | Y |
| Colorado | Colo. Rev. Stat. § 25-4-902 | ✓ | ✓ | ✓ | ✓ | ✓ | ✓ | § 25-4-903 | N |
| Connecticut | Conn. Gen. Stat. § 10-204a | ✓ | ✓ | ✓ | ✓ | ✓ | ✓ | § 10-204a | N |
| Delaware | Del. Code Ann. tit. 14, § 131 | ✓ | ✓ | ✓ | | ✓ | | § 14-131 | N |
| D.C. | D.C. Code Ann. § 31-501 | ✓ | ✓ | ✓ | ✓ | ✓ | | § 31-506 | N |
| Florida | Fla. Stat. Ann. § 232.032 | ✓ | ✓ | ✓ | ✓ | ✓ | ✓ | § 232.032 | N |
| Georgia | Ga. Code Ann. § 20-2-771 | ✓ | ✓ | ✓ | ✓ | ✓ | ✓ | § 20-2-771 | N |
| Hawaii | Haw. Rev. Stat. § 302A-1154 | ✓ | ✓ | ✓ | ✓ | ✓ | ✓ | § 302A-1156 | N |
| Idaho | Idaho Code § 39-4801 | ✓DT | ✓ | ✓ | ✓ | ✓ | | § 39-4802 | Y |
| Illinois | 105 Ill. Comp. Stat. § 5/27-8.1 | ✓ | ✓ | ✓ | ✓ | ✓ | | 410 ILCS § 315/2 | N |
| Indiana | Ind. Code Ann. § 20-8.1-7-9.5 | ✓ | ✓ | ✓ | | ✓ | | § 20-8.1-7-2 | Y |
| Iowa | Iowa Code Ann. § 139.9 | ✓ | ✓MR | ✓ | | | | § 139.9 | N |
| Kansas | Kan. Stat. Ann. § 72-5209 | ✓ | ✓ | ✓ | | | | § 72-5209 | N |
| Kentucky | Ky. Rev. Stat. Ann. § 214.034 | ✓ | ✓ | ✓ | ✓ | ✓ | ✓ | § 214.036 | N |
| Louisiana | La. Rev. Stat. Ann. § 17:170(A) | ✓ | ✓ | ✓ | | ✓ | | § 17:170(E) | Y |
| Maine | Me. Rev. Stat. Ann. tit. 20-A, § 6355 | ✓DT | ✓ | ✓ | | | | tit. 20-A, § 6355 | Y |

| State | Citation | | | | | | | Citation | |
|---|---|:-:|:-:|:-:|:-:|:-:|:-:|---|:-:|
| Maryland | MD. CODE ANN. EDUC. § 7-403 | ✓ | ✓ | | ✓ | ✓ | ✓ | § 7-403 | N |
| Massachusetts | MASS. GEN LAWS ch. 76, § 15 | ✓ | ✓ | | ✓ | ✓ | ✓ | ch. 76, § 15 | N |
| Michigan | MICH. COMP. LAWS ANN. § 333.9208 | ✓ | ✓ | | ✓ | ✓ | ✓ | § 333.9215 | Y |
| Minnesota | MINN. STAT. ANN. § 121A-15 | ✓ | ✓ | | ✓ | ✓ | | § 121A.15 | Y |
| Mississippi | MISS. CODE ANN. § 41-23-37 | ✓ | ✓ | | ✓ | ✓ | | N | N |
| Missouri | MO. REV. STAT. § 167.181 | ✓ | ✓ | | ✓ | | | § 167.181 | N |
| Montana | MONT. CODE ANN. § 20-5-403 | ✓ | ✓ | | ✓ | ✓ | | § 20-5-405 | N |
| Nebraska | NEB. REV. STAT. ANN. § 79-217 | ✓ | ✓ | | ✓ | ✓ | | § 79-220 | Y |
| Nevada | NEV. REV. STAT. § 392.435 | ✓ | ✓ | | ✓ | ✓ | | § 392.437 | N |
| New Hampshire | N.H. REV. STAT. ANN. § 141-C:20-a | ✓ | ✓ | | ✓ | ✓ | | § 141-C:20-c | N |
| New Jersey | N.J. STAT. ANN. § 26:1A-9 | ✓ | ✓ | | ✓ | ✓ | | § 26:1A-9 | N |
| New Mexico | N.M. STAT. ANN. § 24-5-1 | ✓[D] | ✓ | | ✓ | ✓ | ✓ | § 24-5-2dd | N |
| New York | N.Y. PUB. HEALTH LAW § 2164 | ✓ | ✓ | | ✓ | ✓ | | § 2164 | N |
| North Carolina | N.C. GEN. STAT. § 130A-155 | ✓ | ✓ | | ✓ | ✓ | | § 130A-157 | N |
| North Dakota | N.D. CENT. CODE § 23-07-17.1 | ✓ | ✓ | | ✓ | ✓ | ✓ | § 23-07-17.1 | Y |
| Ohio | OHIO REV. CODE ANN. § 3313.671 | ✓ | ✓ | | ✓ | ✓ | | § 3313.671 | Y |
| Oklahoma | OKLA. STAT. ANN. tit. 70, § 1210.191 | ✓ | ✓ | | ✓ | ✓ | ✓ | § 1210.192 | Y |
| Oregon | OR. REV. STAT. § 433.267 | ✓[DT] | ✓ | | ✓ | ✓ | | § 433.267 | N |
| Pennsylvania | 21 PA. CONS. STAT. ANN. § 13-1303a | ✓ | ✓ | | ✓ | ✓ | ✓ | § 13-1303a | N |
| Rhode Island | R.I. GEN. LAWS § 16-38-2 | ✓ | ✓ | | ✓ | ✓ | ✓ | § 16-38-2 | N |
| South Carolina | S.C. CODE ANN. § 44-29-180 | ✓ | ✓ | | ✓ | ✓ | ✓ | § 44-29-180 | N |
| South Dakota | S.D. CODIFIED LAWS § 13-28-7.1 | ✓ | ✓ | | ✓ | ✓ | ✓ | § 13-28-7.1 | N |
| Tennessee | TENN. CODE ANN. § 49-6-5001 | ✓ | ✓ | | ✓ | ✓ | | § 49-6-5001 | N |
| Texas | TEX. EDUC. CODE ANN. § 38.001 | ✓ | ✓ | | ✓ | ✓ | ✓ | § 38.001 | N |
| Utah | UTAH CODE ANN. § 53A-11-301 | ✓ | ✓ | | ✓ | ✓ | ✓ | § 53A-11-302 | N |

TABLE 6 (*continued*)

| State | Statutory Source(s) | DPT | MMR | Polio | Hib† | Hep B | Var | Religious Exemptions | Philosophical Exemptions |
|---|---|---|---|---|---|---|---|---|---|
| Vermont | Vt. Stat. Ann. tit. 18, § 1121 | ✓ | ✓ | ✓ | | ✓ | | § 1122 | Y |
| Virginia | Va. Code Ann. § 22.1-271.2 | ✓ | ✓ | ✓ | | ✓ | ✓ | § 22.1-271.2 | N |
| Washington | Wash. Rev. Code Ann. § 28A.210.080 | ✓ | ✓ | ✓ | | ✓ | | § 28A.210.080 | Y |
| West Virginia | W. Va. Code § 16-3-4 | ✓DT | ✓MR | ✓ | | | | N | N |
| Wisconsin | Wis. Stat. Ann. § 252.04 | ✓DT | ✓ | ✓ | | ✓ | | § 252.04 | Y |
| Wyoming | Wyo. Stat. Ann. § 21-4-309 | ✓ | ✓ | ✓ | | ✓ | ✓ | § 21-4-309 | N |

DPT: Diphtheria/pertussis/tetanus vaccine  
Hep B: Hepatitis B vaccine  
Polio: Poliomyelitis (OPV or IPV) vaccine  
MMR: Measles-mumps-rubella vaccine  
Hib: *Haemophilus influenzae* vaccine  
Var (varicella): Chicken pox vaccine  
†Hib vaccine is required only for children under five years of age.  
DTThese states allow children to enter or attend school if they have received the requisite doses of the Td (diphtheria-tetanus toxoid).  
DThese states allow children to enter or attend school if they have received the requisite doses of the diphtheria toxoid.  
MRThese states require measles and rubella vaccination, but not the mumps vaccine.

laws among states (as of July 2001) according to specific diseases, as well as exemptions for each state.

Despite its unquestionable importance in preventing infectious disease, compulsory immunization often provokes popular resistance. Some people object because they distrust scientists and health officials, fearing that vaccines lack effectiveness or induce injury; others object on grounds of religion or principle; and still others object because they perceive unwarranted governmental interference with autonomy and liberty.

In the following selection, Garrett Hardin, a professor of biology at the University of California–Santa Barbara, argues that individuals acting in their own interests will lead to a "tragedy of the commons." Thus, if each person is left free to pursue his or her own personal aspirations, the individual may benefit but the population will suffer. The solution, Hardin argues, is "mutual coercion mutually agreed upon" (i.e., coercion through democratic decision making). Hardin's argument is highly relevant to vaccination policy. It may be that a parent benefits if his or her child remains unvaccinated because of the risk of adverse effects. This assumes, however, that there is herd immunity in the population. If enough parents resist vaccination, the population loses herd immunity, resulting in a tragedy of the commons.

---

### The Tragedy of the Commons*
*Garrett Hardin*

The rebuttal to the invisible hand in population control is to be found in a scenario first sketched in a little-known pamphlet in 1833 by a mathematical amateur named William Forster Lloyd (1794–1852). We may well call it "the tragedy of the commons," using the word "tragedy" as the philosopher Whitehead (1948, 17) used it: "The essence of dramatic tragedy is not unhappiness. It resides in the solemnity of the remorseless working of things." He there goes on to

---

*Reprinted from *Science* 162 (1968): 1234–48 with permission. © 1968 American Association for the Advancement of Science.

say, "This inevitableness of destiny can only be illustrated in terms of human life by incidents which in fact involve unhappiness. For it is only by them that the futility of escape can be made evident in the drama."

The tragedy of the commons develops in this way. Picture a pasture open to all. It is to be expected that each man will try to keep as many cattle as possible on the commons. Such an arrangement may work reasonably satisfactorily for centuries because tribal wars, poaching, and disease keep the numbers of both man and beast well below the carrying capacity of the land. Finally, however, comes the day of reckoning, that is, the day when the long-desired goal of social stability becomes a reality. At this point, the inherent logic of the commons remorselessly generates tragedy.

As a rational being, each herdsman seeks to maximize his gain. Explicitly or implicitly, more or less consciously, he asks, "What is the utility *to me* of adding one more animal to my herd?" This utility has one negative and one positive component.

(1) The positive component is a function of the increment of one animal. Since the herdsman receives all the proceeds from the sale of the additional animal, the positive utility is nearly +1.

(2) The negative component is a function of the additional overgrazing created by one more animal. Since, however, the effects of overgrazing are shared by all the herdsmen, the negative utility for any particular decision-making herdsman is only a fraction of −1.

Adding together the component partial utilities, the rational herdsman concludes that the only sensible course for him to pursue is to add another animal to his herd. And another; and another. . . . But this is the conclusion reached by each and every rational herdsman sharing a commons. Therein is the tragedy. Each man is locked into a system that compels him to increase his herd without limit— in a world that is limited. Ruin is the destination toward which all men rush, each pursuing his own best interest in a society that believes in the freedom of the commons. Freedom in a commons brings ruin to all.

Some would say that this is a platitude. Would that it were! In a sense, it was learned thousands of years ago, but natural selection favors the forces of psychological denial. The individual benefits as an individual from his ability to deny the truth even though society as a whole, of which he is a part, suffers. Education can counteract the natural tendency to do the wrong thing, but the inexorable succession of generations requires that the basis for this knowledge be constantly refreshed. . . .

## POLLUTION

In a reverse way, the tragedy of the commons reappears in problems of pollution. Here it is not a question of taking something out of the commons, but of putting something in—sewage, or chemical, radioactive, and heat wastes into water; noxious and dangerous fumes into the air; and distracting and unpleasant advertising signs into the line of sight. The calculations of utility are much the same as before. The rational man finds that his share of the cost of the wastes he discharges into the commons is less than the cost of purifying his wastes before releasing them. Since this is true for everyone, we are locked into a system of "fouling our own nest," so long as we behave only as independent, rational, free-enterprisers.

The tragedy of the commons as a food basket is averted by private property, or something formally like it. But the air and waters surrounding us cannot readily be fenced, and so the tragedy of the commons as a cesspool must be prevented by different means, by coercive laws or taxing devices that make it cheaper for the polluter to treat his pollutants than to discharge them untreated. We have not progressed as far with the solution of this problem as we have with the first. Indeed, our particular concept of private property, which deters us from exhausting the positive resources of the earth, favors pollution. The owner of a factory on the bank of a stream—whose property extends to the middle of the stream—often has difficulty seeing why it is not his natural right to muddy the waters flowing past his door. The law, always behind the times, requires elaborate stitching and fitting to adapt it to this newly perceived aspect of the commons. . . .

## MUTUAL COERCION MUTUALLY AGREED UPON

The social arrangements that produce responsibility are arrangements that create coercion, of some sort. . . . Coercion is a dirty word to most liberals now, but it need not forever be so. As with the four-letter words, its dirtiness can be cleansed away by exposure to the light, by saying it over and over without apology or embarrassment. To many, the word "coercion" implies arbitrary decisions of distant and irresponsible bureaucrats; but this is not a necessary part of its meaning. The only kind of coercion I recommend is mutual coercion, mutually agreed upon by the majority of the people affected.

To say that we mutually agree to coercion is not to say that we are required to enjoy it, or even to pretend we enjoy it. Who enjoys taxes? We all grumble about them. But we accept compulsory taxes because we recognize that voluntary taxes would favor the conscienceless. We institute and (grumblingly) support taxes and other coercive devices to escape the horror of the commons. . . .

Every new enclosure of the commons involves the infringement of somebody's personal liberty. Infringements made in the distant past are accepted because no contemporary complains of a loss. It is the newly proposed infringements that we vigorously oppose; cries of "rights" and "freedom" fill the air. But what does "freedom" mean? When men mutually agreed to pass laws against robbing, mankind became more free, not less so. Individuals locked into the logic of the commons are free only to bring on universal ruin; once they see the necessity of mutual coercion, they become free to pursue other goals. I believe it was Hegel who said, "Freedom is the recognition of necessity."

---

\*     \*     \*     \*     \*

The judiciary has supported mandatory vaccination laws for more than a century, emphasizing the overriding importance of communal well-being. For a brief history of judicial opinions regarding vaccination law and policy, see Table 7, which provides a time line of selected federal and state vaccination cases. Recall the expression of "social contract" in the Supreme Court's seminal opinion in *Jacobson v. Massachusetts* (see chapter 7). *Jacobson* stands firmly for the proposition that states possess the police power to compel vaccination for the public good.

The power of states and localities to require children to be vaccinated as a condition of school entrance has been widely accepted and judicially sanctioned. In *Zucht v. King* (excerpted next), the Supreme Court upheld a local government mandate for vaccination as a prerequisite for attendance in public school.

Antagonists of vaccination often frame their objections in terms of the First Amendment freedom of religion. As discussed earlier, forty-eight states currently grant religious exemptions from compulsory vaccination (see Table 6). Most courts uphold the constitutionality of religious exemptions, but the Mississippi Supreme Court in *Brown v. Stone* (excerpted later) found that these exemptions unfairly threaten the health of all school children.

TABLE 7

TIME LINE OF SELECTED FEDERAL AND STATE COURT
DECISIONS REGARDING VACCINATION LAW AND POLICY

| Year | Case Decision and Citation | Major Holding |
|---|---|---|
| 1830 | Hazen v. Strong, 2 Vt. 427 | Local town council had authority to pay for vaccination of persons exposed, even though there were no cases of smallpox in the community. |
| 1894 | Duffield v. School Dist. of City of Williamsport, 29 A. 742 (Pa.) | School Board regulation that prohibited children not vaccinated for smallpox from attending school was reasonable based on a current outbreak and expert opinions on vaccination's efficacy. |
| 1904 | Viemester v. White, 84 N.Y.S. 712, aff'd, 72 N.E. 97 | No constitutional right to an education exists under the New York Constitution and thus, there is no limit on the type of reasonable regulation (including vaccination requirements) that may be imposed on public education by the legislature. |
| 1905 | Jacobson v. Massachusetts, 197 U.S. 1 | The city of Cambridge may require its citizens to be vaccinated against smallpox, provided the regulations are reasonable and the vaccine does not pose a hazard to the individual. |
| 1910 | McSween v. Board of School Trustees, 129 S.W. 206 (Tex. Civ. App.) | School vaccination laws do not constitute an illegal search and seizure violating the Fourth Amendment. |
| 1913 | Adams v. Milwaukee, 228 U.S. 572 | Vaccination laws do not discriminate against school children to the exclusion of others in violation of the equal protection clause of the Fourteenth Amendment. |
| 1922 | Zucht v. King, 260 U.S. 174 | States may delegate to a municipality the power to order vaccination, and the municipality may then give broad discretion to the board of health to apply and enforce the regulation. |
| 1927 | Cram v. School Bd. of Manchester, 136 A. 263 (N.H.) | A father's claim that vaccination of his daughter should not be required because it will "endanger her health and life" by "performing a surgical operation by injecting a poison . . . into [her] blood" is rejected based on Jacobson. |

TABLE 7 (continued)

| Year | Case Decision and Citation | Major Holding |
|------|---------------------------|---------------|
| 1944 | Prince v. Massachusetts, 321 U.S. 158 | A mother can be prosecuted under child labor laws for using her children to distribute religious literature. The First Amendment's free exercise clause does not allow for the right to expose the community or one's children to harm. |
| 1951 | Seubold v. Fort Smith Special Sch. Dist., 237 S.W.2d 884 | School vaccination requirements do not deprive individuals of liberty and property interests without due process of the law. |
| 1963 | State ex rel. Mack v. Board of Educ. of Covington, 204 N.E.2d 86 (Ohio Ct. App.) | A child does not have an absolute right to enter school without immunization against polio, smallpox, pertussis, and tetanus on the basis of his parents' objections to his vaccination. The school board has authority to make and enforce rules and regulations to secure immunization. |
| 1964 | Cude v. State, 377 S.W.2d 816 (Ark.) | Parents have no legal right to prevent vaccination of children when required to attend school even if their objections are based on good-faith religious beliefs in accordance with Prince. |
| 1965 | Wright v. DeWitt Sch. Dist., 385 S.W.2d 644 (Ark.) | A compulsory vaccination law with no religious exemption is constitutional because the right of free exercise is subject to reasonable regulation for the good of the community as a whole. |
| 1968 | McCartney v. Austin, 293 N.Y.S.2d 188 | New York's vaccination statute did not interfere with the freedom to worship in the Roman Catholic faith because the religion does not proscribe vaccination. |
| 1971 | Dalli v. Board of Educ., 267 N.E.2d 219 (Mass.) | State exemption for objectors who believe in the "tenets and practices of a recognized church of religious denomination" violates the equal protection clause by giving preferential treatment to certain groups over others who have sincere, though unrecognized, religious objections. |
| 1976 | Kleid v. Board of Educ., 406 F. Supp. 902 (W.D. Ken.) | Requirement that parents be members of a "nationally recognized and established church or religious denomination" to qualify for religious exemption to vaccination mandate does not violate the establishment clause. |

| 1979 | Brown v. Stone, 378 So. 2d 218 (Miss.), cert. denied, 449 U.S. 887 (1980) | Religious exemption violates the equal protection clause because it "discriminates against the great majority of children whose parents have no such religious convictions." |
| 1985 | Hanzel v. Arter, 625 F. Supp. 1259 (S.D. Ohio) | Parents' objections to vaccination based on "chiropractic ethics" did not fall under the protection of the establishment clause and, therefore, their children were not exempt from the statutory mandates. |
| 1987 | Shear v. Northmost-East Northmost Union Free Sch. Dist., 672 F. Supp. 81 (E.D.N.Y.) | Requirement that parents be "bona fide members of a recognized religious organization" to be exempt on religious grounds from the school vaccination requirement violates the establishment clause. |
| | Maricopa County Health Dept. v. Harmon, 750 P.2d 1364 (Ariz.) | Health Department had authority to exclude unvaccinated children from school even if there were no reported cases of the disease in question and did so without violating the right to public education in the Arizona Constitution. |
| 1988 | Mason v. General Brown Cent. Sch. Dist., 851 F.2d 47 (2d Cir.) | Parents' sincerely held belief that immunization was contrary to "genetic blueprint" was a secular, not religious, belief, and thus their children's required vaccination did not violate the establishment clause. |
| 1994 | Berg v. Glen Cove City Sch. Dist., 853 F. Supp. 651 (E.D.N.Y.) | Jewish parents had sincere religious belief regarding vaccinations even though nothing in their religion prohibited vaccination. |
| 2000 | Farina v. Board of Educ. of the City of New York, 116 F. Supp. 2d 503 (S.D.N.Y) | Catholic parents' beliefs regarding vaccinations were personal and medical, and therefore not adequate basis to recover damages from the City Board of Education based on its refusal to accept their religious exemption. |
| 2001 | Jones v. State Dep't of Health, 18 P.3d 1189 (Wyo.) | Health Department had no authority to require a student to receive a hepatitis B immunization or to require a student applying for a waiver from immunization requirements to provide a reason for a medical contraindication to immunizations. |
| | Bowden v. Iona Grammar School, 726 N.Y.S.2d 685 (App. Div.) | Parents who followed the practices of Temple of the Healing Spirit were entitled to a religious exemption to vaccination requirements for their children because the state statute did not qualify which religions were eligible. |

### Zucht v. King*
*Supreme Court of the United States*
*Decided November 13, 1922*

Justice BRANDEIS delivered the opinion of the Court.

Ordinances of the city of San Antonio, Texas, provide that no child or other person shall attend a public school or other place of education without having first presented a certificate of vaccination. Purporting to act under these ordinances, public officials excluded Rosalyn Zucht from a public school because she did not have the required certificate and refused to submit to vaccination. They also caused her to be excluded from a private school. Thereupon Rosalyn brought this suit against the officials in a court of the state. The bill charges that there was then no occasion for requiring vaccination; that the ordinances deprive plaintiff of her liberty without due process of law, by, in effect, making vaccination compulsory; and also that they are void, because they leave to the board of health discretion to determine when and under what circumstances the requirement shall be enforced, without providing any rule by which that board is to be guided in its action, and without providing any safeguards against partiality and oppression. The prayers were for an injunction against enforcing the ordinances, for a writ of mandamus to compel her admission to the public school, and for damages. . . .

Long before this suit was instituted, *Jacobson v. Massachusetts* [excerpted in chapter 7] had settled that it is within the police power of a state to provide for compulsory vaccination. That case and others had also settled that a state may, consistently with the federal Constitution, delegate to a municipality authority to determine under what conditions health regulations shall become operative. And still others had settled that the municipality may vest in its officials broad discretion in matters affecting the application and enforcement of a health law. A long line of decisions by this court had also settled that in the exercise of the police power reasonable classification may be freely applied, and that regulation is not violative of the equal protection clause merely because it is not all-embracing. In view of these decisions we find in the record no question as to the validity of the ordinance. . . . Unlike *Yick Wo v. Hopkins* [see *Jew Ho*, excerpted in chapter 7] these ordinances

*260 U.S. 174 (1922).

confer not arbitrary power, but only that broad discretion required for the protection of the public health. . . .

Writ of error dismissed.

---

**Brown v. Stone\***
*Supreme Court of Mississippi*
*Decided December 19, 1979*

Judge SMITH delivered the opinion of the court.

This is an appeal by Charles H. Brown, father and next friend of Chad Allan Brown, a six-year-old boy, from a [decision] of the Chancery Court of Chickasaw County [denying Brown's request for] injunction to compel the Board of Trustees of the Houston [Mississippi] Municipal Separate School District to admit his son as a student without compliance with the immunization requirements of MISS. CODE ANN. § 41-23-37 (Supp. 1972). This statute provides (among other things):

> Except as provided hereinafter, it shall be unlawful for any child to attend any school . . . unless they shall first have been vaccinated against those diseases specified by the State Health Officer. A certificate of exemption from vaccination for medical reasons may be offered on behalf of a child by a duly licensed physician and may be accepted by the local health officer when, in his opinion, such exemption will not cause undue risk to the community. A certificate of religious exemption may be offered on behalf of a child by an officer of a church of a recognized denomination. This certificate shall certify that parents or guardians of the child are bona fide members of a recognized denomination whose religious teachings require reliance on prayer or spiritual means of healing.

There was filed with the bill the following certificate, signed by a minister of the Church of Christ:

> Be it known that the church of Christ as a religious body does not teach against the use of medicines, immunizations or vaccinations as prescribed by a duly physician. However, Dr. Charles Brown, our local chiropractor, who is a member of the North Jackson Street Church of Christ in Houston, Mississippi, does have strong convictions against the use of any kind of medications and we respect his views.
>
> Charles E. Bland
> Minister

---

\*378 So. 2d 218 (1979).

[Brown's] bill recited (a) that six-year-old Chad Allan Brown was of sufficient age and residence to qualify for admission to the first grade of the Houston Elementary School, but had not been [properly] vaccinated. . . , (b) Charles H. Brown, the father, has not permitted his son to be vaccinated because of "strong and sincere religious beliefs actively practiced and followed" by Charles H. Brown, (c) Charles H. Brown is a member of the Church of Christ, a religious body which does not teach against the use of medicines, immunizations or vaccinations prescribed by a physician, (d) Charles H. Brown has sought a religious exemption from vaccination (of his son) but it was denied because the certificate did not comply with [state law], (e) Chad Allan Brown was denied admission to the school because of the failure to be immunized . . . , (f) . . . Mississippi [laws] are invalid "insofar as they force complainants to join a religious organization in order to practice their religious tenants freely," and the denial of admission of Chad Allan Brown violates complainants' rights protected by the First Amendment to the United States Constitution. . . .

Appellants concede that mandatory immunization against dangerous diseases, without exemptions based on religious beliefs or convictions, has been held constitutionally valid as a reasonable exercise of police power. They contend, however, that the provision for religious exemption violates the First Amendment . . . protecting the free exercise of religion. . . .

The fundamental and paramount purpose of the Mississippi Legislature . . . was to afford protection for school children against crippling and deadly diseases by immunization. That this can be done effectively and safely has been incontrovertibly demonstrated over a period of a good many years and is a matter of common knowledge of which this Court takes judicial notice.

If the religious exemption from immunization is to be granted only to members of certain recognized sects or denominations whose doctrines forbid it, and, as contended by appellants, to individuals whose private or personal religious beliefs will not allow them to permit immunization of their children, . . . the protection of school children generally comprising the school community is defeated.

Is it mandated by the First Amendment . . . that innocent children, too young to decide for themselves, are to be denied the protection against crippling and death that immunization provides because of a religious belief adhered to by a parent or parents? . . .

[W]e have concluded that the statute in question, requiring immunization against certain crippling and deadly diseases particularly dangerous to children before they may be admitted to school, serves an overriding and compelling public interest, and that such interest extends to the exclusion of a child until such immunization has been effected, not only as a protection of that child but as a protection of the large number of other children comprising the school community and with whom he will be daily in close contact in the school room. . . . It must not be forgotten that a child is indeed himself an individual, although under certain disabilities until majority, with rights in his own person which must be respected and may be enforced. Where its safety, morals and health are involved, it becomes a legitimate concern of the state.

The protection of the great body of school children attending the public schools in Mississippi against the horrors of crippling and death resulting from poliomyelitis or smallpox or from one of the other diseases against which means of immunization are known and have long been practiced successfully, demand that children who have not been immunized should be excluded from the school community until immunization has been accomplished. That is the obvious overriding and compelling public purpose of [the state's vaccination law]. To the extent that it may conflict with the religious beliefs of a parent, however sincerely entertained, the interests of the school children must prevail. [The state's vaccination law] is a reasonable and constitutional exercise of the police power of the state insofar as it provides for the immunization of children before they are to be permitted to enter school.

The exception, which would provide for the exemption of children of parents whose religious beliefs conflict with the immunization requirements, would discriminate against the great majority of children whose parents have no such religious convictions. To give it effect would result in a violation of the Fourteenth Amendment to the United States Constitution which provides that no state shall make any law denying to any person within its jurisdiction the equal protection of the laws, in that it would require the great body of school children to be vaccinated and at the same time expose them to the hazard of associating in school with children exempted under the religious exemption who had not been immunized as required by the statute. . . .

We have no difficulty here in deciding that the statute is "complete in itself" without the provision for religious exemption and that it serves a compelling state interest in the protection of school children. Therefore, we hold that the provision providing an exception from the operation of the statute because of religious belief is in violation of the Fourteenth Amendment to the United States Constitution and therefore is void. As the United States Supreme Court said in *In re Gault*, 387 U.S. 1 (1967): "Whatever may be their precise impact, neither the Fourteenth Amendment nor the Bill of Rights is for adults alone."

---

## II. CASE FINDING: POPULATION-BASED SCREENING

Although the terms are often used interchangeably, a distinction exists between "testing" and "screening." Clinical testing refers to a medical procedure that determines the presence or absence of disease, or its precursor, in an individual patient. In contrast, screening is the systematic application of a medical test to a defined population with the objective of identifying persons with infectious diseases. Public health authorities can then offer education, counseling, or treatment. They can also help monitor the epidemic and devise more precisely targeted prevention programs.

Disease screening is a basic tool of modern public health and preventive medicine, but it is not always beneficial and can be intrusive and unjust. First, screening can be unreliable if the test is technically deficient. If the test instrument is not sufficiently "sensitive," it will fail to detect most cases of infection in a population. If the text instrument is not sufficiently "specific," it will produce false positives (i.e., persons will test positive although they are not actually infected). Even technically proficient tests will have poor predictive value in populations with a low prevalence of infection. Screening in low-prevalence populations is likely to identify few cases of infection because relatively few cases exist. (For further discussion of the predictive value of screening, see chapter 7 in the companion text.)

Second, screening can be intrusive unless the person is fully informed and provides consent. Screening without informed consent undermines personal autonomy and bodily integrity. Additionally, screening reveals sensitive medical information. If this information is revealed without permission, people's privacy is invaded and they may experience discrimination in employment and insurance.

Third, screening can be unjust if it is targeted against vulnerable populations. Suppose TB screening were targeted only toward the homeless or syphilis screening were targeted only toward commercial sex workers. The targeted groups would have a claim that the screening program was unjust. Even if screening programs target "high-risk" groups, they can be unjust. For example, the IOM (1999) and CDC (2000e) recommend universal HIV screening of pregnant women rather than targeted screening in high-risk communities. Their reason is that targeted screening would disproportionately burden racial minorities, which would appear to be unfair (Kass 2000).

The readings in this section discuss the ethical and legal aspects of screening. Ruth R. Faden and her colleagues at the Johns Hopkins University and Georgetown University examine the ethical foundations of screening. Thereafter, the section examines the constitutionality of government screening programs.

---

## Warrants for Screening Programs:
## Public Health, Legal, and Ethical Frameworks*
*Ruth R. Faden, Nancy Kass, and Madison Powers*

When a screening program is designed, it is necessary to decide how participation in the program is to be determined. Conventionally, this decision is viewed as a choice between two options: participation in the program is to be either compulsory or voluntary. Often, however, it is difficult to categorize programs simply as one or the other; some elements of the program make participation appear voluntary, while others seem to include some level of compulsion. As a step toward better organizing this issue for the purpose of analysis, we propose dividing programs into five, rather than two, categories: (1) completely mandatory programs; (2) conditionally mandatory programs; (3) "routine without notification" programs; (4) "routine with notification" programs; and (5) voluntary programs. . . . [T]hese categories are not mutually exclusive or exhaustive. . . . [A]lthough for government programs these categories may approximate a continuum of legal compulsoriness, they do not necessarily represent a continuum either of autonomous choice on the part of participants or of protection of the public's health, issues to which we will return shortly.

---

*Reprinted from *AIDS, Women and the Next Generation: Towards a Morally Acceptable Public Policy for HIV Testing of Pregnant Women and Newborns,* edited by Ruth R. Faden, Gail Geller, and Madison Powers (New York: Oxford Univ. Press, 1991), 3–24.

The most stringent level of testing in terms of legal compulsoriness is a *completely mandatory program*, in which, typically, a government agency requires citizens to undergo an intervention, with sanctions imposed on those who do not comply. . . .

In a *conditionally mandatory program*, either government or an institution in the private sector makes access to a designated service or opportunity contingent on participating in the program. These could be rules either established by government (such as having to be screened for syphilis in order to obtain a marriage license, . . . or privately authorized (such as . . . having to undergo a general health screening for certain health or life insurance policies). In each of these instances, the individual has the right not to participate in the activities or services offered by the institution; however, . . . participation in the program is mandatory for eligibility. . . .

In a *routine without notification* program, the intervention is routinely and automatically implemented unless an individual expressly asks that it not be done. However, participants are not notified about the intervention or their right to refuse. Thus as a practical matter, refusals rarely occur. . . .

In a *routine with notification* program, participants are informed of the intervention and their right to refuse before the intervention is implemented. This approach has been proposed for newborn testing for PKU but rarely has been adopted.

In a *voluntary* program, the intervention is not implemented without the authorization of participants. In some instances, written informed consent is solicited; in others, authorization or consent is considered to be implied in that participants must ask for or seek out the program. Current examples of voluntary screening programs are programs that screen for the antibody to HIV or those that offer mammograms for screening of breast cancer.

At first, it might appear that these five categories of programs . . . represent a rank ordering, with completely mandatory programs being the most restrictive and voluntary programs being the least restrictive in terms of their impact on autonomous choice. However, depending on the circumstances, conditionally mandatory programs can be as restrictive of choice as completely mandatory ones. The penalties imposed for failing to comply with some completely mandatory programs may be easier to resist than the consequences of forgoing a conditionally mandatory program. For example, in communities where jobs are scarce and needs are great, individuals may have no choice but to submit to preemployment testing. Similarly, routine programs that do not require prior notification may be equally restrictive of choice if the target individuals are unaware that the interventions are being implemented and thus have no opportunity to choose to refuse. Even routine programs with notification requirements and completely voluntary programs provide no guarantees that participation reflects autonomous choice. Questions of manipulation, understanding, and adequacy of information necessarily remain. Clearly, issues of compulsoriness understood narrowly in terms of legal mandates must be distinguished from the impact of a specific program on issues of choice. . . .

## PUBLIC HEALTH FRAMEWORK

Public health is concerned with the prevention and reduction of morbidity and mortality. At the core of a public health framework for evaluating screening programs is a single criterion—the program's harm-to-benefit ratio, where harms and benefits are understood in terms of impact on a community's morbidity and mortality. Although not sufficient in itself, it is always necessary to use the public health framework in assessing the acceptability of a screening program. An acceptable ratio of benefits to harms is, at minimum, a threshold consideration, and, as we shall see, both the legal and ethical frameworks incorporate a public health assessment of harms and benefits in their analyses. No screening program can be justified either legally or morally without first satisfying public health criteria. . . .

Consistently, screening programs have as their goal the reduction of morbidity or mortality in either the general population or a specific population. Screening programs can be justified only if they effect a positive outcome that would not have occurred without the screening. . . . The degree to which a screening program can be successful in reducing morbidity and mortality depends on the prevalence of the condition in the population to be screened, the validity and reliability of the screening tool, the availability of a treatment or intervention for the condition, and the follow-up plans for those detected to be positive. . . . Wilson and Junger (1968) [have identified] . . . nine specific requirements for the establishment of a screening program: (1) the condition for which the screening is done should be an important health problem; (2) there should be an accepted treatment for patients detected; (3) facilities for diagnosis and treatment should be available; (4) there should be a recognizable latent or early symptomatic stage so that detection can prove beneficial; (5) there should be a suitable screening test; (6) the test should be acceptable to the population; (7) the natural history of the condition should be adequately understood; (8) there should be agreement as to who will treat the patients; [and] (9) the cost of case finding, diagnosis, and treatment should be economically balanced in relation to possible expenditure on medical care as a whole.

Only after a given type of screening program has been thoroughly examined in terms of the degree to which it satisfies the public health criteria is it appropriate to examine the . . . ethical justifications for accepting or rejecting that program as a public policy choice. . . .

## ETHICAL FRAMEWORK

Central to [a] framework of ethical analysis is the notion that moral deliberation and justification ordinarily rest on principles, rules, and rights understood as abstract action guides. These action guides, the choice and analysis of which are inherently controversial, together with questions of their relationship both to one another and to a theory of human virtues, constitute the heart of modern ethical theory. . . . [The authors discuss three general moral principles: beneficence, respect for autonomy, and justice.]

### Balancing Moral Principles

Controversial problems about moral principles such as respect for autonomy, beneficence, and justice inevitably arise over how much these principles demand and how to handle situations of conflict among them. Whatever the prominence of these principles, we must acknowledge that if they conflict—as they do on occasion—a serious weighting or priority problem is created. . . . Many problems about policies governing program participation take this form. Primarily they involve whether to override the obligation to respect the autonomy of individuals, as when programs are made completely mandatory. . . .

[T]he decision of whether to implement a screening program requires a balancing of the goals of the three frameworks described. In an important respect, the public health framework is the most fundamental. No screening program can be justified without satisfying at least some public health criteria. . . .

It is our belief that how completely the public health criteria must be satisfied depends on the degree to which the specific type of program proposed compromises other criteria. When a program poses a conflict between public health interests and other interests, greater fulfillment of the public health criteria is necessary in order to justify public health interests taking precedence. For this reason, analyses of the five types of programs must include the degree to which they satisfy public health criteria, understanding that the more programs challenge legal and ethical mandates, the greater will be the requirement that the public health criteria be satisfied.

*   *   *   *   *

Since the guarantees of the Constitution constrain principally actions by the state, the legal battleground over screening has centered on government agencies, as well as private entities acting on federal or state rules that require or authorize screening. (It is important to emphasize that the Americans with Disabilities Act also contains important limits on screening undertaken by employers, as discussed in Feldblum [1991].) The primary constitutional impediment to testing is the Fourth Amendment's right of people to be "secure in their persons" and not subjected to "unreasonable searches and seizures." While the Fourth Amendment is popularly perceived as applying solely to personal or residential searches (as for administrative searches, see chapter 8), the Supreme Court has long recognized that the collection and subsequent analysis of biological samples are "searches." Schmerber v. California, 384 U.S. 757, 767–68 (1966). Privacy and security interests are generated by the invasion of bodily integrity involved in collecting the sample and the ensuing chemical analysis that extracts personal information. The constitutional issue is whether the analysis of blood, urine, or other tissue is "unreasonable." The Supreme Court, in the companion cases of *Skinner v. Railway Labor Executives' Association* (excerpted next) and *Treasury Employees Union v. Von Raab*, 489 U.S. 656 (1989), formulated the modern standard of review for screening programs needed for special purposes other than law enforcement (see Walsh, Chapman, Elinson, and Gostin 1992).

---

## Skinner v. Railway Labor Executives' Association*
*Supreme Court of the United States*
*Decided March 21, 1989*

Justice KENNEDY delivered the opinion of the Court.

[Based on evidence indicating that alcohol and drug abuse by railroad employees had caused or contributed to a number of significant

---

*489 U.S. 602 (1989).

train accidents, the Federal Railroad Administration (FRA) promulgated regulations under petitioner Secretary of Transportation's statutory authority to adopt safety standards for the industry. Subpart C of the regulations requires railroads to conduct blood and urine tests of covered employees following certain major train accidents or incidents. Subpart D authorizes, but does not require, railroads to administer breath or urine tests to covered employees who violate certain safety rules. Respondents, the Railway Labor Executives' Association and various member labor organizations, brought suit.]

We have long recognized that a "compelled intrusio[n] into the body for blood to be analyzed for alcohol content" must be deemed a Fourth Amendment search. Schmerber v. California, 384 U.S. 757 (1966). In light of our society's concern for the security of one's person, it is obvious that this physical intrusion, penetrating beneath the skin, infringes an expectation of privacy that society is prepared to recognize as reasonable. The ensuing chemical analysis of the sample to obtain physiological data is a further invasion of the tested employee's privacy interests. Much the same is true of the breath-testing procedures required under Subpart D of the regulations. Subjecting a person to a breathalyzer test, which generally requires the production of alveolar or "deep lung" breath for chemical analysis, implicates similar concerns about bodily integrity and should also be deemed a search. . . . [T]hese intrusions must be deemed searches under the Fourth Amendment. . . .

To hold that the Fourth Amendment is applicable to the drug and alcohol testing prescribed by the FRA regulations is only to begin the inquiry into the standards governing such intrusions. For the Fourth Amendment does not proscribe all searches and seizures, but only those that are unreasonable. What is reasonable, of course, "depends on all of the circumstances surrounding the search or seizure and the nature of the search or seizure itself." United States v. Montoya de Hernandez, 473 U.S. 531, 537 (1985). Thus, the permissibility of a particular practice "is judged by balancing its intrusion on the individual's Fourth Amendment interests against its promotion of legitimate governmental interests." Delaware v. Prouse, 440 U.S. 648, 654 (1979).

In most criminal cases, we strike this balance in favor of the procedures described by the Warrant Clause of the Fourth Amendment. Except in certain well-defined circumstances, a search or seizure in such a case is not reasonable unless it is accomplished pursuant to a judicial warrant issued upon probable cause. We have recognized exceptions to this rule, however, when "special needs, beyond the normal need for law enforcement, make the warrant and probable-cause requirement impracticable." Griffin v. Wisconsin, 483 U.S. 868, 873 (1987). When faced with such special needs, we have not hesitated to balance the governmental and privacy interests to assess the practicality of the warrant and probable-cause requirements in the particular context.

The Government's interest in regulating the conduct of railroad employees to ensure safety . . . "presents 'special needs' beyond normal law enforcement that may justify departures from the usual warrant and probable-cause requirements." *Griffin*, 483 U.S. at 873–74. The hours of service employees covered by the FRA regulations include persons engaged in handling orders concerning train movements, operating crews, and those engaged in the maintenance and repair of signal systems. It is undisputed that these and other covered employees are engaged in safety-sensitive tasks. . . .

The FRA has prescribed toxicological tests, . . . "to prevent accidents and casualties in railroad operations that result from impairment of employees by alcohol or drugs." 49 C.F.R. § 219.1(a) (1987). This governmental interest in ensuring the safety of the traveling public and of the employees themselves plainly justifies prohibiting covered employees from using alcohol or drugs on duty, or while subject to being called for duty. . . . The question that remains, then, is whether the Government's need to monitor compliance with these restrictions justifies the privacy intrusions at issue absent a warrant or individualized suspicion.

An essential purpose of a warrant requirement is to protect privacy interests by assuring citizens subject to a search or seizure that such intrusions are not the random or arbitrary acts of government agents. A warrant assures the citizen that the intrusion is authorized by law, and that it is narrowly limited in its objectives and scope. . . . In the present context, however, a warrant would do little to further these aims. Both the circumstances justifying toxicological testing and the permissible limits of such intrusions are defined narrowly and specifically in the regulations that authorize them, and doubtless are well known to covered employees. Indeed, in light of the standardized nature of the tests and the minimal discretion vested in those charged with administering the program, there are virtually no facts for a neutral magistrate to evaluate.

We have recognized, moreover, that the government's interest in dispensing with the warrant requirement is at its strongest when, as here, "the burden of obtaining a warrant is likely to frustrate the governmental purpose behind the search." Camara v. Municipal Ct. of San

Francisco [excerpted in chapter 8]. As the FRA recognized, alcohol and other drugs are eliminated from the bloodstream at a constant rate, and blood and breath samples taken to measure whether these substances were in the bloodstream when a triggering event occurred must be obtained as soon as possible. Although the metabolites of some drugs remain in the urine for longer periods of time and may enable the FRA to estimate whether the employee was impaired by those drugs at the time of a covered accident, incident, or rule violation, the delay necessary to procure a warrant nevertheless may result in the destruction of valuable evidence. . . . We do not believe that a warrant is essential to render the intrusions here at issue reasonable under the Fourth Amendment.

Our cases indicate that even a search that may be performed without a warrant must be based, as a general matter, on probable cause to believe that the person to be searched has violated the law. When the balance of interests precludes insistence on a showing of probable cause, we have usually required "some quantum of individualized suspicion," United States v. Martinez-Fuente, 428 U.S. 543, 560 (1976), before concluding that a search is reasonable. . . . In limited circumstances, [however,] where the privacy interests implicated by the search are minimal, and where an important governmental interest furthered by the intrusion would be placed in jeopardy by a requirement of individualized suspicion, a search may be reasonable despite the absence of such suspicion. We believe this is true of the intrusions in question here. . . .

To the extent transportation and like restrictions are necessary to procure the requisite blood, breath, and urine samples for testing, this interference alone is minimal given the employment context in which it takes place. . . . Any . . . interference with a railroad employee's freedom of movement that occurs in the time it takes to procure a blood, breath, or urine sample for testing cannot, by itself, be said to infringe significant privacy interests. Our decision in Schmerber indicates that the same is true of the blood tests required by the FRA regulations. . . . We said also that the intrusion occasioned by a blood test is not significant, since such "tests are a commonplace in these days of periodic physical examinations and experience with them teaches that the quantity of blood extracted is minimal, and that for most people the procedure involves virtually no risk, trauma, or pain. . . ." *Id.* at 771.

The breath tests . . . are even less intrusive than the blood tests. . . . Unlike blood tests, breath tests do not require piercing the skin and may be conducted safely outside a hospital environment and with a minimum of inconvenience or embarrassment. Further, breath tests reveal the level of alcohol in the employee's bloodstream and nothing more. . . . In all the circumstances, we cannot conclude that the administration of a breath test implicates significant privacy concerns.

A more difficult question is presented by urine tests. . . . [T]he procedures for collecting the necessary samples, which require employees to perform an excretory function traditionally shielded by great privacy, raise concerns not implicated by blood or breath tests. . . . The regulations do not require that samples be furnished under the direct observation of a monitor, despite the desirability of such a procedure to ensure the integrity of the sample. The sample is also collected in a medical environment, by personnel unrelated to the railroad employer, and is thus not unlike similar procedures encountered often in the context of a regular physical examination.

More importantly, the expectations of privacy of covered employees are diminished by reason of their participation in an industry that is regulated pervasively to ensure safety, a goal dependent, in substantial part, on the health and fitness of covered employees. . . .

By contrast, the Government interest in testing without a showing of individualized suspicion is compelling. Employees subject to the tests discharge duties fraught with such risks of injury to others that even a momentary lapse of attention can have disastrous consequences. . . . [E]mployees who are subject to testing under the FRA regulations can cause great human loss before any signs of impairment become noticeable to supervisors or others. . . . While no procedure can identify all impaired employees with ease and perfect accuracy, the FRA regulations supply an effective means of deterring employees engaged in safety-sensitive tasks from using controlled substances or alcohol in the first place. . . .

We conclude that the compelling Government interests served by the FRA's regulations would be significantly hindered if railroads were required to point to specific facts giving rise to a reasonable suspicion of impairment before testing a given employee. In view of our conclusion that, on the present record, the toxicological testing contemplated by the regulations is not an undue infringement on the justifiable expectations of privacy of covered employees, the Government's compelling interests outweigh privacy concerns. . . .

\* \* \* \* \*

In *Skinner*, did the Court engage in a sufficiently rigorous inquiry of the government's public health objectives? Also, by focusing on the intrusive nature of the blood, breath, and urine tests, did the Court sufficiently weigh the informational privacy interests entailed in compelled disclosure of sensitive information?

Since most screening programs are not conducted for law enforcement purposes, they fall within the Supreme Court's "special needs" doctrine. For example, courts have upheld compulsory sexually transmitted disease (STD) screening for persons accused or convicted of sexual assaults (*see, e.g., In re* Juveniles A, B, C, D, E, 847 P.2d 455 (Wash. 1993)). The judiciary believes these screening programs are justified by the "special need" to inform rape victims of their potential exposure to STDs (Gostin et al. 1994).

In *Ferguson v. City of Charleston*, the Supreme Court considered the "special needs" doctrine in an intriguing case involving drug testing of pregnant women.

---

**Ferguson v. City of Charleston***
*Supreme Court of the United States*
*Decided March 21, 2001*

Justice STEVENS delivered the opinion of the Court.

[In 1988 a task force made up of the Medical University of South Carolina (MUSC), police, and local officials developed a policy that set procedures for identifying and testing pregnant patients suspected of drug use without obtaining the individuals' consent. The policy also included police procedures and criteria for arresting patients who tested positive and prescribed prosecutions for drug offenses and/or child neglect, depending on the stage of the defendant's pregnancy. Petitioners, MUSC obstetrical patients arrested after testing positive for cocaine, filed this suit challenging the policy's validity on the theory that warrantless and nonconsensual drug tests conducted for criminal investigatory purposes were unconstitutional searches. Respondents argued that the searches were reasonable under the "special needs" doctrine, even absent consent, because they were justified by special non–law-enforcement purposes.]

---

*121 S. Ct. 1281 (2001).

Because the hospital seeks to justify its authority to conduct drug tests and to turn the results over to law enforcement agents without the knowledge or consent of the patients, this case differs from previous cases [including *Skinner*] in which we have considered whether comparable drug tests "fit within the closely guarded category of constitutionally permissible suspicionless searches." Chandler v. Miller, 520 U.S. 305, 309 (1997). . . . In those cases, we employed a balancing test that weighed the intrusion on the individual's interest in privacy against the "special needs" that supported the program. As an initial matter, we note that the invasion of privacy in this case is far more substantial than in those cases. . . . The reasonable expectation of privacy enjoyed by the typical patient undergoing diagnostic tests in a hospital is that the results of those tests will not be shared with nonmedical personnel without her consent. In none of our prior cases was there any intrusion upon that kind of expectation.

The critical difference between those [previous] drug-testing cases and this one, however, lies in the nature of the "special need" asserted as justification for the warrantless searches. In each of those earlier cases, the "special need" that was advanced as a justification for the absence of a warrant or individualized suspicion was one divorced from the State's general interest in law enforcement. . . . In this case, however, the central and indispensable feature of the policy from its inception was the use of law enforcement to coerce the patients into substance abuse treatment.

Respondents argue in essence that their ultimate purpose—namely, protecting the health of both mother and child—is a beneficent one. . . . [H]owever, we [do] not simply accept the State's invocation of a "special need." Instead, we carry out a "close review" of the scheme at issue before concluding that the need in question was not "special," as that term has been defined in our cases. *Chandler*, 520 U.S. at 322. In this case, a review of the policy plainly reveals that the purpose actually served by the MUSC searches "is ultimately indistinguishable from the general interest in crime control." Indianapolis v. Edmond, 531 U.S. 32, 44 (2000).

In looking to the programmatic purpose, we consider all the available evidence in order to determine the relevant primary purpose. . . . Tellingly, the document codifying the policy incorporates the police's operational guidelines. It devotes its attention to the chain of custody, the range of possible criminal charges, and the logistics of police notification and arrests. Nowhere, however, does the document discuss different courses of medical treatment for either mother or infant, aside from treatment for the mother's addiction.

Moreover, throughout the development and application of the policy, the Charleston prosecutors and police were extensively involved in the day-to-day administration of the policy. Police and prosecutors decided who would receive the reports of positive drug screens and what information would be included with those reports. Law enforcement officials also helped determine the procedures to be followed when performing the screens. In the course of the policy's administration, they had access to . . . medical files on the women who tested positive, routinely attended the substance abuse team's meetings, and regularly received copies of team documents discussing the women's progress. Police took pains to coordinate the timing and circumstances of the arrests with MUSC staff. . . .

While the ultimate goal of the program may well have been to get the women in question into substance abuse treatment and off of drugs, the immediate objective of the searches was to generate evidence for law enforcement purposes in order to reach that goal. The threat of law enforcement may ultimately have been intended as a means to an end, but the direct and primary purpose of MUSC's policy was to ensure the use of those means. In our opinion, this distinction is critical. Because law enforcement involvement always serves some broader social purpose or objective, under respondents' view, virtually any nonconsensual suspicionless search could be immunized under the special needs doctrine by defining the search solely in terms of its ultimate, rather than immediate, purpose. Such an approach is inconsistent with the Fourth Amendment. Given the primary purpose of the Charleston program, which was to use the threat of arrest and prosecution in order to force women into treatment, and given the extensive involvement of law enforcement officials at every stage of the policy, this case simply does not fit within the closely guarded category of "special needs."

The fact that positive test results were turned over to the police does not merely provide a basis for distinguishing our prior cases applying the "special needs" balancing approach to the determination of drug use. It also provides an affirmative reason for enforcing the strictures of the Fourth Amendment. While state hospital employees, like other citizens, may have a duty to provide the police with evidence of criminal conduct that they inadvertently acquire in the course of routine treatment, when they undertake to obtain such evidence from their patients for the specific purpose of incriminating those patients, they have a special obligation to make sure that the patients are fully informed about their constitutional rights, as standards of knowing waiver require.

As respondents have repeatedly insisted, their motive was benign rather than punitive. Such a motive, however, cannot justify a departure from Fourth Amendment protections, given the pervasive involvement of law enforcement with the development and application of the MUSC policy. . . . While respondents are correct that drug abuse both was and is a serious problem, "the gravity of the threat alone cannot be dispositive of questions concerning what means law enforcement officers may employ to pursue a given purpose." *Edmond*, 531 U.S. at 32–33. The Fourth Amendment's general prohibition against nonconsensual, warrantless, and suspicionless searches necessarily applies to such a policy.

---

## III. MANDATORY TREATMENT

Medical treatment has transformed public health approaches to disease epidemics. Treatment not only benefits individuals by ameliorating symptoms, but also benefits society by reducing or eliminating infectiousness. But these benefits cannot occur unless individuals take their medication. Similarly, inconsistent treatment can result in drug resistance, making diseases difficult to cure. Because of the benefits to individuals and the community, and the problem of drug resistance, public health authorities have an abiding interest in compulsory treatment. However, mandatory treatment represents a serious intrusion on a person's bodily integrity. The courts are faced with the task of balancing the benefits of treatment against the autonomy of individuals (Eastman and Hope 1988).

Most public health statutes authorize mandatory treatment of contagious diseases, whether or not the person is competent to make the decision for himself. The courts consistently affirm the constitutionality of compulsory treatment of persons with infectious diseases (City of New York v. Antoinette R., excerpted in chapter 13). Although the right to refuse treatment is generally protected by the Constitution, the Supreme Court balances a person's liberty interests against relevant state interests. The Court has held that health authorities may mandate serious forms of treatment, such as antipsychotic medication, if the person poses a danger to himself or others. The treatment must be medically appropriate so that the person benefits. Washington v. Harper, 494 U.S. 210 (1990). The same constitutional standard would likely apply to mandatory treatment for an infectious disease. The state could compel such therapy, but only if the treatment reduces a significant risk of transmission and affords medical benefits to the patient.

## A. DIRECTLY OBSERVED THERAPY

The state's interest in ensuring the completion of treatment may not always require compulsory hospitalization. Treatment in the community often can be assured through directly observed therapy (DOT), commonly used in the management of TB. DOT is a compliance-enhancing strategy in which the taking of each dose of medication is observed by a family member, peer advocate, community worker, or health care professional. Supervised therapy can take place in a variety of locations, ranging from a personal residence or place of employment to a clinic, physician's office, or even a street corner. Ronald Bayer and David Wilkinson of the Columbia University School of Public Health examine the history of DOT.

## Directly Observed Therapy for Tuberculosis: History of an Idea*

*Ronald Bayer and David Wilkinson*

DOT has emerged as the standard of care in the treatment of TB in the USA. In response to the dismal record of assuring that those with TB complete their treatment, the problems of TB in persons with HIV infection, and the public alarm that attended the emergence of multidrug-resistant TB in New York, the Advisory Council for the Elimination of Tuberculosis (ACET) has recommended that DOT be considered for all patients in locales that do not achieve at least a 90% completion rate for treatment. What is so striking about these developments in public health practice is that they were so long in coming. Indeed, the idea of using DOT for all, or virtually all, patients with TB emerged more than three decades ago as a result of work in Madras and Hong Kong. [The authors discuss the history of DOT in Madras, India, and Hong Kong during the late 1950s and 1960s.] . . .

---

*Reprinted from *Lancet* 345 (June 17, 1995): 1545–48. © 1995 by The Lancet, Ltd.

## SUPERVISED THERAPY IN THE USA

While the evidence from abroad suggested that a broad application of supervised therapy was necessary, TB-control efforts in the USA all but ignored the relevance of such findings and remained focused on what insights might be relied upon to predict patient behavior and medication use, and on the importance of fashioning clinical structures and practices that would overcome noncompliance. . . .

DOT remained the exception rather than the rule in the face of evidence to support this approach in problem patients and recommendations from the CDC and the American Thoracic Society that difficult patients be placed on twice weekly supervised therapy.

What accounted for the failure to use directly supervised therapy despite the fact that at least 20–30% of patients throughout the USA failed to complete treatment within 24 months? Many health departments believed that requiring individuals to take their medication in the presence of a responsible party would entail unacceptable assumptions about the prospect of the future behavior of those under care. Rather than a service, DOT was often viewed as an imposition that could be justified only in the presence of evidence that the patient would behave in a way that posed a threat to the public health. At a later date, some argued that widespread application of DOT entailed an inversion of a basic human right by treating TB patients as guilty until proven innocent. But the most important factor was the assumption that the widescale use of supervised therapy would entail an extraordinary and unjustifiable expense. Certainly questions of cost and severe limitations on available resources were among the factors that played a part in the failure of the CDC to press publicly for the wider adoption of DOT as a practice even when some believed such a move would have salutary consequences.

There were, however, examples of successful application of DOT in the 1980s. . . . [I]n Denver, . . . an average of 60% of TB patients treated between 1973 and 1983 were supervised. More striking, there were a few locales where DOT was adopted as a universal or near universal approach in TB. . . . That these developments occurred despite limited support from federal authorities makes clear the fact that resource constraints explained only a part of the resistance in the USA to DOT. Where there was a political commitment to instituting such an approach to TB control it was possible to make substantial changes. Such commitment also required a cultural climate within which supervision of all, or nearly all, patients was not offensive. . . .

The availability of resources and the political and cultural climate surrounding TB control underwent a radical transformation in the early 1990s as a result of a rising number of cases, an increase in drug-resistance disease, and nosocomial outbreaks in hospitals. As a result of the fear that what had been a treatable disease might become an untreatable danger to middle-class populations that had in recent years been spared the threat of TB, concern took hold about the rate at which patients failed to complete their TB therapy in cities such as New York, Chicago, Newark, and Washington. Public concern and a demand for remedial action provoked Congress to greatly increase funding for TB-control efforts. . . . Central to the new commitment was a striking determination to place DOT for most if not all patients at the center of public-health efforts.

When in 1993, the ACET made DOT the standard of care, as a matter of federal policy, it turned from the decades-long efforts to identify individuals at high risk for non-compliance and more recent attempts to designate groups as being at high risk for failure to complete their TB treatment. ACET (1993, 3) stated that "DOT should be considered for all patients because of the difficulty in predicting which patients will adhere to a prescribed regimen. Decisions regarding the use of expanded or universal DOT should be based on a quantitative evaluation of local treatment completion rates." . . .

The embrace of the principle of universal or near-universal DOT by federal, state, and local health departments, has, not surprisingly, provoked opposition from some public-health officials, who believe that their own programs were effective without the need to devote resources to so labor-intensive an effort. More striking has been the criticism from those for whom civil liberties are of pre-eminent importance. Such criticisms have not opposed the universal offer of DOT, making it available to all patients as a service. Nor have they opposed the imposition of DOT by court order after patients have shown that they cannot adhere to the prescribed treatment regimen. What civil liberties groups have found appalling—a violation of the constitutional requirement that the state use the least restrictive alternative in pursuit of public-health goals—is the notion that all or nearly all patients, irrespective of behavior, should be required to ingest their medication in the presence of an observer. The designation of classes of patients—the poor, the homeless, drug users—as being at high risk for noncompliance and as requiring DOT, was viewed as particularly offensive.

Despite such objections we believe that the weight of historical evidence and recent experience make the move to DOT as a standard of care crucial. . . . As DOT programs are started or expanded, it will be necessary to determine the appropriate mix of clinic-based care and care provided by community-based outreach workers; the need for provision of housing for homeless patients; the need for drug and alcohol abuse treatment, and psychiatric services for those who are impaired; the part to be played by financial inducements for remaining in care; and the functions of court mandates and the ultimate threat of compulsory hospitalization for those who refuse to remain in treatment until cured. In short, it will be necessary to examine carefully the role of enablers and incentives. None of these studies will be simple or cheap, and all will require that resources for tuberculosis-control remain adequate, even if the number of new cases declines. Recognizing the centrality of DOT is thus just the beginning of the challenge posed by TB.

* * * * *

Bayer and Wilkinson describe the disagreement between public health advocates and civil libertarians over the use of universal DOT. Suppose that 50 percent of a group of patients with active TB will fail to complete the full course of their medication. Public health authorities could require the entire group to undergo DOT, but this would entail considerable expense and undermine civil liberties. Since half of those who would complete therapy on their own accord are nevertheless required to receive DOT, the policy is substantially overinclusive. Alternatively, the authorities could require only the "nonadherent" to undergo DOT, but this would require a prediction of who will fail to complete their medication. Conceivably, authorities could use certain proxies to make this prediction, such as whether the person is mentally ill, drug or alcohol dependent, or homeless. This approach, however, appears unfair to those who are primarily poor.

Bayer and Wilkinson (1995, 1547) adopt a utilitarian approach: "We believe that the weight of historical evidence and recent experience make the move to DOT as the standard of care crucial to the prevention of drug resistance." In a later article, Bayer and his colleagues (1998, 1056) change their position based on findings that TB medication completion rates of more than 90 percent can be attained without universal supervised therapy:

We began this study with the assumption that the arguments put forth for universal or near-universal supervised therapy possessed a powerful public health logic, one that was of sufficient moment to override some of the ethical and legal objections to the idea of mandatory therapy, the predicate of universal DOT. We assumed that . . . universal supervised therapy was the only method that would resolve the ongoing problem of treatment failure and the attendant problem of drug resistance, and that such efforts would play a crucial role in halting the rise in the incidence of TB. Furthermore, a universal approach would preclude the stigmatizing effect of identifying groups at high risk for noncompletion.

The results of our research reveal a much more nuanced picture. It is a picture that challenges the proposition that universal DOT is a necessary feature of all programs that seek to improve treatment completion rates. Equally important, it is a picture that challenges the assumption that the adoption of universal or near universal DOT is necessary or sufficient in locales that have had a long history of low treatment completion rates.

Considering the arguments on both sides, how important is universal DOT from a public health perspective, and how intrusive is DOT from a civil liberties perspective?

## B. MANDATORY TREATMENT FOR PERSONS LIVING WITH HIV/AIDS

Mandatory treatment is widely regarded as lawful and ethical when applied to persons with multidrug-resistant TB. But suppose a person with HIV infection who engages in high-risk sexual activity persistently refuses to take his medication, leading to drug-resistant strains. Would compulsory treatment be justified? If not, what distinguishes the case of TB from HIV? Consider these possibilities: TB is treatable and potentially curable, and a successful therapeutic regimen renders the person noninfectious. Additionally, the mode of transmission of TB is airborne, whereas the mode of transmission of HIV is bloodborne. How important are these differences? In answering these questions, think about modern treatments for HIV that have the potential to prolong life and reduce infectiousness.

Strong evidence exists that antiretroviral therapy administered to pregnant women can significantly reduce the risk of maternal–infant transmission of HIV (Kass 2000; Moffenson 2000). Suppose a pregnant woman rejects treatment, placing the fetus at a substantially increased risk of being born with HIV infection. Some ethicists maintain that compulsory treatment of pregnant women for HIV disease violates the principle of consent and therefore is unjustified (Bayer 1994). In balancing the bodily integrity of the mother with the health benefits to the fetus, whose interests ought to prevail? Is it fair to separate the fetus's interests from those of the mother, or are their interests inseparable?

## CONCLUSION

This chapter has discussed the central importance of biological approaches to the control of infectious disease. Americans have high confidence in the ability of science and technology to solve their most pressing social problems. But, as we have seen, immunization, screening, and treatment are not sterile scientific pursuits but are highly influenced by politics, law, and values. When these interventions are forced on unwilling individuals or populations, we have to balance public claims for collective well-being against private claims for autonomy and bodily integrity. These are the kinds of tensions that also occur with the equally contested public health interventions discussed in the next chapter: civil confinement and criminal punishment.

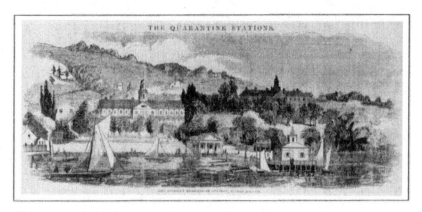

This sketch of a New York quarantine station appeared in *Harper's Weekly* in the late 1880s. It shows the various buildings and structures involved in the quarantining of immigrants and other individuals. The process began when ships entered the harbor, and it ended, for some, with the burying of those who eventually died from infectious disease. (Courtesy of the National Library of Medicine.)

# THIRTEEN

# Restrictions of the Person

*Civil Confinement
and Criminal Punishment*

Measures to control communicable diseases are not limited to biological approaches. Individuals known or suspected of being contagious may be subjected to civil confinement (isolation, quarantine, and compulsory hospitalization) or criminal punishment for knowing or willful exposure to disease. Society's methods of coping with epidemics, therefore, include separation of contagious persons from the rest of the population and punishment for engaging in risk behaviors.

We like to think that these are thoughtful public policies based solely on the sciences of public health and medicine. But the history of infectious disease control teaches a different lesson. Feelings about infectious disease are sometimes visceral—founded on fear, stereotype, and enmity. Individuals with disease are blamed for epidemics, viewed as vectors of infection rather than persons in need of care and support. During various times in history disfavored populations became targets of coercion—for example, racial or religious minorities, commercial sex workers, injecting drug users, and gay men. Animus toward those with infectious disease can be confounded with deep-seated prejudices against marginalized communities.

Even when the exercise of compulsory powers is necessary to prevent the transmission of infectious disease, it is important to consider the effects on individual freedom and dignity. Infectious disease control powers are among society's most coercive measures. Both civil confinement and criminal punishment deprive individuals of their liberty. In a democratic society, therefore, these coercive powers should be carefully justified. We have to balance the public health interests of society against the freedom of the individual.

Personal control measures also raise important issues of justice when they are directed against unpopular individuals or groups. Public health powers, like all benefits and burdens in society, need to be allocated fairly. Power exercised in an arbitrary or discriminatory manner is problematic. Recall the discussion of *Jew Ho v. Williamson* in chapter 7, where San Francisco health officials quarantined an area of the city where the Chinese-American community lived. The city exempted specific homes within the quarantine area that belonged to non-Asians.

Decisions about whether to use compulsory powers, and against which groups, are often influenced by social fears and political pressures. It is difficult to exaggerate the dread caused by disease epidemics and the destabilizing effects on people and their communities. The public places intense political pressure on elected representatives to "do something" to protect the populace. The exercise of compulsory powers represents the most visible expression of government's determination to act decisively, whether or not there is sufficient scientific evidence of effectiveness.

Epidemics, and society's response, can also powerfully affect business interests and the economy. A public health decision that a disease outbreak is the result of contaminated meat or fruit can devastate an industry. In the late 1990s, for example, North America experienced a major outbreak of cyclosporiasis (a parasitic disease that causes gastroenteritis). Public health agencies preliminarily announced that strawberries may have been a vehicle of infection, but later concluded that the source actually was raspberries. Both industries experienced a substantial loss of trade (Herwaldt et al. 1997; Osterholm 1997). Decisions to impose quarantines can also have significant economic effects, with commerce to, and from, the quarantined area significantly impeded.

The authors in this chapter discuss the history of infectious disease control, the legal powers and limits, and the influence of society, politics, and economics. This chapter begins with the most ancient and enduring response to communicable disease—crude separation of the sick from the healthy.


## I. CIVIL CONFINEMENT: ISOLATION, QUARANTINE, AND COMPULSORY HOSPITALIZATION

Public health authorities possess three overlapping powers of detention: *isolation* of known infectious persons, *quarantine* of healthy persons exposed to disease, and *civil commitment* (compulsory hospitalization) for care and treatment. (For definitions of these three forms of detention, see Table 10 in chapter 8 of the companion text [page 216].) These powers, in one form or another, have persisted since the origin of human civilization.

## A. THE HISTORY OF QUARANTINE

The prominent Yale historian David F. Musto (1986, 97) offers this description of early attempts to ward off infectious diseases:

> In ancient times citizens noted that occasionally a disease that had appeared in a distant locale was then sweeping toward them from neighboring villages, or that after a ship from a foreign land reached shore with ill persons aboard, people residing in the port city would take ill. Such temporal sequences cannot be ignored and, if the illness is a serious one, fears escalate as the illness comes closer. Knowing the cause of an illness or its mode of transmission provides some rational approach to interrupting the spread of the disease. Prior to the nineteenth century, however, those were unknowns, and so civil authorities were left with whatever means seemed reasonable in the wisdom of the time to fight the spread of diseases. Protective measures were based upon what we would now consider erroneous explanations for contagion. From this era of scant knowledge comes the origin of the familiar word we use to designate attempts to isolate the sick or contagious from the healthy: "Quarantine."

For a discussion of the historical origins of the term "quarantine," see Tandy (1923b) and Clemow (1929). In the following selection, J. M. Eager describes the ancient practices. The reading is taken from an informative report commissioned by the United States Public Health and Marine-Hospital Service. Many excellent books and articles discuss civil confinement in relation to specific diseases such as tuberculosis (TB) (Rothman 1994), sexually transmitted disease (Brandt 1987), and cholera (Rosenberg 1987).

---

**The Early History of Quarantine:**
**Origin of Sanitary Measures Directed against Yellow Fever\***
*J. M. Eager*

The history of quarantine is closely interwoven with that of medicine in general and of shipping. . . . The story of the beginnings of quarantine is associated particularly with the epidemiology of leprosy, pest, and syphilis. Cholera and yellow fever were later considerations. . . .

---

\*Washington, D.C., Government Printing Office, 1903.

## LEPROSY AND LAND QUARANTINES

The first quarantines of which any mention is made in literature were land quarantines used as a protection against leprosy. The ancients regarded this disease as of African origin, and Lucretius states positively that it first came from Egypt. In the Old Testament the first indications are found of precautions taken against contagious maladies. Leviticus, Numbers, and the First Book of Samuel give directions for the sequestration of lepers, first in the desert, then outside the camp, and afterwards without the walls of Jerusalem. In these books the inspection of persons for the detection of leprosy is detailed. Persons afflicted with skin diseases were directed to present themselves before the priests. An observation of each case was made, and, according to minutely described symptoms, isolation of the patients was ordered for a prescribed period.

The crusaders on their arrival outside the walls of Jerusalem found lazarettoes still in existence, and after taking the city from the Mussulmans sent all contagious maladies to these isolated places. The name Hospital of St. Lazarus was given to the place of sequestration. Returning to Europe, the members of the military expeditions brought back with them not only numerous diseases, but also the word "lazaretto," as applied to a place for the isolation of the victims of communicable maladies. As a result lazarettoes were built outside the gates of nearly all the principal cities of Europe. Leprosy itself had, however, been introduced into Europe many centuries earlier. It is spoken of as a foreign disease by the earlier Greek and Latin writers. . . .

Lepers were not strictly confined to the leper houses. They were, however, required to wear a special costume, to limit their walks to certain roads, to give warning of their approach by sounding a clapper, and to forbear communicating with healthy persons and drinking from or bathing in any running stream.

## PEST AND EARLY VIEWS OF ETIOLOGY

By the word pest is understood not only bubonic plague, but the different epidemic diseases, whatever they may have been, that were formerly included under that term. . . . The word plague as well as pest was given by ancient medical writers to any epidemic disease that wrought in extensive destruction of life. . . . Throughout all this extensive period notions and practices relating to public sanitation were being evolved in accordance with the prevalent tenets of causation. . . .

[The author discusses the various theories of the etiology of disease, ranging from spiritual causes and corruption of the soil or water to the theory of contagion, including the views of Hippocrates, Galen, and Fracastoro.]

## MARITIME QUARANTINE

Maritime quarantine originated in connection with the Levantine trade. Its early history is associated with that of shipping in the Mediterranean, especially with that of the traffic of Venice, Genoa, and Marseille. . . . As has been seen, the practice of isolation was first applied against communicable disease by the Hebrews, but the lazarettoes, it appears, were little used in connection with foreign trade, leaving out of the question commerce by sea. . . .

## EARLY MARITIME SANITARY LAWS

The Venetians were, it is generally admitted, the first to make provision for maritime sanitation. As far back as the year 1000 there were overseers of public health, but at first the office was not a permanent one. The incumbents were appointed to serve during the prevalence of an epidemic only. The first information we have of this kind of public office is under date of 1348, when Nicolaus Venerio, Marinus Querino, and Paulus Belegno (their Christian names given in the Latin of the text) were appointed overseers of public health. These officers were authorized to spend public money for the purpose of isolating infected ships, goods, and persons at an island of the lagoon. A medical man was stationed with the sick. As a later result of these arrangements, the first thoroughly constituted maritime quarantine station of which there is historical record was established in 1403 on the island of Santa Maria di Nazareth, at Venice. . . .

Neighboring States engaged in commerce in the Mediterranean speedily followed the example of Venice. . . . It was not until 1459 that a public bureau of sanitation existed in the Republic of Venice. In that year officers, called conservators of sanitation, were regularly appointed. . . .

During all this period land quarantines were in operation at times of pest. Offenses against quarantine, both land and maritime, were severely punished. Pietro Follerio, a great Neapolitan jurisconsult of the sixteenth century, mentions whipping, the mill, exile, and death as penalties for infringement of sanitary regulations. . . . Torture, long service in the galleys, and work among the sick in a pest hospital are named among the penalties. . . .

## BILLS OF HEALTH

Sanitary bulletins were incident to quarantines and cordons. They were so called because they were stamped with the "bollo" or seal of the authority issuing them. When the system of sanitary bulletins was fully developed these patients, in their connection with ships, were designated as clean, when beyond suspicion; touched, when from a non-infected place in active communication with infected places; suspicious, without sickness aboard, but having received goods from places or from ships or caravans from places where pest prevailed; and dirty, when from a place where disease existed. . . . During the pest at Naples, in the year 1557, citizens, usually merchants, were stationed at the gates of the city to examine bills of health. Corruption and lack of diligence on the part of these persons were punishable by death. Sentinels, some on foot and some on horseback, made a patrol about the city walls to prevent clandestine entrance. Bills of health to be acceptable had to be stamped with the seal of the university of the place from which the traveler came. They gave not only the day but the hour of departure, together with a description of the traveler. Sanitary bulletins were also issued to accompany merchandise, but in times of severe pest all articles except aromatics and medicaments were considered suspicious. . . .

## FURTHER HISTORY OF QUARANTINE

Without touching on quarantine in America, which is another and interesting story, it is profitable to take a view of the further history of quarantine in Europe. Following the discovery by Anthony van Leeuwenhoek, in 1675, of bacteria, called by him "animalcules," there was a wide belief in the casual connection of microscopic creatures with disease, a belief supported by the doctrine of living contagion enunciated by Marcus Antonius Plenciz, of Vienna, in 1762, but it was without marked effect on quarantine procedure. The theory, in fact, lost hold on the public and medical minds to such an extent that in the early part of the nineteenth century the doctrine of a living contagion was looked upon as an absurd assumption. It was not until the middle of the last century, following the investigations of Pasteur, Pollender, and Bavaine, that quarantine practice became established on its modern scientific basis. . . .

[The author discusses quarantine procedure in Europe in the eighteenth century.]

The international sanitary conferences at Paris in 1851 and 1852, in which participated the different European powers having interests in the Mediterranean, marked the close of the old regime of quarantine. . . . England was not signatory. [Lax r]egulations were adopted . . . , it being admitted that the efficacy of many measures formerly practiced was doubtful or negative, science having proclaimed that, for the most part, pestilential maladies are not contagious. This surprising declaration was followed by a revolution in quarantine methods on the Continent and resulted in the general adoption of practices based on the limited communicability of epidemic diseases. These changes, with which the early history of quarantine closes, were brought into effect at the beginning of the new era, during which the doctrine of specific living causes of epidemic diseases have been built up on the substantial basis of experimental medicine.

---

## B. JUDICIAL REVIEW OF CIVIL CONFINEMENT: THE EARLY CASES

As the excerpt by Eager illustrates, the practice of quarantine predates the founding of the republic and continues to modern times. For a discussion of quarantine law in the United States, see Parmet (1985) and Merritt (1986). In the early twentieth century, the courts adopted a permissive approach to quarantine, as the following two state supreme court decisions illustrate. Both cases reveal stereotypical attitudes based on gender and race.

---

### Kirk v. Wyman*
*Supreme Court of South Carolina*
*Decided August 19, 1909*

Judge ALDRICH delivered the opinion of the court.

[The city of Aiken, South Carolina, found that Mary Kirk had contagious leprosy and required her to be isolated in the city hospital for infectious diseases. Kirk claimed that although she had leprosy, she was

---

*65 S.E. 387 (S.C. 1909).

not dangerous to the community. Additionally, she complained that the hospital where she was to be placed was really a "pesthouse, coarse and comfortless" and used for "incarcerating negroes having small-pox and other dangerous infectious diseases." She further objected to her isolation because of the odors coming from the city dumping ground near the hospital. She was granted a temporary injunction. The Board of Health appealed, claiming that she was a danger to community, that they had sought measures to improve the hospital and would eventually provide a private cottage for her, and that the city dump was located nearby but did not contain foul deposits.]

Municipal boards of health . . . are to be considered as deriving their authority to isolate infected persons . . . from section 1099 of the Civil Code, which provides:

> The said board of health shall have power and it shall be their duty to make and enforce all needful rules and regulations to prevent the introduction and spread of infectious or contagious diseases by the regulation of intercourse with infected places, by the arrest, separation, and treatment of infected persons, and persons who shall have been exposed to any contagious or infectious diseases. . . . They shall also have power, with the consent of the town or city council, in case of the prevalence of any contagious or infectious diseases within the town or city, to establish one or more hospitals and to make provisions and regulations for the management of the same. . . .

The principles of constitutional law governing health regulations by statute and municipal ordinance may be thus stated:

First. Statutes and ordinances requiring the removal or destruction of property or the isolation of infected persons, when necessary for the protection of the public health, do not violate the constitutional guaranty of the right of the enjoyment of liberty and property, because neither the right to liberty nor the right of property extends to the use of liberty or property to the injury of others. . . . The individual has no more right to the freedom of spreading disease by carrying contagion on his person, than he has to produce disease by maintaining his property in a noisome condition.

Second. The state must of necessity lodge the power somewhere to ascertain, in the first instance, and act with promptness, when the public health is endangered by the unhealthful condition of the person or the property of the individual; and the creation by legislative authority of boards of health, with the discretion lodged in them of summary inquiry and action, is a reasonable exercise of the police power. . . .

Third. Arbitrary power over persons and property could not be conferred on a board of health, and no attempt is made in the Constitution or statutes to confer such power. . . . It is always implied that the power conferred to interfere with these personal rights is limited by public necessity. From this it follows that boards of health may not deprive any person of his property or his liberty, unless the deprivation is . . . reasonably necessary to the public health; and such inquiry must include notice to the person whose property or liberty is involved, and the opportunity to him to be heard, unless the emergency appears to be so great that such notice and hearing could be had only at the peril of the public safety.

Fourth. To the end that personal liberty and property may be protected against invasion not essential to the public health—not required by public necessity—the regulations and proceedings of boards of health are subject to judicial review, by an action for damages or for injunction or other appropriate proceeding, according to the circumstances. In passing upon such regulations and proceedings, the courts consider, first, whether interference with personal liberty or property was reasonably necessary to the public health, and, second, if the means used and the extent of the interference were reasonably necessary for the accomplishment of the purpose to be attained.

Fifth. . . . [T]he courts must determine whether there is any real relation between the preservation of the public health and the legislative enactment, or the regulations and proceedings of boards of health under authority of the statute. If the statute or the regulations made or the proceedings taken under it are not reasonably appropriate to the end in view, the necessity for curtailment of individual liberty, which is essential to the validity of such statutes and regulations and proceedings, is wanting, and the courts must declare them invalid, as violative of constitutional right. . . .

In applying these principles, it is to be borne in mind that the case under consideration is unusual, imposing upon the Aiken board of health a delicate and unpleasant duty. Miss Kirk is not only a lady of refinement, highly esteemed in the community, but she is quite advanced in years. The proceedings of the board show clearly their solicitude to treat Miss Kirk with courtesy and consideration. . . .

That Miss Kirk is afflicted with anaesthetic leprosy contracted while engaged in missionary work in Brazil is admitted. While there is a strong showing that the anaesthetic form of the disease is only slightly contagious, when the distressing nature of the malady is regarded, it is manifest that the board were well within their duty in requiring the victim of it to be isolated. The case then turns on whether, under the principles above stated, . . . the manner of the isolation was so clearly beyond what was necessary to the public protection that the court ought to enjoin it as arbitrary. . . . [T]here is hardly any danger of contagion from Miss Kirk, except by touch, or at least close personal association. What is more important than these opinions is the uncontroverted fact that Miss Kirk has for many years lived in the city of Aiken, attended church services, taught in the Sunday school, mingled freely with the people in social life, resting on the opinion of Dr. Hutchinson, a distinguished London specialist, that her disease was not contagious, and in all that time there has been nothing to indicate that she has imparted the disease to any other person. Was there any necessity to send such a patient to the pesthouse? The board of health had established a strict quarantine of her dwelling, and there was no evidence that Miss Kirk had made any effort to violate it. The maintenance of this quarantine, we cannot doubt, afforded complete protection to the public. It is true the board could not be expected to maintain a permanent quarantine of a house in the heart of the city of Aiken; but the city council had agreed to build for the purpose of isolation a comfortable cottage outside of the city limits, which could have been completed in a short time.

There is some conflict in the affidavits as to the condition of the pesthouse; but it is not denied that it is a structure of four small rooms in a row, with no piazzas, used heretofore for the isolation of negroes with smallpox, situated within a hundred yards of the place where the trash of the city, except its offensive offal, is collected and burned. The smoke from this pile is blown through the house. The board of health, it is true, have made it less uncomfortable by painting and some other work; but, with this improvement, we are forced to the conclusion that even temporary isolation in such a place would be a serious affliction and peril to an elderly lady, enfeebled by disease, and accustomed to the comforts of life. Nothing but necessity would justify the board of health in requiring it, and we think . . . there was no good reason to conclude that such necessity existed.

---

## Ex parte Company*
Supreme Court of Ohio
Decided December 5, 1922

Judge CLARK delivered the opinion of the court.

[Defendants Martha Company and Irene Irvin were arrested, on separate occasions, on the charge of violating § 13031-13 of the

---

*139 N.E. 204 (Ohio 1922).

Ohio General Code (including prostitution, lewdness, and assignation). While in custody, both were found to have sexually transmitted diseases (syphilis and gonorrhea). The commissioner of health of the city of Akron confined them in their detention home under a quarantine for approximately two months (the time necessary to render each noninfectious through treatment). The defendants filed writs of habeas corpus to protest that their detention violated their constitutional right to due process. Refusing the writs, the Supreme Court of Ohio upheld the state statute permitting the detention of the defendants as a legitimate exercise of the state's police powers.]

Regulation 2 of the Sanitary Code . . . named, classified, and declared dangerous to the public health certain diseases and disabilities, . . . includ[ing] . . . chancroid, gonorrhea, and syphilis. Regulation 18 of the Sanitary Code declares such diseases to be contagious, infectious, communicable, and dangerous to the public health. Regulation 23 empowers the health commissioner of each city to make examination of persons reasonably suspected of having a venereal disease. All known prostitutes and persons associating with them shall be considered as reasonably suspected of having a venereal disease. Regulation 24 provides that the health commissioner may quarantine any person who has, or is reasonably suspected of having, a venereal disease, whenever in his opinion quarantine is necessary for the protection of the public health. . . .

The right of the state through the exercise of its police power to subject persons and property to reasonable and proper restraints in order to secure the general comfort, health, and prosperity of the state is no longer open to question. In the American constitutional system the power to establish the necessary police regulations has been left with the several states. . . . The regulations here under consideration, if otherwise lawful, are not in conflict with any provision of the federal or state Constitutions.

It is urged that the Sanitary Code, and the particular regulations in question, are in opposition to and violative of subsection c of § 13031-17 [which states] . . . :

> Any person charged with a violation of § 13031-13 of the General Code, shall, upon the order of the court having jurisdiction of such case, be subjected to examination to determine if such person is infected with a venereal disease. . . . No person charged with a violation of § 13031-13 of the General Code shall be discharged from custody, paroled or placed on probation if he or she

has a venereal disease in an infective stage unless the court having jurisdiction shall be assured that such person will continue medical treatment until cured or rendered noninfectious.

In the cases here considered it is to be observed that both of the petitioners were charged with violations of § 13031-13. Regulation 24 provides that such infected persons shall be subject to quarantine. The statutory provision is that such infected persons shall not be discharged from custody, paroled, or placed on probation. No inconsistency is found as between the regulations complained of and the provisions of subsection c of § 13031-17. In either event quarantine is established. Quarantine in the sense herein used means detention to the point of preserving the infected person from contact with others. The power to so quarantine in proper case and reasonable way is not open to question. It is exercised by the state and the subdivisions of the state daily. The protection of the health and lives of the public is paramount, and those who by conduct and association contract such disease as makes them a menace to the health and morals of the community must submit to such regulation as will protect the public. . . .

The right to quarantine by exclusion has been upheld in the recent case of *Zucht v. King* [excerpted in chapter 12]. . . .

It is our conclusion that the provisions of §§ 1232, 1234, 1235, and 1236, General Code, creating a state department of health, a public health council, and authorizing such public health council "to make and amend sanitary regulations to be of general application throughout the state," and to provide for the certification, publication, and enforcement of such regulations, is a lawful and valid exercise of legislative power.

---

\*     \*     \*     \*     \*

The Ohio Supreme Court upheld a quarantine regulation that "all known prostitutes and people associated with them shall be considered as reasonably suspected of having a venereal disease." "Suspect conduct and association" were deemed sufficient to justify imposing control measures. An Illinois court accepted similarly unfounded assumptions: "suspected" prostitutes were considered "natural subjects and carriers of venereal disease," making it "logical and natural that suspicion be cast upon them." People *ex rel.* Baker v. Strautz, 54 N.E.2d 441, 444 (Ill. 1944).

## C. JUDICIAL REVIEW OF CIVIL CONFINEMENT: MODERN STANDARDS

Although modern public health authorities exercise compulsory powers much less frequently than those of the past, they sometimes still detain persons with infectious disease. The Gillis W. Long Hansen's Disease Center, called the "Louisiana Leper Home" or "Carville," closed in 1998. The center was used as a place of residence and treatment of persons with leprosy (Jauhar 1998). Additionally, many states still maintain places for the treatment of TB (Gasner et al. 1999; Oscherwitz et al. 1997). Edward W. Campion (1999), an editor of the *New England Journal of Medicine*, comments on the use of legal action, including mandatory detention, in New York City to control multidrug-resistant tuberculosis (MDR-TB):

> To be effective, TB-control programs must be able to get nearly every patient to complete the full course of antituberculosis-drug therapy, but full compliance with a multidrug regimen lasting for months is notoriously difficult. Even with directly controlled therapy, which is now used widely, patients sometimes stop cooperating or just disappear. In response to the resurgence of TB in New York City, the commissioner of health was given added powers, including the power to detain patients, not only while they were infectious but also, if necessary, until they completed a full course of treatment. Sending patients to a locked facility for treatment is an extreme measure, and the threat to civil liberties is particularly serious since most of the patients likely to receive such orders are impoverished and powerless. . . .
>
> Over a period of two years there were more than 8000 patients with active TB, and legal orders to complete treatment were issued to only about 4 percent. Most of those patients had alcoholism or used illicit drugs. Many had histories of homelessness or imprisonment, and most had left hospitals against medical advice in the past. More than half the orders issued were simply for directly observed therapy in the community. But 139 people were detained for treatment of TB, and most of these patients were kept on the secure ward of a hospital for about six months. The special ward has exercise and recreation facilities and is not a prison, but patients are forced to live there, away from their neighborhoods and families. As one of these patients described it, a major hardship of mandatory confinement is "being bored like an oyster."

How would the modern courts review public health practices such as the detention of persons with TB? The judiciary uses a heightened standard of review, but still almost invariably upholds the exercise of public health powers. The Supreme Court, in an analogous context, held that civil commitment of the mentally ill constitutes a "massive curtailment of liberty." Vitek v. Jones, 445 U.S. 480, 491 (1980). To justify confinement the courts probably would require the state to demonstrate a substantial interest in preventing the spread of disease, a well-targeted intervention that was not overinclusive, and that loss of liberty was the least restrictive alternative.

The modern courts are also process oriented and would require fair procedures before permitting civil confinement. As the Supreme Court recognized, "There can be no doubt that involuntary commitment to a mental hospital, like involuntary confinement of an individual for any reason, is a deprivation of liberty which the State cannot accomplish without due process of law." O'Connor v. Donaldson, 422 U.S. 563, 580 (1975) (Berger, C.J., concurring). In *Greene v. Edwards* (excerpted in chapter 7) the West Virginia Supreme Court reasoned that there is little difference between loss of liberty for mental health reasons and loss of liberty for public health rationales. Persons with an infectious disease, therefore, are entitled to similar procedural protections as persons with mental illness facing civil commitment, including the right to counsel and a hearing. Such rigorous procedural protections are justified by the fundamental invasion of liberty occasioned by long-term detention, the serious implications of erroneously finding a person dangerous, and the value of procedures in accurately determining the complex facts that are important to predicting future dangerous behavior (see discussion of *Mathews v. Eldridge* in chapter 7).

In the following case, a New York trial court authorized the isolation of a person with TB. Notice that the court is deferential to public health authorities, but insists that the state must have a substantial public health interest and afford the individual a fair process. *See* New York v. Franklin, 205 A.D.2d 469 (N.Y. App. Div. 1994) (upholding isolation to prevent the spread of MDR-TB, but only after finding that it was the least restrictive alternative).

---

### City of New York v. Antoinette R.*
*Supreme Court, Queens County*
*Decided April 21, 1995*

Judge McGANN delivered the opinion of the court.

[The city health commissioner sought enforcement of order requiring forcible detention in a hospital setting of a person (Antoinette R.) with ac-

---

*630 N.Y.S.2d 1008 (S. Ct. Queens Cty. 1995).

tive, infectious TB. The purpose of the detention was to allow for completion of an appropriate regime of medical treatment. The court found in favor of detention despite evidence regarding Antoinette's recent cooperation in adhering to a voluntary treatment regime.]

Due to a resurgence of TB, New York City recently revised the Health Code to permit the detention of individuals infected with TB who have demonstrated an inability to voluntarily comply with appropriate medical treatment. Thus, effective April 29, 1993, New York City Health Code § 11.47 was amended to give the Commissioner of Health the authority to issue an order for the removal or detention in a hospital or other treatment facility of a person who has active TB. The prerequisite for an order is that there is a substantial likelihood, based on the person's past or present behavior, that the individual cannot be relied upon to participate in or complete an appropriate prescribed course of medication or, if necessary, follow required contagion precautions for TB. Such behavior may include the refusal or failure to take medication or to complete treatment for TB, to keep appointments for the treatment of TB, or a disregard for contagion precautions.

The statute provides certain due process safeguards when detention is ordered. For example, there are requirements for an appraisal of the risk posed to others and a review of less restrictive alternatives which were attempted or considered. Furthermore, there must be a court review within five days at the patient's request, and court review within sixty days and at ninety-day intervals thereafter. The detainee also has the right to counsel, to have counsel provided, and to have friends or relatives notified. . . .

When [TB] initially becomes active, it is often highly infectious, that is, capable of being transmitted to others. A person with infectious TB can normally be rendered non-infectious within days to weeks. Thereafter, the individual must continue to take a full course of medication, generally for six to nine months, to cure the active TB. If a patient stops taking the appropriate medication before the expiration of these six to nine months, however, that patient will likely become infectious again. Moreover, when the medical regime is interrupted, and the TB resurges in an infectious state, the organisms in the individual's system may eventually mutate and become resistant to the original drugs prescribed. The more times medication is suspended, the more likely is the chance of developing a strain of TB which is resistant to drugs.

These multi-drug resistant strains of TB stay infectious and active over longer periods of time and therefore require long-term treatment with more toxic drugs. By comparison, the standard treatment for non-resistant TB consists of administering two drugs, isoniazid and rifampin, for approximately six months until the patient is cured. The cure rate for those completing this treatment is considered 100%. MDR-TB, on the other hand, is resistant to these drugs and to as many as seven other antibiotics. To obtain a cure rate of 60% or less, toxic drugs must be maintained over a minimum period of eighteen to twenty-four months. . . . The most critical characteristic of these MDR strains is that they are capable of being transmitted directly to others during the infectious stage. . . .

The Board recognized that the failure of a TB patient to complete an effective course of therapy creates the likelihood of relapse and facilitates development of drug resistant strains of the disease. The Board therefore decreed that the refusal or failure of TB patients, whether or not infectious, to complete a course of anti-TB therapy creates a significant threat to the public health. Accordingly, the New York City Health Code was amended to allow the Commissioner to issue orders of detention [through] . . . an application to the court for enforcement . . . [based on] clear and convincing evidence [of] the particularized circumstances constituting the necessity for the detention. . . .

The [Commissioner's] request for enforcement of the order . . . is granted. The [Commissioner] has demonstrated through clear and convincing evidence the respondent's inability to comply with a prescribed course of medication in a less restrictive environment. . . . [Antoinette R.] has repeatedly sought medical treatment for the infectious stages of the disease and has consistently withdrawn from medical treatment once symptoms abate. She has also exhibited a pattern of behavior which is consistent with one who does not understand the full import of her condition nor the risks she poses to others, both the public and her family. On the contrary, she has repeatedly tried to hide the history of her condition from medical personnel. Although the court is sympathetic to the fact that she has recently undergone an epiphany of sorts, there is nothing in the record which would indicate that once she leaves the controlled setting of the hospital she would have the self-discipline to continue her cooperation. Moreover, her past behavior and lack of compliance with outpatient treatment when her listed residence was her mother's house, makes it all the more difficult to have confidence that her mother's good intentions will prevail over the respondent's inclinations to avoid treatments. In any event, the court will reevaluate the progress of the respondent's ability to cooperate in a less restrictive setting during its next review of the order in ninety days.

Accordingly, [Antoinette R.] shall continue to be detained in a hospital setting until [she] . . . has completed an appropriate course of medication for TB, or a change in circumstances indicates that the respondent can be relied upon to complete the prescribed course of medication without being in detention.

---

\*          \*          \*          \*          \*

During the first decades of the HIV/AIDS epidemic, commentators urged public health authorities to employ their powers of detention. See, for example, Buckley (1986) and Grutsch and Robertson (1986). At least two forms of detention could have been used: *status-based,* applying to all persons with HIV infection or AIDS, and *behavior-based,* applying only to persons with HIV/AIDS who engage in specified high-risk behaviors. A status-based program would have been highly impractical, potentially affecting hundreds of thousands of Americans. A behavior-based program would have granted public health authorities wide discretion, enabling them to target vulnerable groups such as gay men or commercial sex workers. What are the principal arguments, for and against, isolation of persons living with HIV/AIDS? For a discussion, see Bayer and Fairchild-Carrino (1993), Sullivan and Field (1988), and Gostin (1989).

## II. THE CRIMINAL LAW:
## KNOWING OR WILLFUL EXPOSURE TO INFECTION

---

### Nushawn's Girls*
*Jennifer Frey*

It has been two years since Andrea last gave herself to Nushawn Williams. She has traded the drugs and the parties and the jail cells for a room in her mother's middle-class house. Her belly is eight months swollen. . . .

---

*Reprinted from *Washington Post,* June 1, 1999, C2.

Andrea—who asked that her last name not be revealed—is 19 now, and she has a new boyfriend named Angel, and they are thrilled to have a baby on the way. She is happy, after a lifetime of unhappiness. And she is furious. Furious at [Nushawn] Williams, the man who infected her—and 12 other young women in rural Chautauqua County [New York]—with HIV, the virus that causes AIDS. Furious that he received only a 4-to-12-year sentence for his actions. Furious at herself for taking the risks she took with a drug dealer from Brooklyn, a man she never even loved. "If I could take back one moment in my life," she says, "it would be the moment I laid eyes on him.". . . .

[Andrea] became one of "Nushawn's girls," as the young women now are commonly known here. Nushawn's girls: Four have had babies, two more—including Andrea—are pregnant, and none are sick yet, unless you count the sickness that is regret. The youngest was 13 when she met Williams, the oldest in her mid-twenties. Andrea was 17. He wooed her the way he wooed many of the others: He bought her nice presents. He told her she had pretty eyes. He took her to parties. He let her move in.

He also treated her like a possession, according to Andrea, slapping her around if she so much as went to the store for a soda without his permission. Andrea says, "I hated having sex with him." She says he had sex with other women while she was with him. Still, she stayed for a while. Because it was exciting. Because he made her feel special, if only for a moment.

"There are Nushawns in every city waiting for girls like Andrea," says her mother, Wendy. "This is about frustrated lives festering with all sorts of problems. Once you are hopeless, and have no more dreams, then you don't give a damn about what you do to yourself. You live for the moment." . . .

When the Williams story made national news in October 1997, it became, as one AIDS educator described it, "a teachable moment." What happened here was supposed to serve as proof that AIDS can happen to anyone, anywhere. . . .

This, then, is a story not just about Jamestown [in Chautauqua County] but about the legacy of AIDS. What Jamestown can show is that—no matter the place, no matter the people—AIDS still brings denial, displacement and blame.

It was Oct. 27, 1997, when Richard Berke, the county health commissioner, held a news conference to announce to the world that Chautauqua County had been home to a one-man HIV epidemic named Nushawn Williams. In this county of 141,000, there had been just 60 reported cases of full-blown AIDS since 1981. So when several teenage girls popped up HIV-positive in a short period of time, the health department took notice.

It took a while to trace them back to Williams. He used so many aliases—Face, Shyteek, Headteck, Shoe—that it wasn't until Berke got to the sixth girl that he realized the connection. It's a connection he probably couldn't have made if Chautauqua were a bigger county, with more clinics and more HIV cases and more counselors. It's a place where Berke didn't have to walk more than few hundred yards to talk to the judge who let him publicly reveal Williams's HIV status by deeming Williams a "public health risk."

So Berke held his news conference. Officials papered the county with posters bearing Williams's likeness and the message "Health Alert." And chaos hit. . . . More than 1,400 individuals—many of them teenagers—flocked to local clinics for testing. . . .

Williams had identified 48 sexual partners to Chautauqua County health officials. Of those 48, 41 were eventually tested. Thirteen turned up positive—seven infected by Williams before he knew his own HIV status, according to Berke, and the other six afterward. One man also is believed to have been infected by one of those women. And one baby, thus far, has been born with HIV. . . .

The information about [Nushawn's girls] is sketchy. . . . "They probably fit the profile of the people we've been having trouble reaching all along," Berke says. "Because of the chaos in their own lives—kids who are up all night, alcohol, abuse, all kinds of situations—the message may not be making it. Or the message may be making it, but it's not all that relevant to their life." . . .

Then there are the babies. Four born, two on the way. [O]ne who has tested HIV-positive. . . . It's not so amazing to Heather Watts, a medical officer at the National Institutes of Health who specializes in pediatric and maternal AIDS and has treated numerous pregnant women who are HIV-positive. Watts says that the average rate of infection from mother to child is 25 percent, but that it can be reduced to 5 to 8 percent with proper drug treatments, and in cases like Andrea's, where the mother has a low level of the virus in her blood, it can be as low as 2 percent.

"Many make informed decisions," Watts says. "I think it's analogous to genetic diseases before we had the more sophisticated tests. It's a powerful pull, the desire to procreate. People take risks."

Ask Andrea why she wants a child and she says, "In case I get sick." Ask her to elaborate and she says, "You know, so I have something to leave behind." Mostly though, Andrea refuses to talk about the possibility of getting full-blown AIDS.

Her denial is not uncommon. Two of the other young women have stopped taking their medication. One cut off contact with her doctors after she had a baby, and the baby tested negative. . . .

There were a few concrete changes that came out of what happened here. Youth outreach programs were formed and a daylong teen summit held, and there are plans for a teen center. People no longer go through the back basement door to get to AIDS Community Services in the old mansion at Fifth and Main streets. AIDS is no longer a secret here. But it's still a curse. . . .

Much energy has been directed toward passing laws that will make it easier to punish the Nushawn Williamses of the world (Williams pleaded guilty to one count of statutory rape and one count of reckless endangerment). . . .

This is the legacy of AIDS: People may say, "AIDS can happen to anyone," but deep inside they're still thinking, "It can't happen to me." There's always a way to make it about someone else. Gays. Drug users. People who hang out with gays and drug users. Blacks and Hispanics in big-city ghettos. White trash.

---

\*     \*     \*     \*     \*

There is a powerful appeal in using the criminal law to prosecute individuals who knowingly or willfully risk transmission of an infectious disease. The public views individuals who engage in this behavior as morally blameworthy and supports criminal sanctions for aberrant and irresponsible conduct. The criminal law deters risk behavior and sets a clear standard for behaviors that society will not tolerate.

The criminal law is backward looking, concerned with punishing individuals for dangerous acts that have already occurred. Civil confinement, on the other hand, is forward looking, concerned with averting risk behavior that may occur in the future. Many scholars believe that the criminal law is clearer and more objective than civil detention. Whereas civil confinement often uses broad standards, such as "dangerousness," the criminal law must specify the behavior that is prohibited. Whereas "dangerousness" need only be proved by clear and convincing evidence, each element of a crime must be proved beyond a reasonable doubt. Whereas the period of civil confinement is indefinite, the period of criminal confinement is usually finite and proportionate to the gravity of the offense.

There are two kinds of charges that can be filed against persons who risk transmission of an infectious disease: traditional crimes of violence and public health offenses (Hodge and Gostin 2001). This section discusses each of these aspects of the criminal law and concludes with a critique, arguing that criminal prosecutions often can be both unfair and ineffective as a public health intervention.

## A. TRADITIONAL CRIMES OF VIOLENCE

The traditional crimes of violence that can be read to apply to the transmission of an infectious disease are homicide (actual and attempted) and assault. Murder prosecutions resulting from transmission of an infectious disease are rare because they require the death of the victim. Infectious diseases often do not result in death and, if they do, the length of time from infection to death usually precludes prosecution. Additionally, homicide requires proof of causation, and it may be difficult to demonstrate that the person contracted the infection from the defendant.

Prosecutions for attempted murder also should be rare and difficult to prove. As Kathleen Sullivan and Martha Field (1988, 163) observe, "having sex or sharing needles is a highly indirect modus operandi for the person whose purpose is to kill." Nevertheless, attempted homicide charges have been brought for a broad range of conduct.

The criminal law uses a subjective standard for criminal attempts so that if the facts are as the person believes them to be, it is an offense. This is important in the infectious disease context because a person could be convicted of attempted murder if his intent is to kill, regardless of whether the method used poses a significant risk of transmission. Under this theory, the Indiana Court of Appeals upheld the conviction for attempted murder of a person infected with HIV for splattering emergency workers with his blood. See *State v. Haines*, which follows. Other courts have upheld convictions for attempted murder for other low-risk acts of aggression such as biting and spitting. *See, e.g.,* State v. Smith, 621 A.2d 493 (N.J. Super. Ct. 1993); Weeks v. State, 834 S.W.2d 559 (Tx. Ct. App. 1992).

A simple assault is a purposeful, knowing, or reckless infliction of bodily injury. Defendants with infectious diseases who engage in harmful behavior, such as biting or throwing body fluids, have been convicted of assault instead of attempted murder. The crime becomes aggravated assault if the person causes a "serious" bodily injury or uses a "deadly weapon." In *United States v. Sturgis,* excerpted later, a federal court of

appeals upheld the conviction of an inmate for aggravated assault, holding that teeth, under certain circumstances, can constitute a deadly
weapon. *See also* United States v. Moore, 846 F.2d 1163 (8th Cir. 1988).

---

### State v. Haines*
*Indiana Court of Appeals*
*Decided October 31, 1989*

Judge BUCHANAN delivered the opinion of the court.

On August 6, 1987, in Lafayette, Indiana, two police officers went to
Haines' apartment in response to a possible suicide. The officers found
Haines face down in blood, unconscious, with both writs slashed and
bleeding. Haines then stood and ran towards one officer, Dennis, screaming that he should be left to die because he had AIDS. The police officers
tried to subdue him but Haines continued to fight and stated he would
"give it to him" and "use his wounds" as he jerked his arms, causing blood
to go into the officers mouth and eyes. He repeatedly yelled that he had
AIDS and could not deal with it and would make Dennis deal with it.

Haines also struggled with emergency medical technicians, threatening to infect them with AIDS and continued to spit, bite, scratch, and
grab the personnel until several were bleeding from scratches and
scrapes on their arms and hands. Upon arrival to the hospital, Haines
was still kicking, screaming, throwing blood, and spitting and again announced he had AIDS and was going to show everyone else what it was
like to have the disease and die, again biting a person.

Haines' homosexual [partner] recalled that a doctor had informed
Haines that he had the virus and Haines told him he knew it was a fatal
disease and at the time warned medical staff not to touch him because
he was diseased.

Haines was charged with three counts of attempted murder. At trial,
medical experts testified that the virus could be transmitted through
blood, tears, and saliva. They also observed that policemen, firemen, and
other emergency personnel are generally at risk when they are exposed to
body products. One medical expert observed that Dennis was definitely
exposed to the HIV virus and others acknowledged that exposure of in-

---

*545 N.E.2d 834 (Ind. Ct. App. 1989).

fected blood to the eyes and the mouth is dangerous, and that it is easier for the virus to enter the blood stream if there is a cut in the skin. . . .

[The State of Indiana appeals from the trial court's grant of Haines' motion for judgment on the evidence, claiming that the trial judge erred in vacating the jury's verdicts of three counts of attempted murder and entering judgments of conviction as to three counts of battery, a class D felony. The State also alleges that the trial court erred in excluding the testimony of two physicians.]

The only issue before us is whether the trial court erred in granting Haines' motion for judgment on the evidence vacating the three counts of attempted murder. . . . When the trial judge sentenced Haines on February 2, 1988, [he] made this statement:

> I believe my decision in this case was made easier by the State's decision to not introduce any medical expert scientific evidence. . . . All of us know that the conduct of spitting, throwing blood and biting cannot under normal circumstances constitute a step, substantial or otherwise, in causing the death of another person, regardless of the intent of the defendant. More has to be shown, more has to be proven, in my judgment. And the more in this case was that the conduct had to be coupled with a disease, a disease which by definition is inextricably based in science and medicine. . . .
>
> [I]n this case, the State took the position that everyone has heard of AIDS; that everybody has read about the disease of AIDS; and that everyone knows that this disease can be lethal or that it is lethal; that AIDS, if you will, is as common a killer as a gun or a knife, which by their very nature are deadly weapons. All of the medical evidence . . . shows conclusively that this medical condition and what it means is not very clear. And this is especially true when the [u]ncontroverted evidence in this case was that the defendant did not, in fact, have what the doctors consider . . . AIDS; but, having instead, as set out in the charges that were filed in this case, an AIDS Related Complex [(ARC)], which is a preliminary stage of the disease of AIDS. . . . There was no medical expert evidence that the person with ARC or AIDS can kill another by transmitting bodily fluids as alleged in this case. And there was no medical evidence from any of the evidence that the defendant had any reason to believe that he could transmit his condition to others by transmitting bodily fluids as are alleged in this case. . . . I find that the State failed in its burden of establishing that the defendant had a medical disease of ARC as alleged, that ARC can lead to AIDS, that AIDS or ARC is a disease that can be or is lethal and that spitting, biting or throwing blood at the victims is a method of transmitting AIDS or ARC. . . .
>
> Record at 699–703 (emphasis supplied). . . .

Contrary to Haines' contention that the evidence did not support a reasonable inference that his conduct amounted to a substantial step toward murder, the record reflects otherwise. At trial, it was definitely established that Haines carried the AIDS virus, was aware of the infection, believed it to be fatal, and intended to inflict others with the disease by spitting, biting, scratching, and throwing blood. His biological warfare with those attempting to help him is akin to a sinking ship firing on its rescuers. . . .

[T]he State was not required to prove that Haines' conduct could actually have killed. It was only necessary for the State to show that Haines did all that he believed necessary to bring about an intended result, regardless of what was actually possible. . . . [S]ome jurisdictions provide for the dismissal of a charge or reduction in sentence on the basis of "inherent impossibility" if the defendant's conduct was so inherently unlikely to result or culminate in the commission of a crime, inasmuch as neither the conduct nor the action taken would present a public danger. . . .

While we have found no Indiana case directly on point, the evidence presented at trial renders any defense of inherent impossibility inapplicable in this case. . . . In addition to Haines' belief that he could infect others there was testimony by physicians that the virus may be transmitted through the exchange of bodily fluids. It was apparent that the victims were exposed to the AIDS virus as a result of Haines' conduct. Ernest Drucker, an epidemiologist, knew of at least one case involving a health-care worker who became infected when a tube of blood containing the virus exploded, and the contaminated blood splashed on her skin and into her eyes and mouth. . . . Paul Balson, a professor of medicine at Louisiana State, testified that infection through "skin to skin" contact is possible, and that risk of infection exists when blood is splattered into the eyes or other mucous membranes. . . .

From the evidence in the record before us we can only conclude that Haines had knowledge of his disease and that he unrelentingly and unequivocally sought to kill the persons helping him by infecting them with AIDS, and that he took a substantial step towards killing them by his conduct believing that he could do so, all of which was more than a mere tenuous, theoretical, or speculative "chance" of transmitting the disease. From all of the evidence before the jury it could have concluded beyond a reasonable doubt that Haines took a substantial step toward the commission of murder. . . .

The trial court's judgment is reversed with instructions to reinstate the jury's verdict and resentence Haines accordingly.

---

*     *     *     *     *

*State v. Haines* is a difficult and troubling case. The jury returned a verdict of attempted murder in under 60 minutes, viewing Mr. Haines as morally blameworthy. Another way to see this case is that Mr. Haines was making a "cry for help." He had just attempted suicide and was in despair over the diagnosis of AIDS, which at the time was an invariably fatal disease. Mr. Haines asked the emergency workers to leave him alone and let him "die from AIDS." His behavior, while highly concerning, was unlikely to have transmitted the infection. In these circumstances, did Mr. Haines deserve criminal punishment, and would use of the criminal law in these kinds of cases deter others from risk behavior?

---

## United States v. Sturgis*

*Fourth Circuit Court of Appeals*
*Decided February 21, 1995*

Judge WILKINSON delivered the opinion of the court.

Jeffrey Wayne Sturgis appeals his conviction for assault with a dangerous weapon. . . . Sturgis, who is HIV positive, bit two correctional officers who were attempting to restrain him during an altercation at the Lorton Reformatory. We conclude that the evidence was sufficient to establish Sturgis' intent to harm the correctional officers. The question of whether Sturgis' teeth qualified as a dangerous weapon was also one of fact for the jury. Here the jury could reasonably have concluded that Sturgis used his mouth and teeth as a "dangerous weapon" during the incident. Accordingly, we affirm Sturgis' conviction.

On July 15, 1993, Jeffrey Wayne Sturgis went to Lorton Reformatory in Virginia to visit an inmate and upon entering was required to . . . submit to a search of his person and belongings. . . . During the search, one officer discovered a foreign object in Sturgis' pants. Upon questioning, Sturgis declared he wanted to end the search and forgo the visit. He then took the object from his pants and placed it in his mouth. Suspicious that Sturgis had contraband, one officer tried to force his jaws open to retrieve the object. Sturgis began to struggle and finally spit out the object (pink bubble gum) and as the officer tried to retrieve the

---

*48 F.3d 784 (4th Cir. 1995).

object Sturgis attacked him by biting him on the thumb, causing bleeding. As the struggle escalated, more officers tried to help restrain Sturgis, who was kicking and flailing and eventually bit another officer on the arm with substantial bleeding. Once subdued, Sturgis was then transferred to DeWitt Army Hospital for treatment and observation (for fear that he had actually swallowed narcotics).

While at the hospital, Sturgis continued to be combative by struggling, shouting, biting, spitting, and threatening the medical personnel trying to treat him. He was told to stop because he was HIV positive but he stated he knew of his condition and was trying to infect the staff.

Sturgis' stomach was pumped at the hospital. Although no foreign objects were found, a drug screen revealed traces of cocaine and marijuana in his bloodstream. A blood test performed at DeWitt Army Hospital also confirmed Sturgis' HIV positive status. . . .

At Sturgis' trial, the government presented medical records compiled while Sturgis was an inmate at Lorton. Those records contained eight references to Sturgis' HIV positive status and indicated that he had been informed of that status in 1991. The United States also offered expert testimony to establish that HIV, which is found in human saliva, can be transmitted through a bite. . . .

Sturgis . . . insisted that he was unaware of his HIV positive status until counsel informed him of the results of the test taken at DeWitt Army Hospital in July of 1993. . . .

Conviction for assault with a dangerous weapon under 18 U.S.C. § 113(c) requires proof of (1) an assault, (2) with a dangerous weapon, (3) with intent to do bodily harm. . . .

Sturgis claims that the evidence fails to establish that he acted with the requisite intent to do bodily harm to the correctional officers. Rather, he maintains that he acted wholly in self-defense. . . . [T]he evidence amply establishes Sturgis' intent to inflict harm. The record demonstrates that Sturgis acted in a violent and aggressive manner throughout the confrontation with the correctional officers and continued to kick, scream, and thrash about even after being taken to DeWitt Army Hospital. . . . Moreover, Sturgis' own statements, specifically his threats against the medical personnel who treated him, indicate that he was aware he was infected with HIV and wanted to infect others. Finally, evidence that Sturgis held each of the bites on the correctional officers for several seconds indicates intent to inflict serious bodily harm, not merely to defend himself from attack.

We next address whether Sturgis' use of his teeth to bite the correctional officers amounted to use of a "dangerous weapon." . . . [W]hat constitutes a dangerous weapon depends not on the object's intrinsic character but on its capacity, given "the manner of its use," to endanger life or inflict serious physical harm. United States v. Johnson, 324 F.2d 264, 266 (4th Cir. 1963). In *United States v. Moore,* 846 F.2d 1163 (8th Cir. 1988), the Eighth Circuit reached a similar conclusion: "Almost any weapon, as used or attempted to be used, may endanger life or inflict great bodily harm; as such, in appropriate circumstances, it may be a dangerous and deadly weapon." *Id.* at 1166. Thus an object need not be inherently dangerous to be a dangerous weapon. Rather, innocuous objects or instruments may become capable of inflicting serious injury when put to assaultive use. . . .

[T]eeth may also be a dangerous weapon if they are employed as such. . . . Parts of the human body have been held dangerous weapons under circumstances in which the body part was employed to inflict death or serious physical injury. . . . Here a jury could reasonably have concluded that Sturgis' use of his teeth to inflict potentially lethal bite wounds amounted to use of a dangerous weapon. . . .

Finally, there is at least a substantial possibility that HIV, which causes AIDS, can be transmitted via a human bite. . . . Sturgis' attack may not only have inflicted serious injury on the officers but endangered their lives as well. In sum, the jury could have found that the wounds inflicted by Sturgis' teeth were in essence indistinguishable from punctures caused by a knife or an ice pick. The assertion that human teeth can never qualify as a dangerous weapon ignores the harm to those on whom these bites were inflicted. . . . For the foregoing reasons, Sturgis' conviction and sentence are affirmed.

---

*            *            *            *            *

Certainly, persons who engage in assaultive behavior deserve criminal punishment. However, should individuals be convicted of more serious offenses (e.g., assault with a deadly weapon) *because* of their infectious state? From a public health perspective, the answer may be "no" because prevention of negligible risks represents a low priority. From a criminal justice perspective, are persons with infectious disease more culpable if they engage in assaultive behavior knowing that there is a small possibility of transmitting the infection?

## B. PUBLIC HEALTH OFFENSES

Despite the spate of prosecutions for traditional crimes of violence, the mental elements of "purpose" or "knowledge" can be difficult to prove. Partly in frustration with the difficulty of proof, and partly in response to political pressure, legislatures have sought other avenues to criminalize the risk of transmission. Infectious disease statutes create public health offenses that vary from state to state. A few states have broad provisions that criminally punish behavior that risks transmission of *any* contagious disease. Most statutes, however, create "disease-specific" offenses that were often enacted in waves in response to public misapprehensions about epidemics of the day. In the early twentieth century, states enacted statutes directed at TB, followed by STDs, and, in the latter part of the century, HIV/AIDS.

Public health offenses can differ depending on the state, but they often contain the following elements: (1) knowledge of an infectious condition (e.g., the person tests positive for an STD or HIV), (2) behavior risking transmission of the infection (e.g., sexual intercourse or the sharing of drug injection equipment), and (3) failure to disclose the risk to a partner or contact. While most STD and TB statutes carry mild sanctions, many HIV statutes are highly punitive. Courts have upheld the constitutionality of HIV-specific statutes against challenges based on vagueness, overbreadth, and the absence of a *mens rea* or specific-intent requirement. [*See, e.g.,* State v. Mahan, 971 S.W.2d 307 (Mo. 1998).]

Public health offenses can have advantages over traditional crimes of violence, making them much easier to prosecute. If narrowly written, they can be more precise than the traditional criminal law: individuals are forewarned of the prohibited behaviors and prosecutors are vested with less discretion. Society may also value public health offenses because they declare a public interest in responsible behavior and encourage disclosure to persons at risk of infection. Despite these benefits, are public health offenses useful prevention strategies? Are they likely to deter high-risk behavior? Alternatively, is it possible that they may create the *wrong* incentive? Consider the possibility that persons at risk may be better off not knowing their serologic status because only those who are aware of their status can be prosecuted. Additionally, by creating a specific offense legislatures implicitly invite the interest of police, prosecutors, and the apparatus of the criminal justice system. Does this create problems of potentially intrusive surveillance and selective enforcement?

Whether society should resort to the criminal law when a person risks transmission of an infectious disease depends on the severity of the case prosecuted. Think about the preferred public policy response to the following four scenarios involving persons with infectious conditions. In case 1, the person truly intends to kill and uses a means reasonably calculated to achieve that end (e.g., a father injects his son with an HIV-contaminated needle to avoid paying child support). In case 2, the person acts with reckless disregard for life, such as Nushawn Williams in Chautauqua County, who hid his HIV status from multiple sexual partners. In case 3, the person engages in epidemiologically low-risk behavior such as biting, spitting, or donating blood. Finally, in case 4, the person engages in epidemiologically higher-risk behavior, but the conduct is common among the population (e.g., failure to inform a sexual partner of the risk of infection). In discussing these scenarios, inquire whether prosecution would achieve its traditional goals: deterrence, retribution, incapacitation, and rehabilitation.

## CONCLUSION

In this and the previous chapter, we considered interventions to control infectious disease—biological approaches and deprivations of liberty. The final chapter of this *Reader* provides case studies on important problems facing our society: emerging infectious diseases, bioterrorism, and public health genetics.

# PART FOUR

# The Future of Public Health

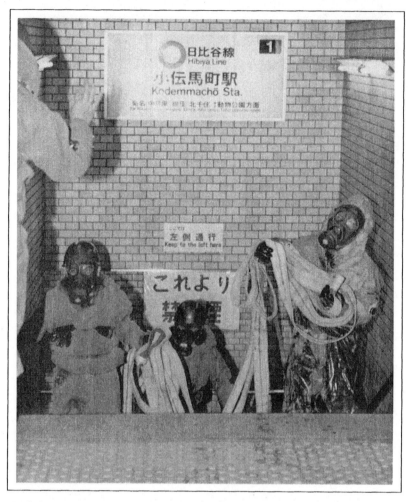

Firefighters wearing gas masks and protective suits emerge after cleaning toxic gas–contaminated cars at Tokyo's Kodemmacho subway station on March 21, 1995. A dozen people were killed and more than 5,500 became ill as a result of the attack by the Aum Shinrikyo cult. (Atusushi Tsukada, AP/Wide World Photos, 3/21/95.)

# FOURTEEN

# Vision and Challenges

*Case Studies on Emerging Infections,*
*Bioterrorism, and Public Health Genetics*

The field of public health helped vastly to improve the health and well-being of populations during the twentieth century, leading to substantial increases in life expectancy, improved sanitation and living conditions, and reductions in infectious diseases. Nevertheless, major problems, as well as remarkable opportunities, confront the field in a new century. (Compare the ten greatest public health achievements in the twentieth century [Table 8] with current and future public health challenges [Table 9].)

This chapter offers case studies on three of the most complex and important challenges: emergent and reemergent infectious diseases (including the problem of drug-resistant organisms), biological warfare and bioterrorism, and public health genetics.

## I. EMERGENT AND REEMERGENT INFECTIOUS DISEASES

One can think of the middle of the 20th century as the end of one of the most important social revolutions in history—the virtual elimination of the infectious disease as a significant factor in social life.

> *Sir F. McFarland Burnet*
> *and David O. White (1962)*

TABLE 8

TEN GREAT PUBLIC HEALTH ACHIEVEMENTS:
UNITED STATES, 1900–1999

1. Vaccination
2. Motor vehicle safety
3. Safer workplaces
4. Control of infectious diseases
5. Decline in deaths from coronary heart disease and stroke
6. Safer and healthier foods
7. Healthier mothers and babies
8. Family planning
9. Fluoridation of drinking water
10. Recognition of tobacco use as a health hazard

SOURCE: Centers for Disease Control and Prevention. "Ten Great Public Health Achievements—United States, 1900-1999." *Morbidity and Mortality Weekly Report* 48 (50) (December 24, 1999): 1141–98.

TABLE 9

CURRENT AND FUTURE PUBLIC HEALTH CHALLENGES

To position the nation for the century ahead, we believe that the medical, scientific, and public health communities must do the following:
1. Institute a rational health care system
2. Eliminate health disparities among racial and ethnic groups
3. Focus on children's emotional and intellectual development
4. Achieve a longer "healthspan" for the rapidly growing aging population
5. Integrate physical activity and healthy eating into daily lives
6. Clean up and protect the environment
7. Prepare to respond to emerging infectious diseases
8. Recognize and address the contributions of mental health to overall health and well-being
9. Reduce the toll of violence in society
10. Use new scientific knowledge and technological advances wisely

SOURCE: Koplan, Jeffrey P., and David W. Fleming. "Current and Future Public Health Challenges." *JAMA* 284 (October 4, 2000): 1696–98.

During the twentieth century, North America and Europe experienced a substantial decline in mortality and an increase in life expectancy. According to Gregory L. Armstrong and colleagues (1999, 61) at the CDC, the "theory of epidemiologic transition attributes these trends to the transition from an 'age of pestilence and famine,' in which the mortality pattern was dominated by high rates of infectious disease deaths, to the current 'age of degenerative and man-made diseases,' in which mortality from chronic diseases predominates." Infectious diseases now account for only 4.2 percent of all disability-adjusted life years lost in countries like the United States, with established market economies, whereas chronic and neoplastic diseases account for 81 percent (Murray and Lopez 1997).

Until recently, public health experts assumed that the epidemiologic transition brought about a permanent reduction in infectious disease mortality in the United States. However, infectious diseases have emerged or reemerged in the United States. Mortality due to infectious diseases increased 58 percent from 1980 to 1992 (Armstrong, Conn, and Pinner 1999), emphasizing the dynamic nature of infectious diseases and the need for preparedness to address them.

The Institute of Medicine (IOM) (1992) defines emerging infections as new, reemerging, or drug-resistant infections whose incidence in humans has increased within the past two decades or threatens to increase in the near future. Michael T. Osterholm (2000, 1280) explains the difficulty of combating emerging infections: "The task of public health is a lot like trying to swim against the current of a raging river. Even with intelligent and extensive efforts, the rapidly changing world we live in tends to favor infectious agents."

In the 1980s the United States experienced new epidemics (e.g., HIV/AIDS, Lyme disease, and Hantavirus) and resurgent epidemics (e.g., multidrug-resistant tuberculosis) (Small and Fujiwara 2001). In the 1990s the United States experienced major outbreaks of waterborne disease (e.g., *Cryptosporidium*), food-borne disease (e.g., *E. coli*), and mosquito-borne disease (e.g., West Nile virus infection) (Craven and Roehrig 2001; Desselberger 2000). The burden of infectious diseases in the twenty-first century is still unknown, but there are many reasons to believe that epidemics will take their toll on populations around the world. (For a national strategy to prevent emerging infections in the twenty-first century, see CDC [1998] and Binder et al. [1999].)

The primary factors contributing to this resurgence of infectious disease include societal changes (e.g., migration and population growth); economic changes (e.g., disparities in socioeconomic status); health care system changes (e.g., widespread use of antibiotics); globalization of the food supply and changes in farming practices; human behavior (e.g., international travel); environmental changes resulting in flood, drought, and famine; decay in the public health infrastructure; and microbial adaptation resulting in changes in virulence and development of resistance to antibiotics (IOM 1992; Farmer 1996; Gostin 1998). Mary E. Wilson, of the Harvard School of Public Health, offers an ecologic perspective of emerging infectious diseases.

## Infectious Diseases: An Ecologic Perspective*
*Mary E. Wilson*

Microbes have played a decisive role in human history. Between 1348 and 1352 in many European countries plague was estimated to have killed a third to a half of the population. It was not swords and guns but imported microbes, carried by explorers over oceans, that defeated native populations in the Americas, and in Australia and southern Africa the arrival of Europeans killed off local populations by introducing infectious diseases. Local flora and fauna were also irreversibly altered. Many of these fertile, temperate, and now less populated lands were subsequently settled by Europeans.

By the middle of the 20th century, infectious diseases were no longer the major causes of mortality in developed countries. The eradication of smallpox reinforced the perception that infectious diseases could be eliminated. Improved sanitation, clean water, and better living conditions, along with vaccines and antimicrobial agents, brought many infectious diseases under control in industrialized countries, but infections continued to kill millions each year in the developing world. Infectious diseases remain the most common single cause of death in the world today. . . .

Increasingly humans have changed the earth in ways that make it easier for microbes to move and to reach vulnerable populations. Widespread use of antimicrobial agents and chemicals produces selective pressure for the survival and persistence of more resistant populations of microbes, and also of more resilient insect vectors. Patterns of infectious diseases are changing globally and on a massive scale. . . .

Diseases such as Lassa fever, AIDS, and Ebola disease have focused attention on viral infections, but pathogens involved in these changed

---

*Reprinted from *British Medical Journal* 311 (1995): 1681–84.

infectious diseases also include bacteria, fungi, protozoa, and helminths. Drug resistance is increasingly reported not only in bacteria but also in viruses, fungi, protozoa, and helminths. Arthropods, such as mosquitoes, lice, and ticks, are becoming more resistant to pesticides. Outbreaks of infectious diseases have caused die offs in species as diverse as beans, rice, seals, dolphins, lions, chickens, and horses. . . .

## MORE THAN MERE MICROBES

Today we understand that the concept of the microbe as the cause of an infection is inadequate and incomplete because it ignores the influence of the host, the milieu, and the social and physical environment. Yet medical science still tends to focus on the microbe as the foe, and our response has often been to seek and destroy the invader.

A more enlightened understanding would embrace an ecological perspective. Humans have reached such numbers and have developed such technologies that human activities have a global impact and have changed the earth for all other biological life. Humans are part of a vast evolutionary process and all life is interdependent. Students of human health must look at the health and resilience of the ecosystem and approach analysis at a systems level.

Three general forces can affect the burden of infectious diseases in humans: change in abundance, virulence, or transmissibility of microbes; an increase in probability of exposure of humans to microorganisms; and an increase in the vulnerability of humans to infection and to the consequences of infection. A wide range of biological, physicochemical, behavioral, and social factors influence one or more of these forces. Many are interrelated, and multiple synergies exist.

## MIGRATION

Migration of people has always played a large part in introducing infections into new populations. . . . The magnitude and speed of migration today is unparalleled in history. . . . Much migration is unplanned and unwanted and leads to settlement in areas or under conditions that place people at increased risk of infectious diseases.

Because of political conflict or instability, economic pressures, and environmental changes, masses of people are being displaced. Many refugees seek asylum in developing countries. Refugee camps, resettlement areas, and temporary shelters are often characterized by crowded living conditions, poor sanitation, limited access to clean water, little medical care, poor nutrition, and lack of separation from insects and animals in the environment. These features increase the probability of exposure to infections in such vulnerable populations. . . .

The massive movement occurring in the world today includes animals, plants, seeds, insects, and all manner of biological life in addition to humans. Through their conveyances by air, water, and land, humans have given wings to plants, animals, and microbes, extending and speeding up their spread. Air travel accelerated the spread of HIV around the globe. Introductions of new species of plants and animals can change the ecology in an area, sometimes extinguishing local species because of predation, disease, competition, and changes in the habitat. Introducing insect vectors can affect human health if the vector is capable of transmitting pathogens to humans. . . .

## CLIMATIC EFFECTS

Changes in climate and the environment have many direct and indirect effects on human health. Temperature and humidity influence the abundance and distribution of vectors and intermediate hosts. Global warming can reshape vegetation zones and can be expected to change the distribution and abundance of vector borne infections, such as malaria. Warmer temperatures may allow insects and pests to survive winters that normally would have limited their populations. An increase in malaria in Rwanda coincided with record high temperatures and rainfall. In 70 communities in Mexico, median temperature during the rainy season was the strongest predictor of dengue fever: higher temperatures increased vector efficiency. . . .

Extreme climatic events, such as droughts and floods, are expected to increase with predicted global climate changes. Many disease outbreaks have occurred after extreme climatic conditions. These include vector borne infections such as malaria and Venezuelan encephalitis, animal borne infections such as hantaviruses, and water borne infections such as cholera and hepatitis E.

## SETTLEMENT PATTERNS

Climatic and environmental changes also lead humans to migrate, to develop new lands, and to live in settings that favor the spread of infectious diseases. Simultaneously we are seeing increased urbanization and exploration and clearing of new lands. Both carry risks for infectious diseases. The huge periurban settlements that have grown, especially in tropical regions, have risks for infectious diseases similar to those precipitated by resettlement. . . .

Population growth means people are living in higher densities, heightening the risk for rapid spread of infections. An estimated 1.3 billion people in the developing world lack access to clean water and nearly 2 billion lack an adequate system for disposing of feces. More people are being pushed to the margins of habitable land. Much of the increased urban growth is in areas within 75 miles of the sea, which are at risk for hurricanes and floodings, and in areas at increased risk for earthquakes. Increased density of populations and inadequate resources also make for social and political instability. These multiple vulnerabilities often converge in a population or geographical region.

## NEW VULNERABILITIES

Technological gains are often offset by new vulnerabilities. Interventions can often have unintended and unexpected consequences. Wide use of antimicrobials has led to high rates of resistance among many bacteria. Mass processing and distribution of food has resulted in occasional massive outbreaks of infections, such as salmonellosis and *Escherichia coli* O157:H7, that could not have occurred without the wide distribution networks. Large municipal water systems made it possible to infect more than 400,000 people with *Cryptosporidium parvum* within a few days. Modern medical techniques applied with inadequate training and resources have had disastrous consequences, as shown by dramatic outbreaks of nosocomial Lassa fever in Nigeria and Ebola disease in Zaire. Transmission of virus to patients and medical staff resulted from exposure to contaminated needles and from lack of adequate barriers during surgery.

Changes in climate lead to creation of new habitats that are energy expensive and provide new avenues for spread of infection. Air and water cooling systems have been associated with outbreaks of Legionnaires' disease. The natural habitat for *Legionella pneumophila*, the cause of the disease, is streams, lakes, and other bodies of water, where it is present in small numbers. Human inventions such as water cooling towers and water distribution systems provide favorable conditions for the survival and proliferation of the bacteria and the means for dissemination. . . .

## FATAL MIXTURES

The world today is in a state of turbulence and rapid change. The emergence of infections in many geographical areas is but one manifestation of instability and stress in the system. Today there are unprecedented opportunities for mixing of people, animals, and microbes from all geographical areas in an environment that has been altered by industry, technology, agriculture, chemicals, and climate change and by the demands of population growth. Diverse genetic pools are mixing in rates and combinations and in a time frame too short to allow adaptation through genetic change. Many interventions have been carried out with too narrow an understanding of their impacts.

The invisible weapons of today's conflicts are micro-organisms. In most of the wars throughout history, infectious diseases killed more troops than did the weapons of war. Since the second world war more civilians than combatants have died from war. In recent conflicts the victims have often been those whose lives have been upset by the upheaval—refugees, displaced populations, children without access to immunization and oral rehydration fluids, the hungry and vulnerable masses who succumb to infections that are neither exotic nor new. Earlier in this century mortality from tuberculosis in many European countries showed a striking increase in response to war.

There is an urgent need to integrate knowledge about infectious diseases with knowledge of climate and environmental change, migration and population growth, demography, and the consequences of conflict. All are inextricably linked and play a part in the changed patterns we are seeing in infectious diseases.

We have more scientific data about the present and past than ever before. We have biopsies of the earth, the ice cores, that reveal secrets of past climatic patterns. Frozen bodies, preserved insects, mice, and mummies examined by the polymerase chain reaction and other techniques help to create a fuller knowledge of life in past centuries. Will this translate into understanding and changed behavior in a way that preserves the health of humans and the biosphere? Many events suggest that there is a mismatch between what we know and what we have been able to do. The barriers to identifying and intervening in infectious diseases are more often social and political than scientific.

Much recent attention has focused on exotic and previously unrecognized lethal pathogens. While it is important to study these pathogens and to identify the events that lead to their appearance and spread, it is essential not to ignore pathogens that are familiar and thus often less feared. Influenza, which killed 20 million people in the year after the end of the first world war, is still a killer and has the capacity to change rapidly and spread widely throughout the world. . . .

## PROGRESS WITHOUT BREAKTHROUGHS?

What can be done? . . . We should recognize the links between population growth, climatic and environmental change, global migration, and human health and security; develop databases that combine information about climate, demography, population movements, and diseases in humans, animals, and plants; identify markers for regions or populations at high risk of epidemic disease so that we can intervene to reduce the impact of disease; continue efforts to slow population growth; take steps to reduce mass migration and displacement of populations; reduce consumption; pay more attention to land use and production and disposal of toxins and chemicals; take a broader view and longer time frame when analyzing the potential impact of interventions; and view human life as part of a constantly evolving biosphere. . . . Any meaningful response must integrate knowledge from multiple disciplines and approach the problem at the systems level. To be successful, we must apprehend infectious diseases in their evolutionary and ecological context.

---

\*     \*     \*     \*     \*

The discovery of potent antimicrobial agents was one of the greatest contributions to public health in the twentieth century. For the first time, health care and public health professionals could not only effectively treat persons with infectious diseases, but they could also reduce their infectiousness, breaking the cycle of contagion. Shortly after the mass production of penicillin in the 1940s, microbiologists were already aware that antibiotics had an Achilles' heel. Alexander Fleming (1946), who discovered penicillin, wrote that "the administration of too small doses . . . leads to the production of resistant strains of bacteria."

Antibiotic-resistant strains of bacteria are a problem that vexes public health to this day, contributing to increased morbidity and mortality as well as higher health care costs. Yearly expenditures arising from drug resistance in the United States are estimated at $4 billion and are rising (File 1999). Robert C. Moellering, Jr. (1998, S135), observes that the problem has progressed to the point where it is "now far easier to list the unusual organisms that have remained susceptible to first-line antimicrobial agents than to list the organisms that are multidrug-resistant." For example, approximately two million people annually contract difficult-to-treat infections in hospitals (CDC 2000c). Stuart B. Levy, of the Alliance for the Prudent Use of Antibiotics, explains the phenomena of drug-resistant organisms.

## Antibiotic Availability and Use:
## Consequences to Man and His Environment*
*Stuart B. Levy*

Antibiotics are unique as pharmacological agents since they treat not only the patient but also the patient's environment. In the process of killing the targeted pathogen, antibiotics also kill other susceptible strains of bacteria sharing the immediate ecosystem. This creates a potential for long-range problems because there is a selection for uncommon (sometimes rare) resistant strains which survive. These strains multiply in the luxury of no competitors. With repeated antibiotic "treatments," environments can become havens for high numbers of resistant bacterial strains. This strong and steady selective force of antibiotics, combined with the intrinsic genetic properties of bacteria, has led, after 40–50 years of antibiotic use, to antibiotic resistant variants of common bacteria, many of which cause severe infections in man.

Although resistance does not increase virulence, the chances that an illness will be caused by a resistant strain will increase as the numbers of resistant pathogens (and resistance genes) increase in the environment. Moreover, as shown in the outbreaks of *Salmonella* infections, patients who are receiving antibiotics for other reasons are at increased risk of colonization and infection with small numbers of *Salmonella*, presumably because the normal flora is altered.

The problem today is not as simple as it was following the initial use of antibiotics. Instead of resistance to single agents, bacteria are now appearing with resistance to multiple drugs. Such a situation may leave the clinician with only a single useful agent, with dozens of others ineffective because of bacterial resistance to them.

### RESISTANCE IS A WORLDWIDE PROBLEM

The resistance problem has been aggravated by the misuse and overuse of antibiotics throughout the world in the treatment of man, animals, and agriculture. The effect of such usage is a general ecological selection of those resistant bacteria which survive. In some parts of the world, mainly developing countries, inadequate supplies of antibiotics

---

*Reprinted from *Journal of Clinical Epidemiology* 44: 83S–87S with permission from Elsevier Science. © 1991.

are available and partial treatments are given. This fails to cure the disease and, instead, aids in the emergence and spread of resistant bacteria. These resistant strains become part of the microbial community which, if they cause infections, cannot be treated by current and available antibiotics.

Developing countries have another situation which aggravates the problem. Antibiotics are available over the counter, without prescription. The use of a particular antibiotic is touted for a number of symptomatic problems, from diarrhea to cough. . . . The selling of multiple antibiotics in fixed combination is another practice which not only threatens harm to patients because of combined potential side effects, but also aids in the selection of multiresistant organisms.

Even in the U.S., with legislative constraints on antibiotic availability, these agents are misused. The ease of procuring a prescription through a physician, and the practice of storing unused antibiotics for later use have allowed them to be grossly overused for inappropriate treatment of common viral illnesses and for non-specific symptoms.

Antibiotic resistance may be more readily handled in developed countries, because of the apparent continued availability of newer drugs to which the organisms are susceptible and where cost is not prohibitive. However, in developing countries, with severe constraints on funds, the ability to obtain costlier, effective antibiotics, crucially important in the treatment, is often not possible. Despite resistance prevalence, "old guard" antibiotics which are no longer effective, but readily available and inexpensive, continue to be used. This practice only augments the resistance problem by selecting and propagating the resistant bacteria in the environment. Since these organisms are often multiresistant, use of any one of a number of antibiotics will select for the same resistant strain. In these instances, no antibiotic is preferred, unless it is not subject to the resistance carried by the organism being treated. . . .

## RESISTANCE IS TRANSFERRABLE

Antibiotic resistance is not static. Not only do resistant bacteria travel from place to place and from country to country, but also their resistance genes move among diverse species and genera. This phenomenon occurs because many resistance genes are located on self-replicating genetic elements, called plasmids, which can be transferred among different types of bacteria. The same antibiotic resistance plasmids have been found among different genera. . . .

Today, we see newly resistant pathogens among previously susceptible species. Where and how have they developed resistance so quickly?
Genetic studies show that the resistance determinants . . . have been acquired from existing resistant strains. . . .

## FUTURE PROSPECTS

When faced with this situation, we must seriously take stock of what is
happening with antibiotics. Where must we go to prevent further insult
to their therapeutic armament? On one hand, the situation looks grim
and depressing, but on the other hand, there are more promising findings coming from various studies. Following discontinuation of antibiotics, susceptible organisms do eventually return to colonize the ecologic site, although this process may be slow. Certain groups are trying
to use lactobacillus or other "gentle" enteric strains to displace resistant ones and allow colonization by susceptible strains.

The most effective and least expensive way to prevent and curb resistance is to use antibiotics appropriately and for designated periods of
time (as short as needed), thereby reducing their overall selective effects.
Large amounts of antibiotics are not generally needed—just enough of
the correct drug can go a long way in eradicating a disease problem. Resistance, and in particular multiresistance, propagates where antibiotics
are being overused or misused in the face of resistance already present
and poor public hygiene. In these areas antibiotics are unsuccessful as
therapy, but very successful as selective agents of resistance.

Understanding the genetics of resistance, and understanding the
quantities of antibiotics needed under different circumstances should
allow a rational use from the standpoint of dosage and timing in the
treatment of particular infections. Wise use of antibiotics should include use which is specified for a particular bacterial infection, one that
is narrowed to that particular infectious organism, and one whose duration is sufficient for the treatment of that infection. Obviously this
"ideal" presumes that the disease organism is known, but if not, the microbial epidemiology of the area may provide important information.
For instance, knowing the kinds of common disease agents and their
susceptibility profiles can help in making a successful empiric decision
about which antibiotic to use. . . .

Through increased awareness of the problem and thoughtful rational use, we can save sorely needed health expenses and curb the
mounting problem of antibiotic resistance. The latter problem thwarts
the effectiveness of antibiotics, taking its toll in healthcare costs in areas

of the world where such costs can limit therapy and ultimately lead to loss of lives.

---

                    *      *      *      *      *

Antimicrobial resistance has become a major concern with the interconnected epidemics of tuberculosis (TB) and HIV/AIDS (Cassell and Mekalanos 2001). In several U.S. cities in the 1980s, 25 percent or more of TB infections were resistant to front-line medications (IOM 2000b). Antibiotic resistance is particularly troubling for persons dually infected with *Mycobacterium* tuberculosis (M.TB) and HIV because they have a substantially increased risk of morbidity and mortality from TB (Gostin 1995b).

By the late 1990s, antiretroviral resistance became a significant concern in the HIV epidemic. An increasing proportion of persons living with HIV are resistant to antiretroviral medication, jeopardizing the major advances in treatment (Mayer 1997).

The problem of antimicrobial resistance is caused by several factors, including overprescribing by physicians, feeding antibiotics to farm animals, and inconsistent or incomplete courses of medication taken by patients. Given these factors, what are the most promising and innovative policies to combat this problem? Many policy makers place the responsibility squarely on patients, arguing for mandatory treatment or directly observed therapy (see chapter 12). Even if patients could be forced to take the full course of their medication, society would still be faced with the problems of overprescribing and agricultural use of antibiotics.

## II. BIOLOGICAL WARFARE AND BIOTERRORISM: "PUBLIC HEALTH IN REVERSE"

Picture the following. Over a period of about one week, increasing numbers of patients report to their general practitioners and emergency departments with fever, malaise, and myalgia, and other symptoms in keeping with a viral respiratory-tract infection. Increasing numbers of patients become septicaemic and then deaths start to occur. By the time the diagnosis of anthrax is made, each patient will have been in contact with many family members as well as with colleagues and people in hospitals.

[*Editor's comment:* Anthrax is not transmissible person-
to-person.] The initial exposure of, say several hundred
people, to the organism has now spread to many tens of
thousands. Panic would ensue and hospitals would be
overwhelmed—the clamour for antibiotic prophylaxis and
mass vaccination is the stuff of nightmares.

*Richard Wise (1998, 1387)*

The nation experienced the devastating effects of civilian mass casualties within our borders from the terrorist attacks at New York's World
Trade Towers, at the Pentagon, and in Pennsylvania on September 11,
2001. These events placed in stark perspective the massive task of prevention, early detection and containment of health threats, and the care
and treatment of large populations that suffer from injury, disease, and
death (Garrett 2000).

This section examines the timely and important problems of biological warfare and bioterrorism. Biological warfare is defined as the deliberate release of microorganisms or toxins of biological origin against
armed forces in a time of war. Bioterrorism is the deliberate release of
microorganisms or toxins of biological origin against civilian populations for the purposes of destabilization of social and political structures. The U.S. Public Health Service has called biological warfare and
bioterrorism "public health in reverse" because of the potentially devastating effects on populations (Department of Health, Education, and Welfare 1959; Cohen, Gould, and Sidel 1999).

Biological warfare has evolved from the crude use of cadavers to con-
taminate water supplies to the development of specialized munitions for
battlefield and covert use. Documented episodes of bioterrorism, although
rare, have been dramatic. In 1995 the Aum Shinrikyo ("Supreme Truth")
cult released the chemical agent sarin in a Tokyo subway. In 1984 an Ore-
gon cult allegedly contaminated salad bars with the biological agent salmonella (Cole 1995; MacKenzie 1998). In the aftermath of September 11,
2001, public health and criminal justice authorities investigated cases of
intentional dispersal of anthrax.

The agents most likely to be used as biological weapons have the potential to be aerosolized and dispersed over a wide geographic area and
are resistant to sunlight, desiccation, and heat. They also have the potential to cause lethal or debilitating disease, are transmitted person to
person, and are not easily prevented or treated. The agents that best
meet these criteria include smallpox, anthrax, plague, viral hemor-

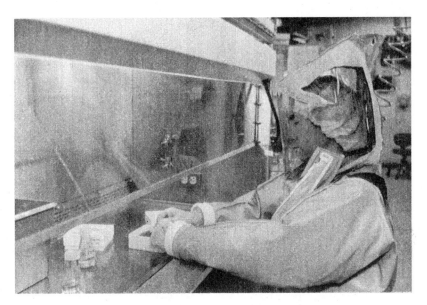

A researcher at the Centers for Disease Control and Prevention examines biological agents in a maximum containment virology lab in 1987.

rhagic fever, and botulism (Leggiadro 2000). See Table 10. For detailed plans to manage these potential biological weapons, see Inglesby and colleagues (1999; 2000) and Henderson and colleagues (1999).

The use of anthrax and smallpox as biological weapons raises particularly fascinating and controversial issues. In 1998 the Department of Defense (DoD) established the Anthrax Vaccine Immunization Program (AVIP), designed to achieve total force protection against anthrax by 2004 (CDC 2000b). The military is concerned about battlefield safety, but the AVIP remains highly controversial. The evidence for the safety and effectiveness of the anthrax vaccine is equivocal. Members of the armed forces are concerned about possible adverse effects in the short and long term. They also question the DoD's decision to compel soldiers to be vaccinated against their will (IOM 2000a).

The public health response to smallpox is equally controversial, but for a different reason. Smallpox vaccination is very effective, but most people today have no immunity. Mass immunization came to an end more than twenty-five years ago, after smallpox had been eradicated. The World Health Organization (WHO) destroyed most of the vaccine stocks in the early 1990s. The smallpox virus (known as variola) is now

TABLE 10

DEADLIEST FIVE BIOLOGICAL AGENTS

| | Description | Symptoms | Fatality Rate | Treatment |
|---|---|---|---|---|
| (Inhalational) Anthrax (*Bacillus anthracis*) | Inhaled spores germinate and release toxins, causing swelling in the chest cavity. Possible blood and brain infection. | Fever, fatigue, and malaise, starting within 2 to 46 days; progresses to chest pain, cough, rapid deterioration of health. | Kills more than 85 percent of those it infects, often within one to three days after symptoms appear. | Antibiotics (preferably ciprofloxacin) should be given before symptoms appear. Vaccine available, though not for civilians. |
| Smallpox (*Variola* virus) | Very contagious, airborne disease. | About 12 to 14 days after infection. Fever, aches, vomiting, rash of small red spots that grow into larger painful pustules covering the body. | Fatal in 30 percent of unvaccinated patients. | No treatment. U.S. had vaccine for about 6 million people. Only a fraction of those vaccinated before 1972 still protected. |
| (Pneumonic) Plague (*Yersinia pestis*) | Natural, flea-borne form causes bubonic plague. Gravest threat is posed by aerosol, leading to pneumonic plague. | High fever, headache, and bloody cough; progresses to labored breathing, bluish-grayish skin color, respiratory failure, and death. | If untreated, a person with pneumonic plague will almost always die within one to two days after symptoms begin. | Various antibiotics, including streptomycin and gentamicin. Isolate patients. |
| Viral Hemorrhagic Fever | Highly infectious RNA viruses including Ebola, Marburg, Lassa, and dengue fever. Spread by rodents, ticks, mosquitoes. | Vary from one type of HFV to the next. Include fever, muscle aches, exhaustion, internal bleeding. | Varies. Death rate from dengue is as low as 1 percent. Ebola fatality rates have reached 90 percent. | Mainly supportive therapy. Antiviral drug ribavirin useful in treating some viruses but not others (Ebola, Marburg). |
| (Inhalational) Botulism (*Clostridium botulinum*) | Produces toxin that blocks nerve signals, inhibits muscle movement. Weapon would most likely aerosolize toxin. | Difficulty swallowing food, mental numbness, muscle paralysis, possible breathing failure. | Inhalational form: Difficult to say since only a handful of cases have been reported. | Patients with respiratory paralysis should be placed on ventilator. Antitoxin given early may prevent progression. |

SOURCE: U.S. Centers for Disease Control and Prevention/U.S. Army Military Research Institute of Infectious Diseases.

classified as a Biosafety Level 4 hot agent (the most dangerous virus) because it is lethal, airborne, and highly contagious.

At present, the variola virus exists officially in only two repositories — at the CDC in Atlanta, Georgia, and a Russian facility in Novosibirsk, Siberia. However, there is growing suspicion that the virus may also live unofficially in clandestine biowarfare laboratories. WHO has struggled with the question of whether to destroy the two official stocks of the virus. Experts are concerned about the accidental or intentional release of the virus because the appearance of a single case of smallpox anywhere on earth would become a global health emergency. However, if official stocks of the virus were destroyed, it would make research and development of a new vaccine exceedingly difficult if unofficial stocks were used as biological weapons (Preston 1999). In November 2001, the United States announced it would not destroy its stock of smallpox virus (Miller 2001).

For an intriguing historical perspective of biological warfare (discussing the 1972 Convention on the Prohibition of the Development, Production, and Stockpiling of Bacteriological [Biological] and Toxin Weapons and on Their Destruction), see Christopher and colleagues (1997). In 2001, President Bush rejected an international accord aimed at enforcing the 1972 treaty (Olson 2001).

In the following section, Donald A. Henderson, from the Johns Hopkins Center for Civilian Biodefense Studies, examines the looming threat of bioterrorism. Next, the CDC provides a strategic plan for preparedness for and response to potential bioterrorism events. For additional scholarship regarding the management of potential bioterrorism events, see Kellman (2001); Lillibridge, Bell, and Roman (1999); Macintyre and colleagues (2000); and Waeckerle (2000).

---

### The Looming Threat of Bioterrorism*
*Donald A. Henderson*

[O]f the weapons of mass destruction (nuclear, chemical, and biological), the biological ones are the most greatly feared, but the country is least well prepared to deal with them. Virtually all federal efforts in

---

*Reprinted from *Science* 283 (February 26, 1999): 1279–82 with permission. © 1999 American Association for the Advancement of Science.

strategic planning and training have so far been directed toward crisis management after a chemical release or an explosion. Should such an event occur, fire, police, and emergency rescue workers would proceed to the scene and, with the FBI assuming lead responsibility, stabilize the situation, deal with casualties, decontaminate, and collect evidence for identification of a perpetrator. This exercise is not unfamiliar. Spills of hazardous materials, explosions, fires, and other civil emergencies are not uncommon events.

The expected scenario after release of an aerosol cloud of a biological agent is entirely different. The release could be silent and would almost certainly be undetected. The cloud would be invisible, odorless, and tasteless. It would behave much like a gas in penetrating interior areas. No one would know until days or weeks later that anyone had been infected (depending on the microbe). Then patients would begin appearing in emergency rooms and physicians' offices with symptoms of a strange disease that few physicians had ever seen. Special measures would be needed for patient care and hospitalization, obtaining laboratory confirmation regarding the identity of microbes unknown to most laboratories, providing vaccine or antibiotics to large portions of the population, and identifying and possibly quarantining patients. Trained epidemiologists would be needed to identify where and when infection had occurred, so as to identify how and by whom it may have been spread. Public health administrators would be challenged to undertake emergency management of a problem alien to their experience and in a public environment where pestilential disease, let alone in epidemic form, has been unknown.

The implicit assumption has frequently been that chemical and biological threats and the responses to them are so generically similar that they can be readily handled by a single "chembio" expert, usually a chemist. This is a serious misapprehension. . . .

PROBABLE AGENTS

Any one of thousands of biological agents that are capable of causing human infection could be considered a potential biological weapon. Realistically, only a few . . . can be cultivated and dispersed effectively so as to cause cases and deaths in numbers that would threaten the functioning of a large community. Other factors also determine which microbes are of priority concern: specifically, the possibility of further human-to-human spread, the environmental stability of the organism, the size of the infectious dose, and the availability of prophylactic or therapeutic measures.

A Russian panel of bioweapons experts reviewed the microbial agents and concluded that there were 11 that were "very likely to be used." The top four were smallpox, plague, anthrax, and botulism. Lower on their list were tularemia, glanders, typhus, Q fever, Venezuelan equine encephalitis, and Marburg and influenza viruses. Each of the four top-rated agents is associated with high case fatality rates when dispersed as an aerosol. The rates range upward from 30% for smallpox to more than 80% for anthrax. Smallpox and anthrax have other advantages in that they can be grown reasonably easily and in large quantities and are sturdy organisms that are resistant to destruction. They are thus especially suited to aerosol dissemination to reach large areas and numbers of people. . . .

## LIKELY PERPETRATORS

Some argue that almost anyone with intent can produce and dispense a biological weapon. It is unlikely, however, that more than a few would be successful in obtaining any of the top-rated agents in a form suitable to be dispensed as an aerosol. Naturally occurring cases of plague, anthrax, and botulism do occur on almost every continent and so provide a potential source for strains. However, there is considerable variation in the virulence of different strains, and a high level of expertise, which is much less obtainable than the agents themselves, is needed to identify an especially pathogenic one. Moreover, producing these particular organisms in large quantity and in the ultra-small particle form needed for aerosolization is beyond the average laboratory. . . .

## GREATEST THREATS: SMALLPOX AND ANTHRAX

Of the potential biological weapons, smallpox and anthrax pose by far the greatest threats, albeit because of different clinical and epidemiological properties. . . .

Smallpox poses an unusually serious threat; in part, because virtually everyone is now susceptible, vaccination having stopped worldwide 20 or more years ago as a result of the eradication of the disease. Because of waning immunity, it is probable that no more than 20% of the population is protected. Among the unprotected, case fatality rates after infection with smallpox are 30%. There is no treatment. Virus, in aerosol form, can survive for 24 hours or more and is highly infectious even at low dosages.

An outbreak in which as few as 100 people were infected would quickly tax the resources of any community. There would be both actual cases and people with a fever and rash for whom the diagnosis was uncertain. In all, 200 or more patients would probably have to be treated in the first wave of cases. Most of the patients would be extremely ill with severe aching pains and high fever and would normally be hospitalized. . . . [P]atients would have to be confined to rooms under negative pressure that were equipped with special filters to prevent the escape of the virus. Hospitals have few rooms so ventilated; there would, for example, probably be less than 100 in the Washington, D.C., metropolitan area.

A vaccination program would have to be undertaken rapidly to protect as many as possible of those who had been in contact with the patients. Vaccination given within 3 to 4 days after exposure can protect most people against a fatal outcome and may prevent the disease entirely. It is unlikely, however, that smallpox would be diagnosed early enough and vaccination programs launched rapidly enough to prevent infection of many of the people exposed during the first wave. Few physicians have ever seen smallpox and few, if any, have ever received training in its diagnosis. . . .

A second wave of cases would be almost inevitable. From experiences with smallpox imported into Europe over the past 40 years, it is estimated that there would be at least 10 secondary cases for every case in the first wave, or 1000 cases in all, appearing some 14 days after the first wave. Vaccination would initially be needed for health workers, essential service personnel, and contacts of patients at home and at work. With mounting numbers of cases, contacts, and involved areas, mass vaccination would soon be the only practical approach. That would not be possible, however, because present vaccine supplies are too limited, there being approximately 5 to 7 million doses currently available. To put this number in perspective, in New York City in 1947, 6 million people were vaccinated over approximately 1 week in response to a total of eight cases of smallpox. Moreover, there are no longer any manufacturers of smallpox vaccine. Best estimates indicate that substantial additional supplies could not be ensured sooner than 36 months from the initial outbreak. [*Editor's comment*: The United States announced a major initiative to increase vaccine supply in November 2001.]

A scenario for an inhalation anthrax epidemic is of no less concern. Like smallpox, the aerosol would almost certainly be unobtrusively released and would drift throughout a building or even a city without being noticed. After 2 to 3 days, infected individuals would appear in emergency rooms and doctors' offices with a variety of nonspecific symptoms such as fever, cough, and headache. Within a day or two, patients would become critically ill and then die within 24 to 72 hours. It is doubtful that antibiotic therapy given after symptoms develop would be of benefit. The case fatality rate is 80% or greater.

Although anthrax does not spread from person to person, it has another dangerous attribute. Individuals who are exposed to an aerosol may abruptly develop illness up to 8 weeks after the initial exposure. Cases can be prevented by the administration of antibiotics, but such treatment would have to be continued daily for at least 60 days. This period might be shortened by the prompt administration of vaccine. Experimental studies suggest that two doses of vaccine given 15 days apart may provide protection beginning 30 days after the initial inoculation. At this time, however, there is no vaccine available for civilian use; building of stockpiles of antibiotics is still in the planning stage, and no city at present has a plan for distributing antibiotics so as to ensure that drugs are given over a 60-day period. [*Editor's comment*: The United States began stockpiling antibiotics in response to the intentional anthrax dispersals in the fall of 2001.]

## A LOOK AT THE FUTURE

At the request of the president and with bipartisan support from Congress, $133 million was appropriated to HHS for fiscal 1999 for countering biological and chemical threats, $51 million of which is for an emergency stockpile of antibiotics and vaccines. Most of the funds are allocated to the CDC, primarily for the strengthening of the infectious disease surveillance network and for enhancing the capacity of federal and state laboratories. This is not a large sum of money, considering the needs of a fragile public health infrastructure extending over 50 states and at least 120 major cities, but it is a beginning.

The most effective step now is to strengthen the public health and infectious disease infrastructure. An augmented full-time cadre of professionals at the state and local level would represent, for biological weapons, a counterpart to the National Guard Rapid Assessment and Initial Detection Teams for chemical weapons. Rather than being on a standby basis, however, the biological cadre would also serve to strengthen efforts directed toward dealing with new and emerging infections and food-borne diseases. . . .

National Institutes of Health– and CDC-administered research agendas are needed to attract both university and private sector talents to address a host of constraints and problems. Among the most critical needs now are improved vaccines, available in large supply, for both smallpox and anthrax. Areas for vaccine improvement include increasing overall efficacy; in the case of smallpox, reducing complications and in the case of anthrax, reducing the number of inoculations. Feasibility studies suggest that substantially improved second-generation vaccines can be developed quickly.

Finally, there is a need both now and in the longer term to pursue measures that will prevent acts of terrorism. . . . The strengthening of our intelligence capabilities so as to anticipate and perhaps interdict terrorists is of the highest priority. The fostering of international cooperative research programs to encourage openness and dialogue as is now being done with Russian laboratories is also important.

---

## Biological and Chemical Terrorism:
## Strategic Plan for Preparedness and Response*
*Centers for Disease Control and Prevention*

### INTRODUCTION

The public health infrastructure must be prepared to prevent illness and injury that would result from biological and chemical terrorism, especially a covert terrorist attack. As with emerging infectious diseases, early detection and control of biological or chemical attacks depends on a strong and flexible public health system at the local, state, and federal levels. In addition, primary health-care providers throughout the United States must be vigilant because they will probably be the first to observe and report unusual illnesses or injuries. . . .

### U.S. VULNERABILITY TO BIOLOGICAL AND CHEMICAL TERRORISM

Terrorist incidents in the United States and elsewhere involving bacterial pathogens, nerve gas, and a lethal plant toxin (i.e., ricin) have demonstrated that the United States is vulnerable to biological and chemical threats as well as explosives. Recipes for preparing "homemade" agents are readily available, and reports of arsenals of military bioweapons raise the possibility that terrorists might have access to highly dangerous agents, which have been engineered for mass dissemination as small-particle aerosols. . . . Responding to large-scale outbreaks caused by these agents will require the rapid mobilization of

---

*Reprinted from *Morbidity and Mortality Weekly Report* 49 (April 21, 2000): 1–13.

public health workers, emergency responders, and private health-care providers. Large-scale outbreaks will also require rapid procurement and distribution of large quantities of drugs and vaccines, which must be available quickly.

## OVERT VERSUS COVERT TERRORIST ATTACKS

In the past, most planning for emergency response to terrorism has been concerned with overt attacks (e.g., bombings). Chemical terrorism acts are likely to be overt because the effects of chemical agents absorbed through inhalation or by absorption through the skin or mucous membranes are usually immediate and obvious. Such attacks elicit immediate response from police, fire, and EMS personnel.

In contrast, attacks with biological agents are more likely to be covert. They present different challenges and require an additional dimension of emergency planning that involves the public health infrastructure. Covert dissemination of a biological agent in a public place will not have an immediate impact because of the delay between exposure and onset of illness (i.e., the incubation period). Consequently, the first casualties of a covert attack probably will be identified by physicians or other primary health-care providers. . . . Only a short window of opportunity will exist between the time the first cases are identified and a second wave of the population becomes ill. During that brief period, public health officials will need to determine that an attack has occurred, identify the organism, and prevent more casualties through prevention strategies (e.g., mass vaccination or prophylactic treatment). As person-to-person contact continues, successive waves of transmission could carry infection to other worldwide localities. These issues might also be relevant for other person-to-person transmissible etiologic agents (e.g., plague or certain viral hemorrhagic fevers). . . .

## FOCUSING PREPAREDNESS ACTIVITIES

Early detection of and response to biological or chemical terrorism are crucial. Without special preparation at the local and state levels, a large-scale attack with variola virus, aerosolized anthrax spores, a nerve gas, or a foodborne biological or chemical agent could overwhelm the local and perhaps national public health infrastructure. Large numbers of patients, including both infected persons and the "worried well," would seek medical attention, with a corresponding need for medical supplies, diagnostic tests, and hospital beds. Emergency responders, health-care workers, and public health officials could be at special risk, and everyday life would be disrupted as a result of widespread fear of contagion. . . .

Steps in Preparing for Biological Attacks

- Enhance epidemiologic capacity to detect and respond to biological attacks.
- Supply diagnostic reagents to state and local public health agencies.
- Establish communications programs to ensure delivery of accurate information.
- Enhance bioterrorism-related education and training for healthcare professionals.
- Prepare educational materials that will inform and reassure the public during and after a biological attack.
- Stockpile appropriate vaccines and drugs.
- Establish molecular surveillance for microbial strains including unusual or drug-resistant strains.
- Support the development of diagnostic tests.
- Encourage research on antiviral drugs and vaccines.

## CONCLUSION

Investment in national defense ensures preparedness and acts as a deterrent against hostile acts. Similarly, investment in the public health system provides the best civil defense against bioterrorism. Tools developed in response to terrorist threats serve a dual purpose. They help detect rare or unusual disease outbreaks and respond to health emergencies, including naturally occurring outbreaks or industrial injuries that might resemble terrorist events in their unpredictability and ability to cause mass casualties (e.g., a pandemic influenza outbreak or a large-scale chemical spill). Terrorism-preparedness activities described in CDC's plan, including the development of a public health communication infrastructure, a multilevel network of diagnostic laboratories, and an integrated disease surveillance system, will improve our ability to investigate rapidly and control public health threats that emerge in the twenty-first century.

*     *     *     *     *

Preparedness for and response to bioterrorism require not only a strong public health infrastructure, but also sound legal foundations. At least three kinds of laws are required to effectively combat bioterrorism: emer-

TABLE 11

LAWS TO COMBAT BIOTERRORISM

| | |
|---|---|
| Emergency Management | Civil preparedness: scarcity, panic, and civil unrest |
| Criminal Sanctions | Possession, manufacture, or distribution of biological weapons<br>Threats, hoaxes, and conspiracies |
| Public Health Powers | Collection and analysis of data<br>Control of property<br>Management of persons |

TABLE 12

PUBLIC HEALTH POWERS NEEDED IN A BIOTERRORISM EVENT

| | |
|---|---|
| Data Collection | Report new diseases, unusual clusters, and suspicious events<br>Access medical records<br>Share data with law enforcement |
| Control of Property | Access suspicious premises<br>Close or decontaminate facilities<br>Seize or destroy property<br>Confiscate, control, or ration property |
| Control of Persons | Detain and question persons<br>Collect lab specimens and perform tests<br>Track exposed persons and contacts and provide follow-up<br>Perform physical examination, vaccination, and medical treatment<br>Isolate and quarantine<br>Manage fatalities |

gency management, criminal sanctions, and public health powers (Table 11).* Emergency management laws enable health and safety officers to respond to the destabilizing effects of terrorism: scarcity of necessities (e.g., food, transportation, medical services), panic, and civil unrest. Criminal sanctions can be used for deterrence and punishment of individuals for possession, manufacture, or distribution of a biological weapon, as well as for threats, hoaxes, and conspiracies. Finally, emergency public health powers may be necessary to collect and analyze data, control property, and control persons in a bioterrorism event (Table 12). For a Model Emergency

---

*I am indebted to Eugene Matthews and Verla Neslund, Office of the General Counsel at the CDC, for this discussion of laws relating to bioterrorism.

Health Powers Act drafted in response to the World Trade Center attack, see the *Reader* web site.

*Data collection.* Public health authorities may need legal authorization to report new diseases, unusual clusters, and suspicious events; to gain access to confidential records held by hospitals, managed care organizations, or health care professionals; and to share data with law enforcement agencies.

*Control of property.* Authorities may need authorization to gain access to suspicious premises; to close or decontaminate facilities (e.g., a building or subway system that harbors a biological agent); to seize or destroy property; and to control, confiscate, or ration property (e.g., health care facilities, pharmaceutical or biotechnology companies, and drug or vaccine stockpiles).

*Control of persons.* Public health officials may need authority to detain and question exposed persons; track and follow up exposed persons and their contacts; collect laboratory specimens and perform tests; compel physical examination, vaccination, and medical treatment; isolate infected persons or quarantine geographic areas; and manage fatalities.

Public health authorities, moreover, may not have the capacity to respond to bioterrorism and may require additional resources. For example, they may need the assistance of the police and military to help enforce public health powers. At the same time, bioterrorism rarely will be confined to a single jurisdiction, but will require the cooperation of various federal, state, and local agencies. It will be important in any given situation to establish clarity as to the agencies and personnel that have primary responsibility.

The powers that government needs to respond to bioterrorism undermine civil liberties: autonomy, bodily integrity, privacy, liberty, and property. The threat to populations is real and substantial, suggesting the need for strong powers. Emergency situations, however, are often used to justify the denial of civil liberties and can lead to overreaction by public officials. How much power should society be prepared to delegate to authorities in a public health emergency? Has that calculation changed since September 11, 2001?

## III. FROM GENES TO PUBLIC HEALTH

For many people, it is difficult to imagine how genetics
and public health intersect. We repeatedly hear that
genetic information is individual, intensely private, indeed

more private than almost any other kind of information,
and in today's environment potentially hazardous to
one's access to employment and insurance. One person's
genetic makeup rarely presents a risk to the health of
others; a woman who has a mutation in BRCA1 and so
is more susceptible to breast cancer cannot transmit the
disease or even the mutation to her best friend. At the
same time, most people think of public health in terms of
the interventions that public health agencies impose on
large groups of people to improve health, ranging from
fluoridation of water to immunization or, in extreme
cases, quarantine. Thinking about the conjunction of private concerns and public actions makes it hard even to
consider genetics and public health at the same time.

*Ellen Wright Clayton (2000, 489)*

The international scientific community mapped the human genome in
2001, commencing the long and arduous task of understanding the relationships between genes and human health. Scientists have long
known about hereditary diseases such as cystic fibrosis, Huntington's
chorea, sickle-cell anemia, and Tay-Sachs disease. The Human Genome
Project now promises to help us understand multifactorial diseases such
as cancer, diabetes, heart disease, and schizophrenia.

Genetic sciences hope to provide many benefits, including informed individual choices through supplying patients predictive information about
their health status, identification of the etiology and physiology of disease,
clinical advances to prevent and treat genetic diseases, and enhanced medical research (Gostin and Hodge 1999). At the same time, increased use of
genetic testing, diagnosis, and clinical intervention raises social concerns,
including privacy invasion through the disclosure of genetic data, stigma
and discrimination (loss of employment or health insurance), inequitable
allocation of benefits and burdens (favoring the rich and powerful), and al-
teration of the "natural" order of life (genetic enhancements, artificial reproduction, and cloning) (Burris, Gostin, and Tress 2000).

Most of these benefits and burdens are cast in individual terms, focusing primarily on clinical decision making, health care policy, and
bioethics. There is, however, another important aspect of genetic science that powerfully affects the health and well-being of populations.
Known as "public health genetics," this field assesses the impact of
genes and their interaction with behavior, diet, and the environment on

the population's health (CDC 1997; Khoury, Burke, and Thomson 2000; Khoury and Genetics Working Group 1996). Public health practitioners and researchers can track the incidence, patterns, and trends of genetic traits and diseases across populations; develop strategies to promote health and prevent disease in populations; and more precisely target interventions based on surveillance and epidemiological investigations.

Public health genetics is an exciting field that brings all the public health sciences to bear on the emerging challenge of interpreting the significance of genetic variation within populations. In research, practice, and policy, both genetics and public health focus on populations. Gilbert S. Omenn (2000, 1–2), of the University of Washington, explains the interdisciplinary nature of public health genetics:

> The sequencing of the human genome and the subsequent demonstration of variation in numerous genes in health and disease will surely stimulate a golden age for the public health sciences. It will be essential to investigate and link other data to information about genetic variation, including data on microbial, chemical, and physical exposures; nutrition, metabolism, growth, and development; lifestyle behaviors; and diagnoses, medications, and health care utilization. Such studies must be conducted on a population basis to interpret the significance of the genetic variation. Laboratory scientists, clinician-investigators, and health care professionals will rely on epidemiologists, biostatisticians, environmental health scientists, behavioral scientists, health economists, and health policy analysts for the collaborative research that will inform evidence-based, cost-effective medical care and public health interventions.

Genetic information contributes to many existing areas of study in public health. For example, marked genetic heterogeneity exists in susceptibility to specific infectious agents (e.g., malaria, TB, HIV/AIDS), exposure to environmental toxins or contaminants, intake of nutrients, and ingestion of prescription medications. In short, exposure to certain pathogens, pollutants, diets, and drugs can affect people quite differently depending on individual genetic traits. Additionally, genetics may have a role in influencing risk behaviors such as smoking, alcoholic beverage consumption, and illicit drug use.

Genetics offers unprecedented promise to change our understanding of how the health of populations is determined and to provide new tools for improving health and reducing disease burden. As scientists learn how nature and nurture interact at the cellular level, policy makers will have important decisions to make about the ecosystem and exposures, the risk/reward ratios of different activities, and even when to alter the genome. In a preface to a major symposium on public health genetics, Jonathan E. Fielding and his colleagues (2000, vi) explain the complex policy issues raised:

> We will need to rethink how standards for environmental and occupational exposures are set, because we will know much more about the variation in human susceptibility to different effects of environmental influences. As one example, will we permit new chemical compounds that cause neurotoxicity in one child per million or the continued manufacture and sale of an existing compound that has this result? Will new laws permit employers to require genetic testing and legally exclude from certain types of jobs those individuals whose genetic predispositions place them at greatly increased risk for adverse health effects? Could an individual who is found to be 10-fold more likely than average to sustain a back injury by lifting heavy objects be legally excluded by a prospective employer from a job that requires these activities? Will prospective employees be required to submit to genetic screening to determine whether they are particularly susceptible to adverse effects of chemicals to which they would be exposed occupationally? Will the FDA change its approach to food labeling based on greater understanding of polymorphism in biotransformational enzymes, which can predispose to cancer, cardiovascular disease, or cerebral degeneration? Although these generic questions of ascertaining risk, workers vs. employer rights, assignment of legal liabilities, and the setting of standards are not new, we will have much better and more quantifiable data to consider in making individual and societal decisions. The looming question is how to translate better data into better decisions.

In the following excerpt, Muin J. Khoury and his colleagues at the CDC's Office of Genetics and Disease Prevention explain the public health approach to genetics.

---

## Challenges in Communicating Genetics: A Public Health Approach*

*Muin J. Khoury, James F. Thrasher, Wylie Burke, Elizabeth A. Gettig, Fred Fridinger, and Richard Jackson*

[A]lmost every day brings a new scientific discovery of a genetic variant that is associated with a specific disease. In the wake of these discoveries,

---

*Reprinted from *Genetics in Medicine* 2 (May/June 2000): 198–202.

the popular press has published numerous articles on how advances in genetic science will radically transform the practice of medicine. These portrayals of the impact of genetics are typified by a recent special issue of Time magazine with headlines reading: "Parenting: Designer Babies," "Genetic Screening: Good Eggs, Bad Eggs," and "Cursed by Eugenics." Rarely, if ever, do these and other articles on genetics cover the public health implications of gene discovery.

The impact of genetic discoveries on public health practice is likely to be felt across all disease areas. . . . [and] has prompted the challenge of finding effective public health interventions based on genetic-epidemiologic information. Public health professionals will increasingly use genetic information to more effectively target behavioral and environmental factors that lead to many diseases. . . .

## HUMAN DISEASES RESULT FROM GENE-ENVIRONMENT INTERACTION

Popular representations of genetics are often deterministic, reinforcing a view of humans as a product of their genes, to the exclusion of nongenetic factors. Early discoveries of severe and often incurable conditions may have raised concerns about genetic determinism (e.g., Tay-Sachs disease, Huntington disease). Indeed, many of these disorders can be traced to a deficiency in the product of one gene that leads to a very high risk of developing some clinical disease. Insights into these single-gene diseases have been extremely important because, collectively, they make up approximately 5–10% of human disease. However, the role of common genetic variants (often called polymorphisms) in susceptibility to common diseases is increasingly understood. As more and more of these genetic variants are discovered, the scope of the public discussion of genetics needs to be broadened beyond single-gene disorders to include almost all human diseases. A useful framework upon which to build discussions about the integration of genetics into public health starts with the idea of gene-environment interaction.

We often tend to think about the spectrum of disease causation as ranging from completely genetic to completely environmental. A common way to summarize and present information about the causes of a specific condition is through a causal pie chart in which all of the causes add up to 100% of the disease. Common methods of genetic analysis (e.g., twin studies) are designed to partition the components of genetic and environmental contributions to disease. However, stating that a condition X is 40% genetic and 60% environmental sets up a misleading dichotomy between genes and the environment and obscures the fact that most if not all human disease results from the interaction between genetic susceptibility and environmental factors (broadly defined to include infectious, chemical, physical, nutritional, and behavioral factors). Even many of the classic single-gene disorders of metabolism result from a deficiency in a gene-produced enzyme that breaks down one or more chemicals in the diet. For example, phenylketonuria (PKU) results from a genetic variant that leads to deficient metabolism of the amino acid phenylalanine; in the presence of normal protein intake, phenylalanine accumulation occurs and is neurotoxic, but the disease can be prevented with a diet low in phenylalanine. The excessive build up of phenylalanine causes the disease, not the gene or dietary exposure by itself. Similarly, the so-called environmentally caused diseases are influenced by genetic susceptibility. For example, even though more than 90% of lung cancer is caused by cigarette smoking, only 10–15% of smokers will develop lung cancer, indicating the interaction of smoking with other factors including genetic ones. Everyone carries genetic variants that increase their susceptibility to some diseases, and, as a result, the same environmental factors will differently affect the development of disease.

If we accept the fundamental premise that variations in genetic make-up are associated with all human disease, there is no compelling reason to label a disease as either genetic or environmental. . . .

For most diseases, there is a large gap between the discovery of a gene and the safe and effective use of genetic information to prevent disease. A simple public health message is that gene discovery is only a beginning. Moving beyond gene discovery to relevant action in the health care system requires research activities in each of the core functions of public health: (1) *assessment*—including epidemiologic research to quantify the impact of a genetic variant and gene-environment interaction on community health; (2) *policy development*—including research to identify and analyze the economic, social, ethical, and psychological implications of advances in human genetics, and the information and communication needs of the general public; and (3) *assurance*—including health service delivery research to identify factors that influence the delivery, utilization, and quality of genetic tests and services. If genetics is not integrated into a public health research agenda, we may not be able to "translate" the numerous gene discoveries into meaningful population-based information that can be used to improve health and prevent disease. . . . Public health professionals will be increasingly involved in monitoring and investigating the impact of genetic variation on the health of communities, developing policy on the appropriate use of genetic tests and services, ensuring the provision of appropriate services, and evaluating the health impact of using genetic information. . . .

When there are proven and cost-effective interventions to prevent disease and disability, the public heath community should take a more active role in promoting the use of genetic tests and services. The need for such public health–driven prevention is more clear-cut for adult-onset multifactorial conditions such as cancer and heart disease, than it is for early-onset, lethal single-gene conditions. Juengst (1995) calls this "phenotypic prevention," the prevention of disease, disability, or death among people with specific genotypes. In its recent strategic plan, CDC endorsed the concept of phenotypic prevention as the strategy for public health–driven programs.

Media coverage of phenotypic prevention concentrates on the medical interventions of gene therapy and pharmacogenomics. Gene therapy refers to replacing the products of nonfunctional genes, and holds great promise for "fixing" many single-gene disorders ranging from cystic fibrosis to thalassemia. Inroads have even been made in the treatment of various cancers by manipulating the genes of malignant cells. Pharmacogenomics may also improve health by identifying genetic factors that contribute to drug metabolism. Researchers in this emerging field will be designing drugs to prevent adverse side effects caused by genetic susceptibility and to enhance therapeutic effectiveness. This approach could include tailoring drug regimens to an individual's genetic profile. . . .

Despite the excitement about new technologies such as gene therapy and pharmacogenomics, it is important to consider that public health interventions based on genetic information are just as likely, if not more likely, to impact disease prevention at the population level. The fact that most human diseases arise from gene-environment interactions leads to the potential for public health interventions on the environmental side. Indeed, many major successes in improving health stem from public health efforts to modify environments. CDC's recent list of the top public health achievements of the 20th century include vaccinations, smoking reduction, prenatal care, food safety, control of occupational exposures, infectious disease control, and water fluoridation [see Table 8]. As we enter the post–human genome project era in the new millennium, it is important to envision the role that environmental interventions could play.

Environmental interventions, medical treatment, diet modification, and behavior modification have already been developed for many single-gene traits that confer a relatively high risk for disease. It is more difficult to devise such precise interventions for common and chronic diseases that have multiple causes. . . . [G]enetic information could more adequately quantify an individual's susceptibility to disease, and, by doing so, could clarify the specific factors that interact with this susceptibility to produce disease. . . . The genetic information that is used to explain such situations will also provide a guide to the most effective targeting of programs for medical, behavioral, and environmental risk reduction.

Genetic information may also provide guidance for targeted screening efforts. For instance, persons who have a first-degree relative with colorectal cancer have an increased risk and earlier onset of colorectal cancer, compared with persons without a family history. Early initiation of colorectal cancer screening in this group represents a public health opportunity. For a small subset of cases in which family history suggests high risk (multiply affected relatives, early age at onset), genetic testing may help determine the most effective recommendations around the frequency, method, and onset of screening. . . .

Knowledge of genetics presents an opportunity to prevent disease and reduce fear over the misuse of genetic information. Qualitative and quantitative research can help determine the best means of communicating about genetics and disease prevention. We hope that these messages can be used to initiate discussions on how scientific advances in genetics will be translated into public health action in the 21st century.

---

\*     \*     \*     \*     \*

The idea of public health genetics, of course, raises profound ethical issues because of its concern with "healthy" genes among the population. This reminds the public of the eugenics movement in the early twentieth century, which sought to "improve" the gene pool by sterilizing persons with mental or physical disabilities. Modern genetics similarly may affect individual or societal decisions concerning reproduction, abortion, and genetic manipulation (e.g., germline therapy or genetic enhancements). Most people do not object to the concept of preventing and treating genetic disease. However, they do object to policies that undermine personal choice or are unfair. In the next reading, four leading bioethicists probe the ethical dimensions of public health genetics and the importance of autonomy and justice.

---

### Two Models for Genetic Intervention*
*Allen Buchanan, Dan W. Brock, Norman Daniels, and Daniel Wikler*

#### THE PUBLIC HEALTH MODEL

Our "ethical autopsy" on eugenics identifies two quite different perspectives from which genetic intervention may be viewed. The first is what we call the public health model; the second is the personal choice model.

The public health model stresses the production of benefits and the avoidance of harms for groups. It uncritically assumes that the appropriate mode of evaluating options is some form of cost-benefit (or cost-effectiveness) calculation. To the extent that the public health model even recognizes an ethical dimension to decisions about the application of scientific knowledge or technology, it tends to assume that sound ethical reasoning is exclusively consequentialist (or utilitarian) in nature. In other words, it assumes that whether a policy or an action is deemed to be right is thought to depend solely on whether it produces the greatest balance of good over bad outcomes.

More important, consequentialist ethical reasoning—like cost-benefit and cost-effectiveness calculations—assumes that it is not only possible but permissible and even mandatory to aggregate goods and bads (costs and benefits) across individuals. Harms to some can be offset by gains to others; what matters is the sum. Critics of such simple and unqualified consequentialist reasoning, including ourselves, are quick to point out its fundamental flaws: Such reasoning is distributionally insensitive

---

*Reprinted from *From Chance to Choice* (Cambridge: Cambridge University Press, 2000), 11–14, 55–60, with the permission of Cambridge University Press. © 2000 Cambridge University Press.

because it fails to take seriously the separateness and inviolability of persons.

In other words, as simple and unqualified consequentialist reasoning looks only to the aggregate balance of good over bad, it does not recognize fairness in the distribution of burdens and benefits to be a fundamental value. As a result, it not only allows but in some circumstances requires that the most fundamental interests of individuals be sacrificed in order to produce the best overall outcome.

Consequentialist ethical theory is not unique in allowing or even requiring that the interests of individuals sometimes yield to the good of all. Any reasonable ethical theory must acknowledge this. But it is unique in maintaining that in principle such sacrifice is justified whenever it would produce any aggregate gain, no matter how small. Because simple and unqualified consequentialism has this implication, some conclude that it fails to appreciate sufficiently that each individual is an irreducibly distinct subject of moral concern.

The public health model, with its affinity for consequentialist ethical reasoning, took a particularly troubling form among some prominent eugenicists. Individuals who were thought to harbor "defective germ plasm" (what would now be called "bad genes") were likened to carriers of infectious disease. While persons infected with cholera were a menace to those with whom they came into contact, individuals with defective germ plasm were an even greater threat to society: They transmitted harm to an unlimited line of persons across many generations.

The only difference between the "horizontally transmitted" infectious diseases and "vertically transmitted" genetic diseases, according to this view, was that the potential harm caused by the latter was even greater. So if measures such as quarantine and restrictions on travel into disease areas that infringed individual freedom were appropriate responses to the former, then they were even more readily justified to avert the greater potential harm of the latter. This variant of the public health model may be called the vertical epidemic model. Once this point of view is adopted and combined with a simple and unqualified consequentialism, the risks of infringing liberty and of exclusion and discrimination increase dramatically.

## THE PERSONAL SERVICE MODEL

Today eugenics is almost universally condemned. Partly in reaction to the tendency of the most extreme eugenicists to discount individual freedom and welfare for the supposed good of society, medical geneticists and genetic counselors since World War II have adopted an almost absolute commitment to "nondirectiveness" in their relations with those seeking genetic services. Recoiling from the public health model that dominated the eugenics movement, and especially from the vertical disease metaphor, they publicly endorse the view that genetic tests and interventions are simply services offered to individuals — goods for private consumption — to be accepted or refused as individuals see fit.

This way of conceiving of genetic interventions takes them out of the public domain, relegating them to the sphere of private choice. Advocates of the personal service model proclaim that the fundamental value on which it rests is individual autonomy. Whether a couple at risk for conceiving a child with a genetic disease takes a genetic test and how they use the knowledge thus obtained is their business, not society's, even if the decision to vaccinate a child for common childhood infectious diseases is a matter of public health and as such justifies restricting parental choice.

The personal service model serves as a formidable bulwark against the excesses of the crude consequentialist ethical reasoning that tainted the application of the public health model in the era of eugenics. But it does so at a prohibitive price: It ignores the obligation to prevent harm as well as some of the most basic requirements of justice. By elevating autonomy to the exclusion of all other values, the personal service model offers a myopic view of the moral landscape.

In fact, it is misleading to say that the personal service model expresses a commitment to autonomy. Instead, it honors only the autonomy of those who are in a position to exercise choice concerning genetic interventions, not all of those who may be affected by such choices. [T]his approach wrongly subordinates the autonomy of children to that of their parents.

In addition, if genetic services are treated as goods for private consumption, the cumulative effects of many individual choices in the "genetic marketplace" may limit the autonomy of many people, and perhaps of all people. Economic pressures, including requirements for insurability and employment, as well as social stigma directed toward those who produce children with "defects" that could have been avoided, may narrow rather than expand meaningful choice. Finally, treating genetic interventions as personal services may exacerbate inequalities in opportunities if the prevention of genetic diseases or genetic enhancements are available only to the rich. It would be more accurate to say, then, that the personal service model gives free reign to some dimensions of the autonomy of some people, often at the expense of others.

## A THIRD APPROACH

Much current thinking about the ethics of genetic intervention assumes that the personal service model is not an adequate moral guide. However, the common response to its deficiencies is not to resurrect the public health model associated with eugenics. Instead, there is a tendency to assume the appropriateness of the personal service model in general and then to erect ad hoc—and less than convincing—"moral firebreaks" to constrain the free choices of individuals in certain areas. For example, some ethicists have urged that the cloning of human beings be strictly prohibited, that there be a moratorium or permanent ban on human germline interventions, or that genetic enhancements (as opposed to treatments of diseases) be outlawed. In each case the proposed moral firebreak shows a distrust of the unalloyed personal service model but at the same time betrays the lack of a systematic, principled account of why and how the choices of individuals should be limited. . . .

We argue that although respect for individual autonomy requires an extensive sphere of protected reproductive freedoms and hence a broad range of personal discretion in decisions to use genetic interventions, both the need to prevent harm to offspring and the demands of justice, especially those regarding equal opportunity, place systematic limits on individuals' freedom to use or not use genetic interventions. . . .

## THE SOCIAL DIMENSION OF GENETICS

In our view, the key issue in appraising the shadow cast by the eugenics movement on clinical genetics is not whether those who build programs of clinical genetics have an individual focus as opposed to a social one. The social goal is not automatically suspect. What matters is whether either goal is pursued justly. In particular, the fact that the prospect of better health—or even enhanced functioning, apart from health—in the next generation is a worthy goal, other things being equal, does not in itself show that this goal would justify restrictions on liberties, social inequalities, or other measures that are suspect from the perspective of justice. Constrained and guided by concerns of justice—the chief focus of this volume—the prospect of healthier and more able generations of human beings in the years to come is an appropriate and defensible goal of public policy on genetics. . . .

The eugenicists were ahead of their time—which was probably a good thing. Since they lacked the means to detect recessive genes in the population, even with full compliance their proposals would hardly make a dent in the distribution of the genes they imagined to be of social importance. More important, their sole instrument of change was the blunderbuss weapon of human breeding (and in extreme cases, sterilization, and euthanasia). Humans are notoriously hard to breed; we are animals with hearts and minds of our own. . . . Our powers are much more impressive, and humankind's future abilities to rewrite our genetic code are apparently limitless. . . . Could eugenicists of the old school make a convincing case for reinstituting their programs, cleansed this time around of bias and pseudoscience and respectful of individual rights? . . .

The core notion of eugenics, that people's lives will probably go better if they have genes conducive to health and other advantageous traits, has lost little of its appeal. Eugenics, in this very limited sense, shines a beacon even as it casts a shadow. Granted, when our society last undertook to improve our genes, the result was mayhem. The task for humanity now is to accomplish what eluded the eugenicists entirely, to square the pursuit of genetic health and enhancement with the requirements of justice. . . .

GENETICS IN PURSUIT OF JUSTICE

Looking to the more distant future, we may entertain the proposition that genetics be used specifically to bring about a more just society. The mainstream eugenicists pursued this goal, in their own fashion, insofar as they believed that the "unfit" were an unfair burden on the fit. We can reject the eugenicists' notions of what is just without disavowing the possibility of using genetics to achieve greater justice. These prospects are largely speculative today, since there is little that we will be able to do in the near future to rectify social injustices. But what if we could distribute genes as readily as we can (but rarely do) distribute wealth? Would justice require that we create a society of equals? Or, if we discovered that greater efficiency and satisfaction were attainable by creating human beings in five distinct grades of overall ability, as in the society in Huxley's *Brave New World*, would this be the better choice—particularly if the added efficiency added to the well-being of even the lowliest members of society? We have a long time, perhaps measured in centuries, to deliberate about such questions. Still, they are of practical importance if they point toward any near-term policies that might affect such dimensions of social justice as overall equality.

---

\*     \*     \*     \*     \*

Buchanan and his colleagues raise fundamental questions about public health genetics. How important is reproductive freedom? Should society strive to increase certain human traits (e.g., intelligence, beauty, strength) within the gene pool? Put another way, should society strive to decrease or eliminate disabilities in the population (e.g., deafness, dwarfism, or Down syndrome)? What effects will genetic sciences have on the enterprise of insurance once future health and disability are far more predictable than at present?

## CONCLUSION

I desire, in closing the series of introductory papers, to
leave this one great fact clearly stated. There is no wealth
but life. Life, including all its powers of love, of joy, and
of admiration. That country is richest which nourishes
the greatest number of noble and happy human beings;
that man is richest, who, having perfected the functions
of his own life to the utmost, has also the widest helpful
influence, both personal, and by possessions, over the
lives of others.

*John Ruskin (1862, 54)*

This chapter, and the *Reader* as a whole, demonstrate the complexity of public health theory and practice. As a society, we want to achieve health and well-being in the community and distribute benefits fairly among all members. At the same time, we want to respect the inviolability of each individual. The values of population health, social justice, and strong personal autonomy are not always in harmony. Society's only sensible course is to search for answers based on rigorous ethical principles, respect for democratic institutions, and adherence to legal doctrine and human rights.

# Bibliography

Advisory Committee on Human Radiation Experiments. *Final Report.* Washington, DC: Department of Energy, 1996.

Advisory Committee on Immunization Practices. "Combination Vaccines for Childhood Immunization." *Pediatrics* 103 (May 1999): 1064–77.

Advisory Council for the Elimination of Tuberculosis. "Initial Therapy for Tuberculosis in the Era of Multidrug Resistance: Recommendations of the Advisory Council for the Elimination of Tuberculosis." *Mortality and Morbidity Weekly Report* 42 (RR7) (1993): 1–8.

Ainslie, Donald C. "AIDS, Sexual Ethics, and the Duty to Warn." *Hastings Center Report* 29 (September–October 1999): 26–35.

Aldana, Steven G. "Financial Impact of Health Promotion Programs: A Comprehensive Review of the Literature." *American Journal of Public Health Promotion* 15 (2001): 296–320.

Allen, Peter Lewis. "AIDS in the U.S.A." In *The Wages of Sin: Sex and Disease, Past and Present.* Chicago: Univ. of Chicago Press, 2000.

American Civil Liberties Union. *HIV Surveillance and Name Reporting.* New York: ACLU, 1998.

Angell, Marcia. "The Ethics of Clinical Research in the Third World." *New England Journal of Medicine* 337 (1997a): 847–49.

———. *Science on Trial: The Clash of Medical Evidence and the Law in the Breast Implant Case.* London: W.W. Norton, 1997b.

Annas, George J. "Burden of Proof: Judging Science and Protecting Public Health in (and out of) the Courtroom." *American Journal of Public Health* 89 (1999): 490–93.

———. "Human Rights and Health—The Universal Declaration of Human Rights at 50." *New England Journal of Medicine* 339 (1998): 1777–81.

Annas, George J., and Michael A. Grodin. *The Nazi Doctors and the Nuremberg Code: Human Rights in Human Experimentation.* New York: Oxford Univ. Press, 1995.

Areen, Judith A., Patricia A. King, Steven Goldberg, Lawrence O. Gostin, and Alexander Morgan Capron, eds. *Law, Science and Medicine.* 2nd ed. New York: Foundation Press, 1996.

Armstrong, Gregory L., Laura A. Conn, and Robert Pinner. "Trends in Infectious Disease Mortality in the United States During the 20th Century." *Journal of the American Medical Association* 281 (1999): 61–66.

Arrow, Kenneth J., Maureen L. Cropper, George C. Eads, Robert W. Hahn, Lester B. Lave, Roger F. Noll, Paul R. Partney, Richard Schmalensee, V. Kerry Smith, and Robert N. Stavins. "Is There a Role for Benefit-Cost Analysis in Environmental, Health and Safety Regulation?" *Science* 272 (1996): 221–22.

Atchison, Christopher, M. A. Barry, N. Kanarek, and Kristine M. Gebbie. "The Quest for an Accurate Accounting of Public Health Expenditures." *Journal of Public Health Management Practice* 6 (2000): 93–102.

Bayer, Ronald. "AIDS Prevention—Sexual Ethics and Responsibility." *New England Journal of Medicine* 334 (1996): 1540–42.

———. "Ethical Challenges Posed by Zidovudine Treatment to Reduce Vertical Transmission of HIV." *New England Journal of Medicine* 331 (1994): 1223–25.

Bayer, Ronald, and Amy Fairchild-Carrino. "AIDS and the Limits of Control: Public Health Orders, Quarantine, and Recalcitrant Behavior." *American Journal of Public Health* 83 (1993): 1471–76.

Bayer, Ronald, and Jonathan D. Moreno. "Health Promotion: Ethical and Social Dilemmas of Government Policy." *Health Affairs* 5 (Summer 1986): 72–85.

Bayer, Ronald, Catherine Stayton, Moise Desvarieux, Cheryl Healton, Sheldon Landesman, and Wei-Yann Tsai. "Directly Observed Therapy and Treatment Completion for Tuberculosis in the United States: Is Universal Supervised Therapy Necessary?" *American Journal of Public Health* 88 (1998): 1052–58.

Bayer, Ronald, and Kathleen E. Toomey. "HIV Prevention and the Two Faces of Partner Notification." *American Journal of Public Health* 82 (1992): 1158–64.

Bayer, Ronald, and David Wilkinson. "Directly Observed Therapy for Tuberculosis: History of an Idea." *Lancet* 345 (1995): 1545–48.

Beaglehole, Robert, and Ruth Bonita. *Public Health at the Crossroads: Achievements and Prospects.* New York: Cambridge Univ. Press, 1997.

Beauchamp, Dan E. *The Health of the Republic: Epidemics, Medicine, and Moralism as Challenges to Democracy.* Philadelphia: Temple Univ. Press, 1998.

———. "Community: The Neglected Tradition of Public Health." *Hastings Center Report* 15 (December 1985): 28–36.

Béchamps, Michon, Ron Bialek, and C. Patrick Caulk. *Privatization and Public Health: A Report of Initiatives and Early Lessons Learned.* Washington, DC: Public Health Foundation, 1999.

Becker, Edmund R., Kris Principe, E. Kathleen Adams, and Steven M. Teutsch. "Returns on Investment in Public Health: Effect of Public Health Expenditures on Infant Health, 1983–1990." *Journal of Health Care Finance* 25 (1998): 5–18.

Becker, Howard. "Whose Side Are We On?" *Social Problems* 14 (1967): 39–47.

Bellah, Robert N., Richard Madsen, William M. Sullivan, Ann Swidler, and Steven M. Tipton. *Habits of the Heart: Individualism and Commitment in American Life.* Berkeley: Univ. of California Press, 1985.

Bennet, Peter, and Kenneth Calman. *Risk Communication and Public Health.* Oxford: Oxford Univ. Press, 1999.

Berkelman, Ruth L., Ralph T. Bryan, Michael T. Osterholm, James W. LeDuc, and James M. Hughes. "Infectious Disease Surveillance: A Crumbling Foundation." *Science* 264 (1994): 368–70.

Berkman, Lisa F., and Ichiro Kawachi, eds. *Social Epidemiology.* Oxford: Oxford Univ. Press, 2000.

Biggs, Hermann M. "Report to Board of Health. December 1911." In "Health Department Control of Venereal Disease," by Ernest J. Lederle. *Social Diseases* 3 (October 1912): 24–27.

Binder, Sue, Alexandra M. Levitt, Jeffrey J. Sacks, and James M. Hughes. "Emerging Infectious Diseases: Public Health Issues for the 21st Century." *Science* 284 (1999): 1311–20.

Bloom, Barry R., and Christopher J. L. Murray. "Tuberculosis: Commentary on a Reemergent Killer." *Science* 257 (1992): 1055–64.

Bowser, René, and Lawrence O. Gostin. "Managed Care and the Health of the Nation." *University of Southern California Law Review* 72 (1999): 1209–95.

Bradely, Peter, and Amanda Burls, eds. *Ethics in Public and Community Health.* New York: Routledge, 2000.

Brandt, Allan M. *No Magic Bullet: A Social History of Venereal Disease in the United States Since 1880.* New York: Oxford Univ. Press, 1987.

———. "Racism and Research: The Case of the Tuskegee Syphilis Study." *Hastings Center Report* 8 (December 1978): 21–29.

Brandt, Allan M., and Martha Gardner. "Antagonism and Accommodation: Interpreting the Relationship between Public Health and Medicine in the United States During the 20th Century." *American Journal of Public Health* 90 (2000): 707–15.

Breakey, William R. "It's Time for the Public Health Community to Declare War on Homelessness." *American Journal of Public Health* 87 (1997): 153–55.

Breyer, Stephen. *Breaking the Vicious Circle: Toward Effective Risk Regulation.* Cambridge, MA: Harvard Univ. Press, 1993.

Buchanan, Allen, Dan W. Brock, Norman Daniels, and Daniel I. Wikler. "Two Models for Genetic Intervention." In *From Chance to Choice: Genetics and Justice.* Cambridge: Cambridge Univ. Press, 2000.

Buchanan, David R. "Disquietudes." In *An Ethic for Health Promotion: Rethinking the Sources of Human Well-Being.* Oxford: Oxford Univ. Press, 2000.

Buckley, Christopher H., and Charles H. Haake. "Separating the Scientist's Wheat from the Charlatan's Chaff: *Daubert*'s Role in Toxic Tort Litigation." *Environmental Law Reporter* 28 (June 1998): 10293–305.

Buckley, William F., Jr. "Identify All the Carriers." *New York Times,* March 18, 1986.

Burnet, F. McFarland, and David O. White. *Natural History of Infectious Disease.* London: Cambridge Univ. Press, 1962.

Burris, Scott. "Studying the Legal Management of HIV-Related Stigma." *American Behavioral Scientist* 42 (April 1999): 1229–43.

———. "Driving the Epidemic Underground? A New Look at Law and the Social Risk of HIV Testing." *AIDS and Public Policy Journal* (Summer 1997a): 66–78.

———. "The Invisibility of Public Health: Population-Level Measures in a Politics of Market Individualism." *American Journal of Public Health* 87 (1997b): 1607–10.

Burris, Scott, Lawrence O. Gostin, and Deborah Tress. "Public Health Surveillance of Genetic Information: Ethical and Legal Responses to Social Risk." In *Genetics and Public Health in the 21st Century: Using Genetic Information to Improve Health and Prevent Disease,* edited by Muin Khoury, Wylie Burke, and Elizabeth Thomson. New York: Oxford Univ. Press, 2000.

Callahan, Daniel, ed. *Promoting Health Behavior: How Much Freedom? Whose Responsibility?* Washington, DC: Georgetown Univ. Press, 2000.

Callahan, Daniel, and Bruce Jennings. "Ethics and Public Health: Forging a Strong Relationship." *American Journal of Public Health* (forthcoming 2002).

Campion, Edward W. "Liberty and the Control of Tuberculosis." *New England Journal of Medicine* 340 (1999): 385–86.

Cassell, Gail, and John Mekalanos. "Development of Antimicrobial Agents in the Era of New and Reemerging Infectious Diseases and Increasing Antibiotic Resistance." *Journal of the American Medical Association* 285 (2001): 601–5.

Cattell, Vicky. "Poor People, Poor Places, and Poor Health: The Mediating Role of Social Networks and Social Capital." *Social Science and Medicine* 52 (2000): 1501–16.

Centers for Disease Control and Prevention (CDC). "National, State, and Urban Area Vaccination Coverage Levels among Children Aged 19–35 Months—United States, 2000." *Morbidity and Mortality Weekly Report* 50 (August 3, 2001): 638–53.

———. "National, State, and Urban Area Vaccination Coverage Levels among Children Aged 19–35 Months—United States, 1999." *Morbidity and Mortality Weekly Report* 49 (July 7, 2000a): 585–89.

———. "Surveillance for Adverse Events Associated with Anthrax Vaccination—U.S. Department of Defense, 1998–2000." *Morbidity and Mortality Weekly Report* 49 (SS3) (April 28, 2000b): 341–45.

———. "Monitoring Hospital-Acquired Infections to Promote Patient Safety—United States, 1990–1999." *Morbidity and Mortality Weekly Report* 49 (March 3, 2000c): 149–71.

——. "Biological and Chemical Terrorism: Strategic Plan for Preparedness and Response." *Morbidity and Mortality Weekly Report* 49 (RR4) (2000d): 1–13.

——. "Recommendations for Human Immunodeficiency Virus Screening of Pregnant Women." *Mortality and Morbidity Weekly Report* 50 (RR19) (2000e): 59–86 .

——. *Public Health's Infrastructure: A Status Report for the Appropriations Committee of the United States Senate.* Washington, DC: Department of Health and Human Services, 2000f.

——. "Achievements in Public Health, 1900–1999: Control of Infectious Diseases." *Morbidity and Mortality Weekly Report* 48 (July 30, 1999a): 621–29.

——. "Ten Great Public Health Achievements—United States, 1900–1999: Impact of Vaccines Universally Recommended for Children—United States, 1990–1998." *Morbidity and Mortality Weekly Report* 48 (April 2, 1999b): 241–48.

——. "Guidelines for National Human Immunodeficiency Virus Case Surveillance, Including Monitoring for HIV Infection and AIDS." *Morbidity and Mortality Weekly Report* 48 (RR13) (1999c): 1–31.

——. "Preventing Emerging Infectious Diseases: A Strategy for the 21st Century." *Morbidity and Mortality Weekly Report* 47 (RR15) (1998): 1–13.

——. *Translating Advances in Human Genetics into Public Health Action—A Strategic Plan.* Atlanta: CDC, 1997.

Chapin, Charles V. "Pleasures and Hopes of the Health Officer." In *Papers of Charles V. Chapin.* New York: Commonwealth Fund, 1934.

Chapman, Audrey R. "Conceptualizing the Right to Health: A Violations Approach." *Tennessee Law Review* 65 (Winter 1998): 389–418.

Christoffel, Tom, and Susan Scavo Gallagher. *Injury Prevention and Public Health: Practical Knowledge, Skills, and Strategies.* Gaithersburg, MD: Aspen, 1999.

Christoffel, Tom, and Stephen P. Teret. "Epidemiology and the Law: Courts and Confidence Intervals." *American Journal of Public Health* 81 (1991): 1661–66.

Christopher, George W., Theodore J. Cieslak, Julie A. Pavlin, and Edward M. Eitzen, Jr. "Biological Warfare: A Historical Perspective." *Journal of the American Medical Association* 278 (1997): 412–17.

Clayton, Ellen Wright. "Genetics, Public Health, and the Law." In *Genetics and Public Health in the 21st Century: Using Genetic Information to Improve Health and Prevent Disease,* edited by Muin Khoury, Wylie Burke, and Elizabeth Thomson. New York: Oxford Univ. Press, 2000.

Clemow, F.G. "The Origin of 'Quarantine.'" *British Medical Journal* 1 (January 19, 1929): 122–23.

Cohen, Hillel W., Robert M. Gould, and Victor W. Sidel. "Bioterrorism Initiatives: Public Health in Reverse?" *American Journal of Public Health* 89 (1999): 1629–30.

Cole, Leonard A. "The Specter of Biological Weapons." *Scientific American* 275 (December 1996): 60–64.

Cole, Philip. "The Moral Bases for Public Health Interventions." *Epidemiology* 6 (January 1995): 78–83.

Coughlin, Steven S., and Thomas L. Beauchamp, eds. *Ethics and Epidemiology.* New York: Oxford Univ. Press, 1996

Coughlin, Steven S., Wendy H. Katz, and Donald R. Mattison. "Ethics Instruction at Schools of Public Health in the United States." *American Journal of Public Health* 90 (2000): 768–70.

Craven, Robert B., and John T. Roehrig. "West Nile Virus." *Journal of the American Medical Association* 286 (2001): 651–53.

Culhane, John G., and Jean Maciarioli Egger. "Defining a Proper Role for Public Nuisance Law in Municipal Suits against Gun Sellers: Beyond Rhetoric and Expedience." *South Carolina Law Review* 52 (2001): 287–329

Daniels, Norman. *Just Health Care.* New York: Oxford Univ. Press, 1985.

Daniels, Norman, Bruce Kennedy, and Ichiro Kawachi. "Justice Is Good for Our Health." *Boston Review* (February/March 2000a): 6–15.

———. *Is Inequality Bad for Our Health?* Boston: Beacon Press, 2000b.

Daynard, Richard A. "Tobacco Liability Litigation as a Cancer Control Strategy." *Journal of the National Cancer Institute* 80 (1988): 9–13.

Daynard, Richard A., and Graham E. Keller, Jr. "The Many Virtues of Tobacco Litigation." *Trial* 34 (November 1998): 34–43.

"Defining 'Disability' Under the ADA: 1997 Update." *National Disability Law Reporter* 2 (1997): 4–8.

Department of Health and Human Services. *Healthy People 2010.* Washington, DC: 2000.

———. *Preventing Tobacco Use among Young People: A Report of the Surgeon General.* Atlanta: U.S. Department of Health and Human Services, 1994.

Department of Health, Education and Welfare. *Effects of Biological Warfare Agents.* Washington, DC: Government Printing Office, 1959.

Desselberger, Ulrich. "Emerging and Re-emerging Infectious Diseases." *Journal of Infection* 40 (2000): 3–15.

Dowdle, Walter. "The 1976 Experience." *Journal of Infectious Diseases* 176 (1997): 69S–72S.

Doxiadis, Spyros A. "Ethics of Health Promotion and Health Education." *International Journal of Bioethics* 2 (July–September 1991): 179–86.

Dubois, René, and Jean Dubois. *The White Plague: Tuberculosis, Man and Society.* New Brunswick, NJ: Rutgers Univ. Press, 1987.

Duffy, John. *The Sanitarians: A History of American Public Health.* Urbana: Univ. of Illinois Press, 1990.

Durkheim, Emile. *Rules of Sociological Method.* Chicago: Univ. of Chicago Press, 1938.

Dworkin, Gerald. "Paternalism." In *Philosophy of Law,* edited by Joel Feinberg and Jules Coleman. 6th ed. Belmont, CA: Wadsworth, 2000.

Eager, John M. *The Early History of Quarantine: Origin of Sanitary Measures Directed against Yellow Fever.* Washington, DC: Government Printing Office, 1903.

Eastman, Nigel L. G., and R. A. Hope. "The Ethics of Enforced Medical Treatment: The Balance Model." *Journal of Applied Philosophy* 5 (1988): 49–59.

Eilbert, Kay W., M. Barry, R. Bialek, and M. Garufi. *Measuring Expenditures for Essential Public Health Services*. Washington, DC: Public Health Foundation, 1996.

Evans, Robert G., Morris L. Barer, and Theodore R. Marmor, eds. *Why Are Some People Healthy and Others Not? Determinants of Health of Populations*. New York: Aldine De Gruyter, 1994.

Faden, Ruth R. "Ethical Issues in Government Sponsored Public Health Campaigns." *Health Education Quarterly* 14 (1987): 27–37.

Faden, Ruth R., Nancy Kass, and Madison Powers. "Warrants for Screening Programs: Public Health, Legal, and Ethical Frameworks." In *AIDS, Women and the Next Generation: Towards a Morally Acceptable Public Policy for HIV Testing of Pregnant Women and Newborns*, edited by Ruth R. Faden, Gail Geller, and Madison Powers. New York: Oxford Univ. Press, 1991.

Farmer, Paul. "Social Inequalities and Emerging Infectious Diseases." *Emerging Infectious Diseases* 2 (October/December 1996): 259–69.

Farrand, Max, ed. *The Records of the Federal Convention of 1787*. Rev. ed., 4 vols. New Haven, CT: Yale Univ. Press, 1966.

Federal Trade Commission (FTC). *Cigar Sales and Advertising and Promotional Expenses for Calendar Years 1996 and 1997*. Washington, DC: Federal Trade Commission, 1999.

Fee, Elizabeth. "The Origins and Development of Public Health in the United States." In *Oxford Textbook of Public Health*. Oxford: Oxford Univ. Press, 1997.

Feinberg, Joel. *The Moral Limits of the Criminal Law*. 4 vols. New York: Oxford Univ. Press, 1987–1990.

Feldblum, Chai R. "The (R)evolution of Physical Disability Anti-discrimination Law: 1976–1996." *Mental and Physical Disability Law Reporter* 20 (September/October 1996): 613–21.

———. "Employment Protections." In *The Americans with Disabilities Act: From Policy to Practice*. New York: Milbank Memorial Fund, 1991.

Fielding, Jonathan E. "Public Health in the Twentieth Century: Advances and Challenges." *Annual Review of Public Health* 20 (1999): xiii–xxx.

Fielding, Jonathan E., Lester B. Lave, and Barbara Starfield. "Preface." *Annual Review of Public Health* 21 (2000).

File, Thomas M., Jr. "Overview of Resistance in the 1990s." *Chest* 115 (March 1999): 3S–8S.

Fleming, Alexander. "Chemotherapy: Yesterday, To-day, To-morrow." *Linacre Lectures* 32 (1946).

Flexner, Abraham. *Medical Education in the United States and Canada: A Report to the Carnegie Foundation for the Advancement of Teaching*. Boston: Merrymount Press, 1910.

Foege, William H. "Challenges to Public Health Leadership." In *Oxford Textbook of Public Health*. Oxford: Oxford Univ. Press, 1997.

Foucault, Michel. "Omnes et Singulatim: Towards a Criticism of 'Political Reason.'" In *The Tanner Lectures of Human Values II*, edited by Sterling M. McMurrin. Salt Lake City: Univ. of Utah, 1979.

Fox, Daniel M. "AIDS and the American Health Polity: The History and Prospects of a Crisis of Authority." In AIDS: The Burdens of History, edited by Elizabeth Fee and Daniel M. Fox. Berkeley, CA: Univ. of California Press, 1988.

———. "From TB to AIDS: Value Conflicts in Reporting Disease." *Hastings Center Report* 11 (December 1986): 11–16.

Freund, Ernst. *The Police Power: Public Policy and Constitutional Rights.* Chicago: Callaghan, 1904.

Frey, Jennifer. "Nushawn's Girls." *Washington Post,* June 1, 1999.

Fried, Charles. *Order and Law: Arguing the Reagan Revolution: A Firsthand Account.* New York: Simon & Schuster, 1991.

Garrett, Laurie. *Betrayal of Trust: The Collapse of Global Public Health.* New York: Hyperion, 2000.

Gasner, M. Rose, Khin Lay Maw, Gabriel E. Feldman, Paula I. Fujiwara, and Thomas R. Frieden. "The Use of Legal Action in New York City to Ensure Treatment of Tuberculosis." *New England Journal of Medicine* 340 (1999): 359–66.

Gebbie, Kristine M. "State Public Health Laws: An Expression of Constituency Expectations." *Journal of Public Health Management Practice* 6 (2000): 46–54.

Gebbie, Kristine M., and Inseon Hwang. *Preparing Currently Employed Public Health Professionals for Changes in the Health System.* New York: Columbia Univ. School of Nursing, 1998.

Gellman, Barton. "World Shunned Signs of the Coming Plague." *Washington Post,* July 5, 2000a.

———. "AIDS Is Declared Threat to Security." *Washington Post,* April 30, 2000b.

Gerzoff, Robert B., Carol K. Brown, and Edward L. Baker. "Full-Time Employees of U.S. Local Health Departments, 1992–1993." *Journal of Public Health Management Practice* 5 (1999): 1–9.

Glantz, Stanton A., Deborah E. Barnes, Lisa Bero, Peter Hanauer, and John Slade. "Looking Through a Keyhole at the Tobacco Industry: The Brown and Williamson Documents." *Journal of the American Medical Association* 274 (1995): 219–24.

Goodrich, Charles B. *The Science of Government.* Boston: Little, Brown, 1853.

Gostin, Lawrence O. "The Human Right to Health: A Right to the 'Highest Attainable Standard of Health.'" *Hastings Center Report* (March-April 2001): 29–30.

Gostin, Lawrence O. "Public Health Law in a New Century: Part I, Law as a Tool to Advance the Community's Health." *Journal of the American Medical Association* 283 (2000a): 2837–41.

———. "Public Health Law in a New Century: Part II, Public Health Powers and Duties." *Journal of the American Medical Association* 283 (2000b): 2979–84.

———. "Public Health Law in a New Century: Part III, Public Health Regulation: A Systematic Evaluation." *Journal of the American Medical Association* 283 (2000c): 3118–22.

——. "Human Rights of Persons with Mental Disabilities: The European Convention of Human Rights." *International Journal of Law & Psychiatry* 23 (2000d): 125–59.

——. "A Proposed National Policy on Health Care Workers Living with HIV/AIDS and Other Bloodborne Pathogens." *Journal of the American Medical Association* 284 (2000e): 1965–70.

——. "Health Legislation and Communicable Diseases: The Role of Law in an Era of Microbial Threats." *International Digest of Health Legislation* 49(1) (1998): 221–33.

——. "Health Information Privacy." *Cornell Law Review* 80 (1995a): 451–528.

——. "The Resurgent Tuberculosis Epidemic in the Era of AIDS: Reflections on Public Health, Law, and Society." *Maryland Law Review* 54 (1995b): 1–131.

——. "The Politics of AIDS: Compulsory State Powers, Public Health, and Civil Liberties." *Ohio Law Journal* 49 (1989): 1017–58.

Gostin, Lawrence O., Scott Burris, and Zita Lazzarini. "The Law and the Public's Health: A Study of Infectious Disease Law in the United States." *Columbia Law Review* 99 (1999): 59–128.

Gostin, Lawrence O., Chai Feldblum, and David W. Webber. "Disability Discrimination in America: HIV/AIDS and Other Health Conditions." *Journal of the American Medical Association* 281 (1999): 745–52.

Gostin, Lawrence O., and James G. Hodge, Jr. "Genetics Privacy and the Law: An End to Genetics Exceptionalism." *Jurimetrics* 40 (1999): 21–58.

——. "The 'Names Debate': The Case for National HIV Reporting in the United States." *Albany Law Review* 61 (1998a): 679–743.

——. "Piercing the Veil of Secrecy in HIV/AIDS and Other Sexually Transmitted Diseases: Theories of Privacy and Disclosure in Partner Notification." *Duke Journal of Law and Gender* 5 (1998b): 9–88.

Gostin, Lawrence O., James G. Hodge, Jr., and Ronald O. Valdiserri. "Informational Privacy and the Public's Health: The Model State Public Health Privacy Act." *American Journal of Public Health* 91 (2001): 1388–92.

Gostin, Lawrence O., and Zita Lazzarini. *Human Rights and Public Health in the AIDS Pandemic.* New York: Oxford Univ. Press, 1997.

——. "Childhood Immunization Registries: A National Review of Public Health Information Systems and the Protection of Privacy." *Journal of the American Medical Association* 274 (1995): 1793–99.

Gostin, Lawrence O., Zita Lazzarini, Dianne D. Alexander, Allan M. Brandt, Kenneth H. Mayer, and Daniel C. Silverman. "HIV Testing, Counseling, and Prophylaxis after Sexual Assault." *Journal of the American Medical Association* 271 (1994): 1436–44.

Gostin, Lawrence O., Zita Lazzarini, Verla S. Neslund, and Michael T. Osterholm. "Water Quality Laws and Waterborne Diseases: *Cryptosporidium* and Other Emerging Pathogens." *American Journal of Public Health* 90 (2000): 847–53.

——. "The Public Health Information Infrastructure: A National Review of the Law on Health Information Privacy." *Journal of the American Medical Association* 275 (1996): 1921–27.

Gostin, Lawrence O., John W. Ward, and A. Cornelius Baker. "National HIV Case Reporting for the United States: A Defining Moment in the History of the Epidemic." *New England Journal of Medicine* 337 (1997): 1162–67.

Gouldner, Alvin. "Anti-Minotaur: The Myth of a Value Free Sociology." In *For Sociology: Renewal and Critique in Sociology Today.* London: Allen Lane, 1973.

Grad, Frank P. *Public Health Law Manual.* 2nd ed. New York: American Public Health Association, 1990.

Graham, John D., and Jonathan Baert Wiener, eds. *Risk versus Risk: Tradeoffs in Protecting Health and the Environment.* Cambridge, MA: Harvard Univ. Press, 1995.

Graham, Mary. "Regulation by Shaming." *Atlantic Monthly* 285 (April 2000): 36–40.

Grant, Jim. *The State of the World's Children.* Oxford: Oxford Univ. Press, 1993.

Granville, Augustus Bozzi. *A Letter to the Right Hon. F. Robinson, M.P., President of the Board of Trade and Treasurer to the Navy, on The Plague and Contagion, with Reference to Quarantine Laws, etc.* London: 1819. In "The Origin of Quarantine," by F. G. Clemow. *British Medical Journal* (January 19, 1929): 122–23.

Green, Lawrence W., and Judith M. Ottoson. *Community and Population Health.* 8th ed. Boston: WCB McGraw-Hill, 1999.

Greenberg, David, and Mary Graham. "Improving Communication about New Food Technologies." *Issues in Science and Technology* (Summer 2000): 42–48.

Grutsch, James F., Jr., and A. D. J. Robertson. "The Coming of AIDS: It Didn't Start with the Homosexuals and It Won't End with Them." *American Spectator* 19 (1986): 12–15.

Guttman, Nurit. *Public Health Communication Interventions: Values and Ethical Dilemmas.* Thousand Oaks, CA: Sage, 2000.

Guttman, Nurit, and W. H. Ressler. "On Being Responsible: Ethical Issues in Appeals to Personal Responsibility in Health Campaigns." *Journal of Health Communications* 6 (2001): 117–36.

Hancock, T. "Healthy Communities Must Also Be Sustainable Communities." *Public Health Reports* 115 (2000): 151–56.

Handler, Arden, Michele Issel, and Bernard Turnock. "A Conceptual Framework to Measure Performance of the Public Health System." *American Journal of Public Health* 91 (2001): 1235–39.

Hardin, Garrett. "The Tragedy of the Commons." *Science* 162 (1968): 1243–48.

Harvard School of Public Health. *Harvard School of Public Health Yearbook.* Cambridge, MA: Harvard School of Public Health, 1965.

Health Resources and Services Administration (HRSA). *The Public Health Workforce.* Washington, DC: U.S. Department of Health and Human Services, 2000.

Heinzerling, Lisa. "The Perils of Precision." *Environmental Forum* (September/October 1998a): 38–43.

———. "Regulatory Costs of Mythic Proportions." *Yale Law Journal* 107 (May 1998b): 1981–2070.

Heinzerling, Lisa, and Frank Ackerman. "The Humbugs of the Anti-Regulatory Movement." *Cornell Law Review* 87 (forthcoming 2002).

Henderson, Donald A. "The Looming Threat of Bioterrorism." *Science* 283 (1999): 1279–82.

Henderson, Donald A., Thomas V. Inglesby, John G. Barlett, Michael S. Ascher, Edward Eitzen, Jr., P. B. Jahrling, Jerome Hauer, M. Layton, Joseph McDade, Michael T. Osterholm, Tara O'Toole, Gerald Parker, Trish M. Perl, Philip K. Russel, and Kevin Tonat. "Smallpox as a Biological Weapon: Medical and Public Health Management." *Journal of the American Medical Association* 281 (1999): 2127–37.

Herwaldt, Barbara L., Marta-Louise Ackers, and the Cyclospora Working Group. "An Outbreak in 1996 of Cyclosporiasis Associated with Imported Raspberries." *New England Journal of Medicine* 336 (1997): 1548–56.

Heywood, Andrew. *Politics.* London: Macmillan, 1997.

Hockheimer, Lewis. "Police Power." *Central Law Journal* 44 (1897): 158–62.

Hodge, James G., Jr. "Implementing Modern Public Health Goals through Government: An Examination of New Federalism and Public Health Law." *Journal of Contemporary Health Law and Policy* 14 (Fall 1997): 93–126.

Hodge, James G., Jr., and Lawrence O. Gostin. "Handling Cases of Willful Exposure through HIV Partner Counseling and Referral Services." *Rutgers Women's Rights Law Reporter* (forthcoming 2001).

Holmes, Oliver Wendell, Jr. "The Common Law." 1881. Reprinted in *Cohen and Cohen's Readings in Jurisprudence and Legal Philosophy,* edited by Philip Schuchman. Boston: Little, Brown, 1979.

Huber, Peter W. *Galileo's Revenge: Junk Science in the Courtroom.* New York: Basic Books, 1991.

Hurt, Richard D., and Channing R. Robertson. "Prying Open the Door to the Tobacco Industry's Secrets about Nicotine." *Journal of the American Medical Association* 280 (1998): 1173–81.

Inglesby, Thomas V., David T. Dennis, Donald A. Henderson, John G. Bartlett, Michael S. Ascher, Edward Eitzen, Jr., A. D. Fine, Arthur M. Friedlander, Jerome Hauer, J. F. Koerner, M. Layton, Joseph McDade, Michael T. Osterholm, Tara O'Toole, Gerald Parker, Trish M. Perl, Philip K. Russell, M. Schoch-Spana, and Kevin Tonat. "Plague as a Biological Weapon: Medical and Public Health Management." *Journal of the American Medical Association* 283 (2000): 2281–90.

Inglesby, Thomas V., Donald A. Henderson, John G. Bartlett, Michael S. Ascher, Edward Eitzen, Jr., Arthur M. Friedlander, Jerome Hauer, Joseph McDade, Michael T. Osterholm, Tara O'Toole, Gerald Parker, Trish M. Perl, Philip K. Russell, and Kevin Tonat. "Anthrax as a Biological Weapon: Medical and Public Health Management." *Journal of the American Medical Association* 281 (1999): 1735–45.

Institute of Medicine (IOM). *Health and Behavior: The Interplay of Cells, Self and Society.* Washington, DC: National Academy Press (2001).

———. *An Assessment of the Safety of the Anthrax Vaccine: A Letter Report.* Washington, DC: National Academy Press, 2000a.

———. *Ending Neglect: The Elimination of Tuberculosis in the U.S.,* edited by Lawrence Geiter. Washington, DC: National Academy Press, 2000b.

———. *Safety of Silicone Breast Implants,* edited by Stuart Bondurant, Virginia Ernster, and Roger Herdman. Washington, DC: National Academy Press, 2000c.

———. *Reducing the Odds: Preventing Perinatal Transmission of HIV in the United States,* edited by Michael A. Stoto, Donna A. Almario, and Marie C. McCormick. Washington, DC: National Academy Press, 1999.

———. *Improving Health in the Community: A Role for Performance Monitoring,* edited by Jane S. Durch, Linda A. Bailey, and Michael A. Stoto. Washington, DC: National Academy Press, 1997.

———. *Growing Up Tobacco Free: Preventing Nicotine Addiction in Children and Youths,* edited by Barbara S. Lynch and Richard J. Bonnie. Washington, DC: National Academy Press, 1994.

———. *Emerging Infections: Microbial Threats to Health in the United States,* edited by Joshua Lederberg, Robert E. Shope, and Stanley C. Oaks, Jr. Washington, DC: National Academy Press, 1992.

———. *The Future of Public Health.* Washington, DC: National Academy Press, 1988.

Jacobson, Peter D., and Kenneth E. Warner. "Litigation and Public Health Policy Making: The Case of Tobacco Control." *Journal of Health Politics, Policy and Law* 24 (August 1999): 769–804.

Jamar, Steven D. "The International Human Right to Health." *Southern University Law Review* 22 (Fall 1994): 1–68.

Jauhar, Sandeep. "Leper Home to Fade but Not Memories of Prejudice." *Houston Chronicle,* June 29, 1998.

John, T. Jacob. "The Final Stages of the Global Eradication of Polio." *New England Journal of Medicine* 343 (September 14, 2000): 806–7.

Juengst, Eric T. "'Prevention' and the Goals of Genetic Medicine." *Human Gene Therapy* 6 (1995): 1595–1605.

Kass, Nancy. "A Change in Approach to Prenatal HIV Screening." *American Journal of Public Health* 90 (2000): 1026–27.

Keane, Christopher, John Marx, and Edmund Ricci. "Perceived Outcomes of Public Health Privatization: A National Survey of Local Health Department Directors." *American Journal of Public Health* 91 (2001a): 611–17.

———. "Privatization and the Scope of Public Health: A National Survey of Local Health Department Directors." *Milbank Quarterly* 79 (2001b): 115–37.

Kellman, Barry. "Biological Terrorism: Legal Measures for Preventing Catastrophe." *Harvard Journal of Law and Public Policy* 24 (2001): 417–88.

Kessel, Reuben A. "The A.M.A. and the Supply of Physicians." *Law & Contemporary Problems* 35 (1970): 267–83.

Kessler, David A. "Regulation of Tobacco: Health Promotion and Cancer Prevention." *Houston Law Review* 36 (September 1999): 1597–1608.

Khoury, Muin J., Wylie Burke, and Elizabeth J. Thomson, eds. *Genetics and Public Health in the 21st Century: Using Genetic Information to Improve Health and Prevent Disease.* Oxford: Oxford Univ. Press, 2000.

Khoury, Muin J., and the Genetics Working Group. "From Genes to Public Health: The Application of Genetic Technology in Disease Prevention." *American Journal of Public Health* 86 (1996): 1717–22.

Khoury, Muin J., James F. Thrasher, Wylie Burke, Elizabeth A. Gettig, Fred Fridinger, and Richard Jackson. "Challenges in Communicating Genetics: A Public Health Approach." *Genetics in Medicine* 2 (May/June 2000): 198–202.

Kinney, Eleanor D. "The International Right to Health: What Does This Mean for Our Nation and World?" *Indiana Law Review* 34 (2001): 1457–75.

Knight, Rebecca M. "Helping Pollack Quit, Even Posthumously." *New York Times,* February 6, 1999.

Knox, Bernard. "Introduction." In *Sophocles: The Three Theban Plays: Antigone, Oedipus the King, Oedipus at Colonus.* New York: Viking Penguin, 1984.

Koplan, Jeffrey P., and David W. Fleming, "Current and Future Public Health Challenges." *Journal of the American Medical Association* 284 (2000): 1696–98.

Krieger, Nancy. "Epidemiology and the Web of Causation: Has Anyone Seen the Spider?" *Social Science and Medicine* 39 (1994): 887–903.

Krieger, Nancy, and Sally Zierler. "What Explains the Public's Health—A Call for Epidemiologic Theory." *Epidemiology* 7 (1996): 107–9.

Kuczewski, Mark G. "The Epistemology of Communitarian Bioethics: Traditions in the Public Debates." *Theoretical Medicine and Bioethics* 22 (2001): 135–50.

Kunz, Josef L. "The United Nations Declaration of Human Rights." *American Journal of International Law* 43 (1949): 316–22.

Lacey, Marc, and Bill Carter. "In Trade-off with T.V. Networks, Drug Office is Reviewing Scripts." *New York Times,* January 14, 2000.

*Lancet* Editorial. "Putting Public Health Back into Epidemiology." *Lancet* 350 (1997): 229.

Lasso, Jose Ayala, and Peter Piot. "Foreword." In *Public Health and Human Rights in the AIDS Pandemic,* by Lawrence O. Gostin and Zita Lazzarini. New York: Oxford Univ. Press, 1997.

Last, John M. *A Dictionary of Epidemiology.* New York: Oxford Univ. Press, 1983.

Lazarus, Richard J. "Putting the Correct 'Spin' on *Lucas.*" *Stanford Law Review* 45 (1993): 1411–32.

Leary, Virginia A. "The Right to Health in International Human Rights Law." *Health & Human Rights* 1 (Fall 1994): 24–56.

Leggiadro, Robert L. "The Threat of Biological Terrorism: A Public Health and Infection Control Reality." *Infection Control and Hospital Epidemiology* 21 (January 2000): 53–56.

Lessig, Lawrence. "The Regulation of Social Meaning." *University of Chicago Law Review* 62 (Summer 1995): 943–1045.

Levy, Barry S., and Victor W. Sidel, eds. *War and Public Health.* New York: Oxford Univ. Press, 1997.

Levy, Stuart B. "Antibiotic Availability and Use: Consequences to Man and His Environment." *Journal of Clinical Epidemiology* 44 (1991): 83S–87S.

Lewin Group. *Assessing Core Capacity for Infectious Diseases Surveillance.* Falls Church, VA: The Lewin Group, 2000.

Lillibridge, Scott R., April J. Bell, and Richard S. Roman. "Centers for Disease Control and Prevention Bioterrorism Preparedness and Response." *American Journal of Infection Control* 27 (December 1999): 463–64.

Locke, John. *The Second Treatise of Government.* 1690. Reprint, New York: Liberal Arts Press, 1952.

Lurie, Peter, and Sidney M. Wolfe. "Unethical Trials of Interventions to Reduce Perinatal Transmission of the Human Immunodeficiency Virus in Developing Countries." *New England Journal of Medicine* 337 (1997): 853–56.

Maantay, Juliana. "Zoning, Equity, and Public Health." *American Journal of Public Health* 91 (2001): 1033–41.

Macintyre, Anthony G., George W. Christopher, Edward Eitzen, Jr., Robert Gum, Scott Weir, Craig DeAtley, Kevin Tonat, and Joseph A. Barbera. "Weapons of Mass Destruction: Events with Contaminated Casualties." *Journal of the American Medical Association* 283 (2000): 242–49.

Macintyre, Sally, Sheila MacIver, and Anne Sooman. "Area, Class and Health: Should We Be Focusing on Places or People?" *Journal of Social Policy* 22 (1993): 213–34.

MacKenzie, Debora. "Bioarmageddon." *New Scientist* 159 (1998): 42–46.

Madison, James. *The Federalist No. 45,* edited by Clinton Rossiter. New York: New American Library, 1961.

Maier, Pauline. *American Scripture: Making the Declaration of Independence.* New York: Vintage Books, 1997.

Mann, Jonathan M. "Medicine and Public Health, Ethics and Human Rights." *Hastings Center Report* 27 (May–June 1997): 6–13.

Mann, Jonathan M., Lawrence O. Gostin, Sofia Gruskin, Troyen Brennan, Zita Lazzarini, and Harvey V. Fineberg. "Health and Human Rights." *Journal of Health and Human Rights* 1 (1994): 6–23.

Mann, Jonathan M., Sofia Gruskin, Michael Grodin, and George Annas, eds. *Health and Human Rights: A Reader.* New York: Routledge, 1999.

Mariner, Wendy K. "Public Confidence in Public Health Research Ethics." *Public Health Reports* 112 (January/February 1997): 33–36.

Marks, Stephen P. "Commentary: A Vision of Health and Human Rights for the 21st Century: A Different View of Mann's Legacy." *Journal of Law, Medicine, and Ethics* 29 (2001): 131–37.

Marmot, Michael, and Richard G. Wilkinson, eds. *Social Determinants of Health.* New York: Oxford Univ. Press, 1999.

Marx, Karl. *Selected Writings in Sociology and Social Philosophy.* New York: McGraw-Hill, 1964.

Mather, Lynn. "Theorizing about Trial Courts: Lawyers, Policymaking and Tobacco Litigation." *Law and Social Inquiry* 23 (1998): 897–940.

Mayer, Douglas L. "Prevalence and Incidence of Resistance to Zidovudine and Other Antiretroviral Drugs." *American Journal of Medicine* 102 (1997): 70–75.

Mays, Glen P., C. Arden Miller, and Paul K. Halverson. *Local Public Health Practice: Trends and Models.* Washington, DC: American Public Health Association, 2000.

McCann, Michael W. "Reform Litigation on Trial." *Law and Social Inequality* 17 (1992): 715–43.

McDonnell, W. Michael, and Frederick K. Askari. "Immunization." *Journal of the American Medical Association* 278 (1997): 2000–2007.

McGinnis, Michael J. "Does Proof Matter? Why Strong Evidence Sometimes Yields Weak Action." *American Journal of Health Promotion* 15 (2001): 391–96.

McGinnis, Michael J., and William H. Foege. "Actual Causes of Death in the United States." *Journal of the American Medical Association* 270 (1993): 2207–12.

McKinlay, John B., and Lisa D. Marceau. "Public Health Matters: To Boldly Go. . ." *American Journal of Public Health* 90 (2000): 25–33.

McKinlay, John B., and Sonja M. McKinlay. "The Questionable Contribution of Medical Measures to the Decline of Mortality in the United States in the Twentieth Century." *Milbank Quarterly* 55 (1977): 405–29.

Merritt, Deborah Jones. "The Constitutional Balance between Health and Liberty." *Hastings Center Report* 16 (Supp.) (December 1986): 2–10.

Meyer, Ilan H., and Sharon Schwartz. "Social Issues as Public Health: Promise and Peril." *American Journal of Public Health* 90 (2000): 1189–91.

Miller, Judith. "Germ Warfare: U.S. Set to Retain Smallpox Stocks." *New York Times* (Novermber 16, 2001).

Moellering, Robert C., Jr., "Antibiotic Resistance: Lessons for the Future." *Clinical Infectious Diseases* 27 (1998): S135–40.

Moffenson, Lynne M. "Perinatal Exposure to Zidovudine—Benefits and Risks." *New England Journal of Medicine* 343 (September 14, 2000): 803–5.

Moore, Joseph E. *The Modern Treatment of Syphilis.* Baltimore: Charles C. Thomas, 1933.

Morrow, Prince. "The Health Department and Control of Venereal Disease." *Social Diseases* 2 (July 1911).

Murray, Christopher J. L., and Alan D. Lopez. "Global Mortality, Disability, and the Contribution of Risk Factors." *Lancet* 349 (1997): 1436–42.

Musto, David F. "Quarantine and the Problem of AIDS." *Milbank Quarterly* 64 (Supp. 1) (1986): 97–117.

National Cancer Institute. *Cigars: Health Effects and Trends,* Smoking and Tobacco Control Monograph No. 9. Bethesda, MD: National Cancer Institute, 1998.

National Center for Environmental Health, National Center for Health Statistics, National Center for Infectious Diseases, and Centers for Disease Control and Prevention. "Achievements in Public Health, 1900–1999 (a Series): Control of Infectious Diseases." *Morbidity and Mortality Weekly Report* 48 (July 30, 1999): 621–29.

National Commission for the Protection of Human Subjects of Biomedical and Behavioral Research. *Belmont Report: Ethical Principles and Guidelines for the Protection of Human Subjects of Research.* Washington D.C.: Government Printing Office, 1978.

National Research Council. *Health Performance Measurement in the Public Sector.* Edited by Edward B. Perrin, Jane S. Durch, and Susan M. Skillman. Washington, DC: National Academy Press, 1999.

———. *Understanding Risk: Informing Decisions in a Democratic Society.* Edited by Paul C. Stern and Harvey V. Fineberg. Washington, DC: National Academy Press, 1996.

National Vaccine Advisory Committee. "Strategies to Sustain Success in Childhood Immunizations." *Journal of the American Medical Association* 282 (1999): 363–70.

Nijhuis, Harry, and Lawrence van der Maesen. "The Philosophical Foundations of Public Health: An Invitation to Debate." *Journal of Epidemiology and Community Health* 48 (1994): 1–3.

Novak, William J. "Governance, Police, and American Liberal Mythology." In *The People's Welfare: Law and Regulation in Nineteenth-Century America.* Chapel Hill: Univ. of North Carolina Press, 1996.

———. "Public Economy and the Well-Ordered Market: Law and Economic Regulation in 19th-Century America." *Law and Social Inquiry* 18 (Winter 1993): 1–32.

Novick, Lloyd F., and Glen P. Mays. *Public Health Administration: Principles for Population-Based Management.* Gaithersburg, MD: Aspen, 2001.

Novotny, Thomas, Charles E. Jennings, Mary Doran, C. R. March, R. S. Hopkins, S. G. Wassilak, and L. E. Markowitz. "Measles Outbreaks in Religious Groups Exempt from Immunization Laws." *Public Health Reports* 103 (1988): 49–54.

Nozick, Robert. *Anarchy, State, and Utopia.* Oxford: Basil Blackwell, 1974.

Olson, Elizabeth. "U.S. Rejects New Accord Covering Germ Warfare." *New York Times,* July 26, 2001.

Omenn, Gilbert S. "Public Health Genetics: An Emerging Interdisciplinary Field for the Post-Genomic Era." *Annual Review of Public Health* 21 (2000): 1–13.

Oscherwitz, Tom, Jacqueline Peterson Tulsky, Steve Roger, Stan Sciortino, Ann Alpers, Sarah Royce, and Bernard Lo. "Detention of Persistently Non-Adherent Patients with Tuberculosis." *Journal of the American Medical Association* 278 (1997): 843–46.

Osterholm, Michael T. "Emerging Infections—Another Warning." *New England Journal of Medicine* 342 (2000): 1280–81.

———. "Cyclosporiasis and Raspberries: Lessons for the Future." *New England Journal of Medicine* 336 (1997): 1597–99.

Osterholm, Michael T., Guthrie S. Birkhead, and Rebecca A. Meriwether. "Impediments to Public Health Surveillance in the 1990s: The Lack of Resources and the Need for Priorities." *Journal of Public Health Management and Practice* 2 (1996): 11–16.

Paine, Thomas. "Common Sense." In *The Complete Writings of Thomas Paine,* edited by Philip S. Foner. New York: Citadel, 1945.

Palmer, Janna. "Hollow Celebration of 50 Years of Human-Rights Campaigning." *Lancet* 351 (1998): 1940.

Pareto, Vilfredo. *The Mind and Society.* New York: Dover, 1963.

Parmet, Wendy E. "Tobacco, HIV, and the Courtroom: The Role of Affirmative Litigation in the Formation of Public Health Policy." *Houston Law Review* 36 (1999): 1663–1712.

———. "Health Care And The Constitution: Public Health and the Role of the State in the Framing Era." *Hastings Constitutional Law Quarterly* (Winter 1992): 267–335.

———. "AIDS and Quarantine: The Revival of an Archaic Doctrine." *Hofstra Law Review* 14 (1985): 53–90.

Parmet, Wendy E., and Richard A. Daynard. "The New Public Health Litigation." *Annual Review of Public Health* 21 (2000): 437–54.

Peckham, Catherine, and Marie-Louise Newell. "Preventing Vertical Transmission of HIV Infection." *New England Journal of Medicine* 343 (October 5, 2000): 1036–37.

Peters, Ronald. *The Massachusetts Constitution of 1780: A Social Compact.* Amherst: Univ. of Massachusetts Press, 1978.

Pope, Thaddeus M. "Balancing Public Health against Individual Liberty: The Ethics of Smoking Regulations." *University of Pittsburgh Law Review* 61 (2000): 419–98.

Potter, John D. "Reconciling the Epidemiology, Physiology, and Molecular Biology of Colon Cancer." *Journal of the American Medical Association* 268 (1992): 1573–77.

Powers, Madison, and Ruth Faden. "Inequalities in Health, Inequalities in Health Care: Four Generations of Discussion about Justice and Cost Effectiveness Analysis." *Kennedy Institute of Ethics Journal* 10 (2000): 109–27.

Presidential Commission on Drunk Driving. *Final Report.* Washington, DC: Presidential Commission on Drunk Driving, 1983.

Preston, Richard. "The Demon in the Freezer." *New Yorker* 75 (July 12, 1999): 44–61.

Rabin, Robert L. "A Sociolegal History of the Tobacco Tort Litigation." *Stanford Law Review* 44 (April 1992): 853–78.

Resnik, David B. "Ethical Dilemmas in Communicating Medical Information to the Public." *Health Policy* 55 (2001): 129–49.

Rice, Ronald E., and Charles K. Atkin, eds. *Public Communication Campaigns.* 3rd ed. Newbury Park: Sage, 2000.

Roettinger, Ruth Locke. *The Supreme Court and State Police Power: A Study in Federalism.* Washington, DC: Public Affairs Press, 1957.

Rose, Geoffrey. "Sick Individuals in Sick Populations." *International Journal of Epidemiology* 14 (1985): 32–38.

———. "Strategy of Prevention: Lessons from Cardiovascular Disease." *British Journal of Medicine* 282 (1981): 1847–51.

Rosenberg, Charles. *The Cholera Years: The United States in 1832, 1849, and 1866.* Chicago: Univ. of Chicago Press, 1987.

Rosenberg, Gerald N. *The Hollow Hope: Can Courts Bring about Social Change?* Chicago: Univ. of Chicago Press, 1991.

Rosenkrantz, Barbara. "Cart Before Horse: Theory, Practice and Professional Image in American Public Health." *Journal of the History of Medicine and Allied Sciences* 29 (1974): 55–73.

Rothenberg, Karen, and Stephen J. Paskey. "The Risk of Domestic Violence and Women with HIV Infection: Implications for Partner Notification, Public Policy, and the Law." *American Journal of Public Health* 85 (1995): 1569–76.

Rothman, Sheila M. *Living in the Shadow of Death: Tuberculosis and the Social Experience of Illness in American History.* New York: Basic Books, 1994.

Rothstein, Laura F. *Disabilities and the Law.* 2nd ed. St. Paul, MN: West Group, 1997.

Roush, Sandra, Guthrie Birkhead, Denise Koo, A. Cobb, and D. Fleming. "Mandatory Reporting of Diseases and Conditions by Health Care Professionals and Laboratories." *Journal of the American Medical Association* 282 (1999): 164–70.

Rowe, John W., and Robert L. Kahn. *Successful Aging.* New York: Pantheon Books, 1998.

Ruskin, John. *Unto This Last: Four Essays on the First Principles of Political Economy.* London: Smith, Elder, 1862.

Russell, Louise, M. R. Gold, J. E. Siegel, Norman Daniels, and M. C. Weinstein. "The Role of Cost-Effectiveness Analysis on Health and Medicine." *Journal of the American Medical Association* 276 (1996): 1172–77.

Ryan, Mary. *Womanhood in America: From Colonial Times to the Present.* New York: Franklin Watts, 1975.

Ryff, Carol D., and Burton Singer. "The Contours of Positive Human Health." *Psychological Inquiry* 9 (1998): 1–28.

Sage, William M. "Regulating through Information: Disclosure Laws and American Health Care." *Columbia Law Review* 100 (1999): 1701–1829.

Salmon, Daniel A., Michael Haber, Eugene J. Gangarosa, L. Phillips, N. J. Smith, and R. T. Chen. "Health Consequences of Religious and Philosophical Exemptions from Immunization Laws: Individual and Societal Risk of Measles." *Journal of the American Medical Association* 282 (1999): 47–53.

Savitt, Todd L. "The Education of Black Physicians at Shaw University, 1882–1918." In *Black Americans in North Carolina and the South,* edited by Jeffrey J. Crow and Flora J. Hatley. Chapel Hill: Univ. of North Carolina Press, 1984.

Schuman, Stanley H., Sidney Olansky, Eunice Rivers, C. A. Smith, and Dorothy S. Rambo. "Untreated Syphilis in the Male Negro: Background and Current Status of Patients in the Tuskegee Study." *Journal of Chronic Diseases* 2 (November 1955): 543–58.

Seidman, Louis, and Mark Tushnet. *Remnants of Belief: Contemporary Constitutional Issues.* New York: Oxford Univ. Press, 1996.

Senate Appropriations Committee. S. Rep. No. 106–166 (1999).

Shattuck, Lemuel. "Introduction and Private Rights and Liberties." In *Report of the Sanitary Commission of Massachusetts.* 1850. Reprint, Cambridge, MA: Harvard Univ. Press, 1948.

Simmons, Marlene. "CDC Says It Erred in Measles Study: Agency Failed to Tell Parents That One of Two Vaccines Used on Infants in L.A. During Epidemic Was Experimental." *Los Angeles Times,* June 17, 1996.

Small, Peter M., and Paula I. Fujiwara. "Management of Tuberculosis in the United States." *New England Journal of Medicine* 345 (2001): 189–200.

Smith, Alwyn. "The Epidemiological Basis of Community Medicine." In *Recent Advances in Community Medicine*. Edinburgh: Churchill Livingstone, 1985.

Snider, Dixie E., and Donna F. Stroup. "Defining Research When It Comes to Public Health." *Public Health Reports* 112 (January/February 1997): 29–32.

Soames, Job R. F. "Effective and Ineffective Use of Fear in Health Promotion Campaigns." *American Journal of Public Health* 78 (1988): 163–67.

Sommer, Alfred, and Mohammad N. Akhter. "It's Time We Became a Profession." *American Journal of Public Health* 90 (2000): 845–46.

Steinbock, Bonnie, and Dan E. Beauchamp, eds. *New Ethics for the Public's Health*. New York: Oxford Univ. Press, 1999.

Steiner, Henry J. "Securing Human Rights: The First Half-Century of the Universal Declaration, and Beyond." *Harvard Magazine* (September/October 1998): 45–46.

Steiner, Henry J., and Phillip Alston. *International Human Rights in Context: Law, Politics, Morals*. New York: Oxford Univ. Press, 2000.

Steinzor, Rena I. "Devolution and the Public Health." *Harvard Environmental Law Review* 24 (2000): 351–463.

Stoddard, Thomas B., and Walter Rieman. "AIDS and the Rights of the Individual: Toward a More Sophisticated Understanding of Discrimination." *Milbank Quarterly* 8 (Supp. 1) (1990): 143–74.

Sullivan, Kathleen, and Martha Field. "AIDS and the Coercive Power of the State." *Harvard Civil Rights—Civil Liberties Law Review* 23 (1988): 139–98.

Sunstein, Cass R. "Health-Health Tradeoffs." *University of Chicago Law Review* 63 (Fall 1996a): 1533–71.

——. "Social Norms and Social Roles." *Columbia Law Review* 96 (1996b): 903–68.

Susser, Mervyn. "The Logic in Ecological, II: The Logic of Design." *American Journal of Public Health* 84 (1994): 830–35.

Syme, S. Leonard. "Social and Economic Disparities in Health: Thoughts about Intervention." *Milbank Quarterly* 76 (1998): 493–505.

Tandy, Elizabeth C. "The Regulation of Nuisances in the American Colonies." *American Journal of Public Health* 13 (1923a): 810–13.

——. "Local Quarantine and Inoculation for Smallpox in the American Colonies (1620–1775)." *American Journal of Public Health* 13 (1923b): 203–7.

Teret, Stephen P. "Litigating for the Public's Health." *American Journal of Public Health* 76 (1986): 1027–29.

Terris, Milton. "The Distinction between Public Health and Community/ Social/ Preventative Medicine." *Journal of Public Health Policy* 6 (1985): 435–39.

Toebes, Brigit C. A. "Towards an Improved Understanding of the International Human Right to Health." *Human Rights Quarterly* 21 (August 1999a): 661–79.

——. *The Right to Health as a Human Right in International Law.* Antwerpen: Intersentia/Hart, 1999b.

Tribe, Laurence. *American Constitutional Law.* 2nd ed. Los Angeles: Foundation Press, 1988.

Teutsch, Steven M., and R. Elliot Churchill, eds. *Principles and Practice of Public Health Surveillance.* 2nd ed. New York: Oxford Univ. Press, 2000.

Turnock, Bernard J. *Public Health: What It Is and How It Works.* Gaithersburg, MD: Aspen, 2001.

United States Public Health Service. *For a Healthy Nation: Returns on Investment in Public Health.* Washington, DC: Department of Health and Human Services and the Public Health Service, 1994.

Varmus, Harold, and David Satcher. "Ethical Complexities of Conducting Research in Developing Countries." *New England Journal of Medicine* 337 (1997): 1003-5.

Vernick, Jon S., and Stephen P. Teret. "New Courtroom Strategies Regarding Firearms: Tort Litigation against Firearm Manufacturers and Constitutional Challenges to Gun Laws." *Houston Law Review* 36 (1999): 1713-54.

Waeckerle, Joseph F. "Domestic Preparedness for Events Involving Weapons of Mass Destruction." *Journal of the American Medical Association* 283 (2000): 252-54.

Waitzkin, Howard. *The Second Sickness: Contradictions of Capitalist Health Care.* New York: Free Press, 1983.

Wall, Susan. "Transformations in Public Health Systems." *Health Affairs* 17 (1998): 64-80.

Walsh, Diana Chapman, Lynn Elinson, and Lawrence O. Gostin. "Worksite Drug Testing." *Annual Review of Public Health* 13 (1992): 197-221.

Walzer, Michael. "Security and Welfare." In *Spheres of Justice: A Defense of Pluralism and Equality.* New York: Basic Books, 1983.

Watson, Jonathan, and Stephen Platt, eds. *Researching Health Promotion.* London: Routledge, 2000.

Weber, Max. *The Theory of Social and Economic Organization.* New York: Oxford Univ. Press, 1947.

*Webster's Third New International Dictionary.* Springfield, MA: Merriam-Webster, 1986.

Weed, Douglas L., and Robert E. McKeown. "Epidemiology and Virtue Ethics." *International Journal of Epidemiology* 27 (1998): 343-49.

Whitehead, A.N. *Science and the Modern World.* New York: Mentor, 1948.

Wikler, Daniel, and Dan E. Beauchamp. "Health Promotion and Education." In *Encyclopedia of Bioethics,* edited by Warren T. Reich. New York: Macmillan, 1995.

Wills, Garry. *Lincoln at Gettysburg: The Words That Remade America.* New York: Simon & Schuster, 1992.

Wilson, James Maxwell Glover, and G. Junger. "Principles and Practice of Screening for Disease," *Public Health Papers,* no. 34. Geneva: WHO, 1968.

Wilson, Mary E. "Infectious Diseases: An Ecological Perspective." *British Medical Journal* 311 (1995): 1681-84.

Winslow, Charles-Edward A. "The Untilled Fields of Public Health." *Science* (1920): 20–30.

Wise, Richard. "Bioterrorism: Thinking the Unthinkable." *Lancet* 351 (1998): 1378.

Wright, Kate, Louis Rowitz, Adelaide Merkele, W. Michael Reid, Gary Robinson, Bill Herzog, Diane Weber, Donna Carmichael, Tom R. Balderson, and Edward Baker. "Competency Development in Public Health Leadership." *American Journal of Public Health* 90 (2000): 1202–07.

Yudof, Mark. *When Government Speaks: Politics, Law, and Government Expression in America.* Berkeley: Univ. of California Press, 1983.

# Table of Cases

# Index

# About the Author

Lawrence Gostin, an internationally recognized scholar in public health law and ethics, is Professor of Law at Georgetown University, Professor of Public Health at the Johns Hopkins University, and Director of the Center for Law & the Public's Health at Georgetown and Johns Hopkins Universities (CDC Collaborating Center "Promoting Public Health Through Law") (http://www.publichealthlaw.net). Professor Gostin is a Member of the Institute of Medicine and serves on the IOM Board on Health Promotion and Disease Prevention, the Institutional Review Board, and expert study committees, including the IOM Committee on Assuring the Health of the Public in the 21st Century. He is also a Fellow of the Kennedy Institute of Ethics and the Hastings Center. He works closely with national and international public health agencies, including the World Health Organization, UNAIDS, the National Institutes of Health, and the Centers for Disease Control and Prevention. Professor Gostin is the Health Law and Ethics Editor of the *Journal of the American Medical Association* (*JAMA*).

Professor Gostin has led major law reform initiatives for the U.S. Department of Health and Human Services (the Model State Public Health Information Privacy Act) and a consortium of states (the "Turning Point" Public Health Statute Modernization Project to draft a Model Public Health Law). In the wake of September 11, 2001, he led the drafting of the Model Emergency Health Powers Act to combat bioterrorism and other emerging health threats.

In the United Kingdom, while head of the National Council of Civil Liberties, Professor Gostin received the Rosemary Delbridge Memorial Award for the person "who has most influenced Parliament and government to act for the welfare of society."

Compositor: Publication Services, Inc.
Text: 10/13 Sabon
Display: Sabon